T0249049

Encyclopedia of Drug Discovery and Development: Research in Pharmacognosy

Volume V

Encyclopedia of Drug Discovery and Development: Research in Pharmacognosy Volume V

Edited by **Ned Burnett**

New Jersey

Published by Foster Academics,
61 Van Reypen Street,
Jersey City, NJ 07306, USA
www.fosteracademics.com

Encyclopedia of Drug Discovery and Development:
Research in Pharmacognosy
Volume V
Edited by Ned Burnett

International Standard Book Number: 978-1-63242-140-1 (Hardback)

Printed in the United States of America.

Contents

Permissions

List of Contributors

Preface

Research-focused information regarding pharmacognosy, the field of medicines derived from natural sources, is provided in this book. The book presents an overview of the developments in the field of pharmacognosy with the aim of drug discovery from natural products, applying traditional knowledge and practices. Several herbs that have been used as food show their potential as chemopreventive agents and the assertions of various medicinal plants used in traditional medicine are now supported by science. This book is an efficient guide which will help us find medicinal solutions for all.

Various studies have approached the subject by analyzing it with a single perspective, but the present book provides diverse methodologies and techniques to address this field. This book contains theories and applications needed for understanding the subject from different perspectives. The aim is to keep the readers informed about the progresses in the field; therefore, the contributions were carefully examined to compile novel researches by specialists from across the globe.

Indeed, the job of the editor is the most crucial and challenging in compiling all chapters into a single book. In the end, I would extend my sincere thanks to the chapter authors for their profound work. I am also thankful for the support provided by my family and colleagues during the compilation of this book.

Editor

Ayurveda the Ancient Science of Healing: An Insight

Manoj Goyal[1], D. Sasmal[2] and B.P. Nagori[1]
[1]Lachoo Memorial College of Science and Technology,
Pharmacy Wing, Jodhpur, Rajasthan,
[2]Department of Pharmaceutical Sciences, BIT Mesra, Ranchi, Jharkhand,
India

1. Introduction

The term Ayurveda, a Sanskrit word, translates into knowledge (*Veda*) of life (*Ayur*); *Veda* also means science. After being transmitted orally for thousands of years, the ancient Ayurvedic texts finally were written and preserved in Sanskrit (an ancient Indian language). Founded on the collective wisdom of ancient Hindu saints and healers, Ayurveda grew into a medicinal science. Ancient Ayurveda was meant essentially to promote health, however, rather than fight disease. The Ayurvedic text, an offspring of the *Atharvaveda*, appeared sometime in 1500 to 1000 BC and described two schools of learning physicians Atreya and surgeons Dhanvantari. *Charak Samhita* (1000 BC) and *Sushrut Samhita* (100 AD) are the main classics. Ayurveda materia medica gives detailed descriptions of over 1500 herbs and 10,000 formulations. Madhav Nidan (800 AD) a diagnostic classic provides over 5000 signs and symptoms. There are eight branches of study in Ayurveda: *Kaya Chikitsa* (General Medicine), *Kaumara Bhruthya* (Paediatrics), *Bhutha Vidhya* (Psychiatry), *Salakya* (ENT and Ophthalmology and dentistry), *Shalya* (Surgery), *Agada Tantra* (Toxicology), *Rasayana* (Rejuvenation Therapy) and *Vajeekarana* (sexual vitality) (Lad, 1995; Agnihotri, 2000; Chopra and Doiphode, 2002; Mukherjee and Wahile, 2006; WHO, 2010; Balasubramani et al., 2011).

1.1 Core concept of ayurveda

In Ayurveda, health is defined as the state where physical body, senses, and psyche are in original or natural state with respect to body and function. Ayurveda believes that both world and human body are made up of five elements earth, water, fire, air, and space (ether) called as *Panch-mahabhuta*. While we are a composite of these five primary elements, certain elements are seen to have an ability to combine to create various physiological functions (Mishra, 2004).

The human body according to Ayurveda is made up of somatic *dosas* (*Vata*, *pitta* and *kapha*) and psychic components (*satogun*, *rajogun* and *tamogun*), body tissues or *dhatus* {*Rasa* (plasma), *Rakta* (blood), *Mansa* (muscular tissue), *Meda* (adipose tissue), *Asthi* (Bone), *Majja* (marrow and myeloid tissue) *and Shukra* (Sperm/Ovum)} and waste products or *malas* { *mutra* (urine), *purisha* (faeces) and *sveda* (sweat)} (Vasant, 2005).

Vata: Ether and air combine to form what is known in Ayurveda as the *Vata dosha, vata* governs the principle of movement and therefore can be seen as the force which directs nerve impulses, circulation, respiration, and elimination. *Vata* is dry, cold and light and correspond to the element *air*.

Pitta: Fire and water are the elements that combine to form the *Pitta dosha*. The *Pitta dosha* is the process of transformation or metabolism. The transformation of foods into nutrients that our bodies can assimilate is an example of a *pitta* function. *Pitta* is also responsible for metabolism in the organ and tissue systems as well as cellular metabolism. *Pitta* is oily, hot and light and correspond to the element *fire*.

Kapha: Water and earth elements combine to form the *Kapha dosha*. Kapha is responsible for growth, adding structure unit by unit. Another function of the *Kapha dosha* is to offer protection. Cerebro-spinal fluid protects the brain and spinal column and is a type of *Kapha* found in the body. Also, the mucousal lining of the stomach is another example of the *Kapha dosha* protecting the tissues. *Kapha* is wet, cold and heavy and corresponds to the element water (Sebastian, 2006; Walter, 2006).

These three *dosas* coexist in a predetermined proportion and function in a complementary manner to overall function of the total organism in spite of their opposite properties and functions. The existence of the *dosas* can be understood at both the macromolecular and micromolecular levels. A balance in the activity of these *dosas* is necessary for health.

2. Pathogenesis of disease

According to Ayurveda, there are three main causes of disease, namely *asatmyendriyartha samyoga* (indiscriminate use of senses and their objects), *prajna-aparadha* (error of intellect resulting in a loss of discrimination between wholesome and unwholesome with subsequent indulgence in unwholesome diets and behaviour) and *kala- parinama* (seasonal variation, cosmic effects and the effects of time) (Frank, 2001).

Pancha lakshana nidana, the five components of the pathology of a disease, assists in diagnosis. They are *nidana* (causative factors), *purvarupa* (prodromal symptoms/ incubatory symptoms), *rupa* (signs and symptoms), *samprapti* (pathogenesis) and *upashaya* (diagnostic tests).

Samprapti: The concept of six stages of pathogenesis is vital for an understanding of the pathological states of the *doshas* that result in disease. First stage is called as *Sanchaya* (accumulation), due to weak digestive power and accumulation of *ama* (toxins) causes imbalance in *doshas*. The second stage is *Prokapa* (aggravation), the accumulated, stagnant doshas are excited by factors as *ahara, vihara* and seasons. Stage three called as *prasara* (overflowing/ spread), in this stage, the toxins accumulated start overflowing. Generally, up to this stage the damage is entirely reversible and restoration of *doshas* balance can be achieved with proper measures.

Sthanasamsraya (localization/ agumentation) is stage four characterized by migration of overflowing toxins in localized weak or defective *dhatus* thereby leading to malfunction and structural damage.

Vyakti (manifestation) and *bheda* (chronic complications) are fifth and sixth stages of pathogenesis, characterized by appearance of symptoms of diseases and chronic manifestation respectively.

3. Diagnosis of disease

The starting place of a successful treatment is a clear diagnosis. ayurvedic diagnostic methods are founded on the three methods of knowing (*pramana*). These are direct *pratyaksa* (perception), *aptopadesa, sabda* (textual authority) and *anumana* (inference). The most clinically useful is direct perception and it includes *Susruta's* threefold methods of diagnosis *trividha pariksa* that includes *sparsana* (palpation), *darsana* (looking), and *prasana* (questioning). Caraka has mentioned that direct perception (*pratyaksa)* includes using the five senses meaning that listening, feeling, looking, smelling and tasting. Later on it became *astasthana pariksa* which includes examination of *nadi* (pulse), *mutra* (urine), *malam* (faeces), *jihva* (tongue), *shabda* (voice), *sparsha* (skin or touch), *drika* (sight or eyes) and *akriti* (appearances, face, overall appearance) (Tirtha, 1998; Mishra, 2004; Vasant, 2005; Sebastian, 2006).

4. Dravyaguna vigyan (ayurvedic pharmacology)

In Ayurveda, substances of natural origin, including whole plants or their parts, animal parts and minerals, are used as medicines, either alone or in combination. In addition, various other measures are used in an attempt to maintain health in a healthy person and alleviate disorders of the body and mind. These substances act on the principles of *samanya* (homologous) and *visesha* (antagonistic) action.

Substances possessing homologous properties and actions increase the relevant elemental properties or constituents of the body while those having antagonistic properties or actions decrease those properties or constituents. In cases of disease or imbalance of *dosha, dhatu* and *mala*, the rational use of naturally available substances aims to restore normality.

The composition of elements in medicines and the diet is studied in terms of various properties, referred to as *rasa, guna, virya, vipaka* and *prabhava*. The effect and action of the medicines or diet depends on these properties.

Rasa (taste): Taste of medicine as perceived by tongue.

There are six different tastes, each with a predominance of two elements and showing the characteristics of these elements. Administration of a medicine featuring a particular *rasa* enhances that property in the body and decreases its opposite. The six tastes are *madhura* (sweet), *amla* (sour), *lavana* (salty), *katu* (pungent), *tikta* (bitter) and *kashaya* (astringent). Tastes provide varying degrees of nourishing strength. Sweet taste is the most nourishing, and as each taste becomes less nourishing, it becomes more bitter, until it is astringent and the least nourishing.

Guna (attributes): Not be measurable but inferred through their pharmacological action, *guna* is property of a medicine detected by sense organs other than the tongue. It appears that *guna* are intimately related to rasa it is a fact that both are separate principles co-existent in the *dravya* (substance). They are 20 in number and represent the characteristics of the elements. There are 10 pairs of contrasting characteristics – *guru* (heavy)/ *laghu* (light), *manda* (dull)/ *tikshna* (sharp), *sita* (cold)/ *ushna* (hot), *snigdha* (unctuous)/ *ruksha* (non-unctuous), *slakshna* (smooth)/ *khara* (rough), *sthira* (immobile)/ *sara* (mobile), *mridu* (soft)/ *kathina* (hard), *visada* (clear)/ *picchila* (slimy), *sandra* (solid)/ *drava* (fluid), *sthula* (bulky)/ *sukshma* (fine).

Virya: Denotes the potency of the medicine. There are eight *virya* namely *mridu, teekshana, guru, laghu, snigdha, ruksha, ushna* and *sita,* representing the active *gunas*. These can be put into two broad categories – *sita* (cooling) and *ushna* (heating).

Vipaka (postdigestive effect): It is the postdigestive effect of *rasas,* the same elements predominate as in the original *rasas,* with the corresponding action. There are three *vipakas*. A sweet taste becomes *madhura vipaka*; sour and salty tastes become *amla vipaka* and pungent, bitter and astringent tastes become *katu vipaka*.

Prabhava (pharmacological action): *Prabhava* has been defined as the special property of a substance which produces actions different from and contrary to those ascribed to *rasa, guna, virya* and *vipaka*. The chemical composition which largely determines the secondary qualities of a *dravya* (substance) such as *rasa, guna, virya* and *vipaka* does not determine a chemical compound. The *rasa, guna, virya* and *vipaka* of Danti (*Baliospermum montanum*.) and Chitraka (*Plumbago zeylanica*) being apparently identical, the former produces purgation, whereas the latter does not produce this action and the specific purgative action of Danti is attributed to its *prabhava* (inexplicable nature) (Paranjpe, 2001; Nishteswar, 2007).

5. Ayurvedic *chikitsa* (therapeutics)

Ayurveda says that healthy of an individual is preserved due to equilibrium of the *doshas*. In diseased people, treatment eliminates the disequilibrium between the *doshas,* and the body is restored to normality. The body has its own intelligence to create balance, ayurvedic treatments helps in that process.

Diseases are treated by nidana *parivarjana,* (avoidance of causative and provocative factors), *shodhana* and *panchakarma* (purifying therapies), *shamana* (palliative therapies) and *rasayana* (rejuvenation) and *vajikarana* (aphrodisiac).

5.1 *Nidana parivarjana* (preventive measures)

The preventive measures or *nidana parivarjana* includes *swastha varta* (personal hygiene), *dinacharya* (daily routine), *ritucharya* (seasonal corrections) and *sadachara* (appropriate behaviour).

5.2 *Shodhana karma* (purifying therapy)

Formation of toxins reduces that natural capacity of body for healing and rejuvenating. The *shodhan* karma such as *panchakarma* enables the body to release excess *doshas* and *ama* (toxins) from cells.

Panchakarma: Is the method of *shodhana*/detoxification or elimination of toxins from the body. It is divided in three stages *poorvakarma* (preparatory procedures) *pradhan karma* (main therapy) and *uttara karma* (post therapy care).

Poorvakarma (preparatory procedures) includes *snehana* (oelation therapy) and *swedana* (fomentation therapy).

Snehana or oelation therapy involves saturation of the body with herbal & medicated oil via external & internal oelation to make body soft and disintegrate the *doshas*. *Shirodhara* is the most commonly employed pre-procedure; it means the dripping of oil like a thread (*dhara*) on the head (*shiro*). This treatment drips warm oil in a steady stream on the forehead, particularly on the brow and in the region between the eyes. It is often added to the *panchakarma* regimen because it pacifies *vata* and calms the central system. It cleans both the mind and the senses which allow the body's natural healing mechanisms to release stress from the nervous systems.

Swedana/ fomentation or sweating is necessarily follows oleation, *Swedana* is induced by heat from different sources it brings sweat on the skin through hair follicles by opening the pores of the skin. Fomentation increases the *agni* (biofire) and the fatty tissue gets mobilised. It also throws out *ama* (toxins/waste) through the skin and helps in liquefying aggravated *doshas*. *Swedana* has two main types, *agni sweda* wherein heat is applied directly as steam and *anagni sweda* where no external heat source is necessary e.g exercises, fighting, walking, lifting heavy loads, exposure to sunlight, putting heavy blankets over the body etc.

Pradhan Karma is consists of the five essential purificatory therapies namely *vamana* (vomiting), virechan (purgation), anuvasana and *niraha* (medicinal enema), *nasya* (nasal insufflation, administration) and *raktamocana* (blood cleansing).

Vamana (emesis): It is therapeutic emesis; done regularly to cleanse the stomach and remove *áma* (toxins) and mucus from chest. It is used for relieving recent fever, diarrhea, pulmonary infections, skin diseases, diabetes mellitus, goiter, and obesity. *Vamana* is induced using herbs such as *vacha* (*Acorus calamus*) and *licorice* (*Glycyrrhiza glabra*).

Virechan (purgation): This is the simplest method of *panchakarma* and has most easily observed effects. It is an excellent method to heal various conditions, including abdominal tumors, hemorrhoids, smallpox, patches of skin discoloration on the face, jaundice, chronic fevers and enlarged abdomen. Strong cathartic and laxative herbs such as *jaiphal* (*Croton tiglium*), *aragwad* (*Cassia fistula*), or *castor oil* (*Ricinus communis*) are used for induction of purgation.

Anuvasana and *niraha* (enemas): For patients emaciated by fever, neither *vamana* nor *virechan* is useful. The mala (digestive waste and toxin) of patients is removed by *nirha* by using decoction enemas. To prevent aggravation of *vata*, an oil enema (anuvasana basti).

Nasya (Nasal cleansing therapy): *Nasya* means nasal administration of medicated powders or liquids. It is a procedure in which medicament administered through the nostrils in order to purify the head and neck region. Nasya is useful in relieving stiffness in the head, neck arteries, throat, and jaw obstructions, *nasya* is useful in disorders of the neck, shoulders, ears, nose, mouth, head, cranium, and scapula.

Raktamokshana (Blood-letting): The small amount of blood is removed intravenously or by leeches, the toxins are removed quickly from systemic circulation. It is useful in blood toxaemia, hypertension and skin disorders. *Raktamokshana* is contraindicated in anemia and pregnancy.

Uttara karma: It is important to resume or establish a diet and lifestyle that is harmonious with one's constitution. If a person returns to old, bad habits, they may worsen their condition by suppressing the renewed healing energies. The toxins may then directly enter cleansed tissues and go deeper than before, causing severe diseases. During convalescence, persons avoid loud talking, bumpy rides, long walks, excessive sitting, and eating, if experiencing indigestion. To avoid aggravating the humors, persons also avoid eating unwholesome food, day naps, and sexual relations (Ojha et al., 1978; Joshi, 2005).

5.3 *Shamana karma* (alleviation therapy)

According to Ayurveda, sh*amana* is the balancing and pacification of bodily *doshas, shamana* is used when *panchakarma* is inappropriate due to the poor strength of the patient. *Shaman*a consists of *dipana, pacana, vrata or ksunnigraha, trsna* or *ernnigraha* Vyayama, Atapasevana and Marutha.

Dipana (enkindling): *Dipana* means enkindling the digestive fire by using warm meals, hot water, eating a small piece of fresh ginger mixed with lime juice and salt before a meal, having a short walk before meals to stimulate the *agni. dipana* is absolutely necessary in *kapha* and *vata* disorders, where the person has low gastric fire.

Pacana (digestion): *Pacana* means digesting of *ama* (toxins) and undigested residues, *pacana* uses many of the same herbs as dipana but instead of taking them before a meal they are taken afterwards and usually at double the dose. These hot herbs literally burn the *ama*. The indication for using *pacana* is when there is hunger but not enough 'fuel' to fan the digestive flames. These spices are the fuel. Of course, when there are already inflammatory conditions, such as ulcers, caution must be taken.

Vrata or ksunnigraha (fasting): *Ksunnigraha* means to 'hold onto your hunger. Fasting inspire a healthy hunger; a true need for food taken in the balanced quantity. Fasting or monodiet are suggested according to *dosha. Vata* people can do a short fast on hot liquid soups, *pitta* constitution can do a liquid fast on fruit juices such as grape or pomegranate and *kapha* types can do a literal fast; although this is a great struggle for them as it challenges their tendency to hold onto things.

Trsna or Ernnigraha (observing thirst): **N**ot drinking water or fasting from water is known as *trsna or ernnigraha. Trsna* is beneficial in water diseases such as oedema, diabetes or kidney problems. It reduces the stress on the water channels in the body *(ambuvahasrotas)*.

Vyayama (exercise and yoga): Ayurveda says exercise has such a quality that it strengthen the *dhatus*, increase agni, improve circulation, accelerates the heart rate, enhances the combustion of calories and also stimulates metabolism, regulates body temperature and maintains body weight. Exercise makes your senses alert and attentive and your mind becomes very sharp and develops keen perception. These qualities of exercise are very important, but again, exercise varies from person to person, *Vata* types should do more relaxing and gentle exercise. *Kapha* people can do more vigorous exercise and *pitta* should exercise regularly but moderate.

Atapa seva (sunbathing): The sun is the source of heat and light. *Atapaseva* is very useful for lightening the body, increasing the *agni* and treating *bhrajaka pitta*. Many conditions are improved by sitting in the sun; certain types of eczema, psoriasis, arthritis, depression and water retention to name a few. Lying in the sun and meditating upon the solar plexus, is a wonderful *shaman* for *kapha* and *vata*. It improves circulation, the absorption of vitamin D, and strengthens the bones.

Maruta/ Marutaseva (wind-bathing): *Marutaseva* is specifically relates to the yogic practice of *pranayama* and of becoming inherently tuned into deep slow breathing using a deep inhalation and long exhalation. It is about imbibing *prana;* the life force surfs on the breath and flows deep into our tissues. Specific problems such as asthma, bronchitis and emphysema greatly benefit from this practice. Also people with a tendency to experience excessive anxiety and fear in their lives benefit from watching the breath flow in and out of themselves.

5.4 *Rasayana* (rejuvenative) and *vajikarana* (aphrodisiac)

Rejuvenation involves *brmhana* (building therapy) using tonic herbs such as ashwagandha (*Withania somnifera*), shatavari (*Asparagus racemosus*) and bala (*Sida cordifolia*) to nourish all the tissues, build the strength, enhance ojas and strengthen immunity. It also involves eating building foods like nuts, ghee and dairy products.

Rasayana (tonic): In Ayurveda tonics are sweet, heavy and oily in quality. The sweet flavour increases the quantity and quality of the tissues as it is anabolic. So many of the modern wonder herbs that boost immunity are full of immune-enhancing saponins and polysaccharides. The sweet flavour is tonifying and rejuvenating, but it must be of a high quality and fully digested to benefit the whole system. Popular ayurvedic tonics are chayawanaprash, ghee and walnuts (*Juglans regia*).

Vajikarana (aphrodisiacs): This refers to herbs that nourish the reproductive organs, increase fertility, promote libido as well as prevent ageing. Herbs such as kapikacchu (*Mucuna pruriens*), ashwagandha (*Withania somnifera*) and amalaki (*Emblica officinalis*) are renowned reproductive tonics as well as being antioxidants (Frawley, 2000; Panda 2000; Acharya, 2005; Sudarshan, 2005; McIntyre, (2005); Murthy and Pandey, 2008).

6. Discussion

Ayurveda has been practiced in India for over 5000 years and is recognized as a complete medical system comparable with allopathic medicine by the government of India. In India, Ayurveda has a complete infrastructure, medical colleges, hospitals integrated with allopathic medicine, research institutes, and scientific journals devoted to Ayurveda. In addition, India's Ayurvedic pharmaceutical industry is governed by the same food and drug laws that regulate conventional drugs. Research in pharmacology, biochemistry, phytochemistry, and clinical trials of Ayurvedic therapies currently constitutes a substantial portion of the total research conducted in government institutes and medical colleges in India (Mishra, 2004).

Ayurveda has the potential to develop into a global health-care system. The concepts of proper lifestyles, personal hygiene, daily routine, seasonal corrections, diet, yoga and herbal therapy can be adopted with suitable modification to different countries in different parts of the globe after giving due consideration to the culture, life style and available medicinal plant resources of the countries.

Name of Category	Meaning in English	Name of Category	Meaning in English
Angamarda-prasamana	Pain relieving	*Purisa-virajaniya*	Faecal depigmenter
Anuvasanopaga	Unctuous enemata	*Sandhaniya*	Healing
Arsoghna	Anti-haemorrhoidal	*Sanjna-sthapana*	Energising
Asthapanopaga	Corrective enemata	*Sirovirecanopaga*	Errhines
Balya	Tonic	*Sita-prasamana*	Calefacient
Bhedaniya	Laxative	*Snehopaga*	Moisturising
Brmhaniya	Bulk-promoting	*Sonita-sthapana*	Haemostatic
Chardi-nigrahana	Anti-emetic	*Srama-hara*	Energy compensator
Daha-prasamana	Refrigerent	*Stanya-janana*	Galactogogue
Dipaniya	Appetite stimulant	*Stanya-sodhana*	Galacto-depurant
Hikka-nigrahana	Anti-hiccough	*Sukra-janana*	Semen promoting
Hrdya	Cordial	*Sukra-sodhana*	Semen depurant
Jivaniya	Vitalising	*Sula-prasamana*	Intestinal antispasmodic
Jwara-hara	Anti-pyretic	*Swasa-hara*	Anti-dyspneic
Kandughna	Anti-pruritic	*Swayathu-hara*	Anti-phlogistic
Kanthya	Beneficial for throat	*Swedopaga*	Diaphoretic
Kasa-hara	Antitussive	*Trptighna*	Thirst-quenching
Krimighna	Anthelmintic	*Trsna-nigrahana*	Anti-dyspepsic
Kusthaghna	Anti-dermatosis	*Udara-prasamana*	Anti-allergic
Lekhaniya	Emaciating	*Vamanopaga*	Emetic
Mutra-sangrahaniya	Anti-diuretic	*Varnya*	Complexion-promoting
Mutra-virajaniya	Urinary depigmentor	*Vayah-sthapana*	Rejuvenating
Mutra-virecaniya	Diuretic	*Vedana-sthapana*	Analgesic
Praja-sthapana	Anti-abortificient	*Virecanopaga*	Purgative
Purisa–samgrahaniya	Intestinal astringent	*Visaghna*	Anti-poison

Table 1. Pharmacological categories of various drugs used in Ayurveda.

7. Acknowledgment

Authors are grateful to all experts of Ayurveda whose work referred in this article.

8. References

Acharya, V., Rao. (2005). Ayurvedic Treatment for Common Diseases. New Delhi: Diamond Pocket Book.

Agnihotri, M.S., (2000). Ayurved (ancient Indian system of medicine) and modern molecular medicine. The Journal of the Association of Physicians of India. 48: 366-367.

Balasubramani, S.P., Venkatasubramanian, P., Kukkupuni, S.K., Patwardhan, B., (2011). Plant-Based Rasayana Drugs from Ayurveda. Chinese Journal of Integrative Medicine. 17: 88-94.

Chopra, A., Doiphode, V.V., (2002). Ayurvedic medicine: Core concept, therapeutic principles, and current relevance. Medical Clinics of North America. 86: 75-89.

Frank, J., N. (2001). An elementary textbook of Ayurveda: medicine with a six thousand year old tradition. Madison, CT: Psychosocial Press.

Frawley, D. (2000). Yoga and Ayurveda: self-healing and self-realization. Delhi: Motilal Banarasidas Publication.

Joshi, S., V. (2005). Ayurveda and Panchakarma: The Science of Healing and Rejuvenation, Motilal Banarasidas Publication, Delhi.

Lad, V., (1995). An introduction to Ayurveda. Alternative Therapies in Health and Medicine. 1: 57-63.

McIntyre, A. (2005). Herbal Treatment of Children: Western and Ayurvedic Perspectives. London: Elsevier Butterworth-Heinemann.

Mishra, L. C. (2004). Scientific basis for Ayurvedic therapies. USA: CRC Press.

Mukherjee, P.K., Wahile, A., (2006). Integrated approaches towards drug development from Ayurveda and other Indian system of medicines. Journal of Ethnopharmacology. 103: 25-35.

Murthy, N., A., Pandey, D., P. (2008). Ayurvedic cure for common diseases. New delhi: Orient Paperbacks.

Nishteswar, K. (2007) Basic Concepts of Ayurvedic Pharmacology Varanasi: Chowkamba Sanskrit Series.

Ojha, D., Kumar, A., Kumar, A. (1978). Panchakarma Therapy in Ayurveda. Varanasi: Chaukhamba Amarabharati Prakashan.

Panda, H. (2000). Handbook On Herbal Medicines. Delhi: Asia Pacific Business Press.

Paranjpe, P. (2001). Indian medicinal plants: forgotten healers : a guide to ayurvedic herbal medicine with identity, habitat, botany, photochemistry, ayurvedic properties, formulations & clinical usage. Varanasi: Chaukhamba Sanskrit Pratishthan.

Sebastian, Pole. (2006). Ayurvedic medicine: the principles of traditional practice. London: Churchill Livingstone Elsevier.

Sudarshan, S., R. (2005). Encyclopaedia of Indian Medicine: Diseases and Their Cures. Mumbai: Popular Prakashan.

Tirtha, S., S. (1998). The Ayurveda encyclopedia: natural secrets to healing, prevention & longevity. Bayville, NY: Ayurveda Holistic Center Press.

Vasant, Lad. (2005). Ayurveda: the science of self-healing : a practical guide. Delhi: Motilal Banarasidas Publication.

Walter, Kacera. (2006). Ayurvedic Tongue Diagnosis. USA: Lotus Press.

World Health Organization. (2010) Benchmarks for training in Ayurveda. Geneva: WHO. Available at:
www.who.int/entity/medicines/.../BenchmarksforTraininginAyurveda.pdf Accessed, 15 April 2011.

2

Standardized Cannabis and Pain Management

A. Paul Hornby
Hedron Analytical Inc.
Canada

1. Introduction

We began our journey researching cannabis as a medicine roughly twelve years ago and have been astounded time and time again at the profound effectiveness of the plant. In this chapter we will describe the usefulness of cannabis in pain management. In so doing we will be describing the *whole plant medicine* such as is dispensed in compassion clubs and medical marijuana dispensaries here in British Columbia, Canada and similarly in California and other parts of the world where cannabis has become legal as a medicine.

We treat cannabis as the herbal medicine that it is. What we do; is apply high tech instrument analysis of the plant and scientific method to members using cannabis therapeutically in attempts to unravel the truth of its efficacy and safety. We have set up research departments, collected membership data, run literally thousands of chromatograms and worked closely with persons with chronic pain at local dispensaries and cannabis clubs here in British Columbia for many years.

What we will describe in the chapter is primarily repeated observation of members of medical marijuana dispensaries who routinely use cannabis to deal with pain. Of the clubs we have worked with over the years most of their members are using cannabis for pain management. Often greater than 70% of the members surveyed will be using cannabis for this purpose. This holds true for medical dispensaries here in B.C. as well as for California, Holland and Switzerland (1). Simply put, most persons frequenting medical cannabis dispensaries are there for pain management.

Many of the people we have worked with over the years have been terribly broken up, either in car accidents, on the job injuries, infection (Reiter's syndrome), surgeries or cancer therapy, plus many other causes, that lead to 24/7 chronic pain. As if the pain isn't bad enough, often cycling with the pain is mood disorder, such as depression, attention deficit disorder and anxiety.

When it is difficult to put on a jacket, climb a flight of stairs or tie shoelaces, normal life is affected and the individual adjusts by changing their life style in attempts to relieve pain. These adjustments can often bring on anxiety (not being able to go out) or depression (relating to friends and family) since now the person's lifestyle is not as it used to be…now it is ruled by pain.

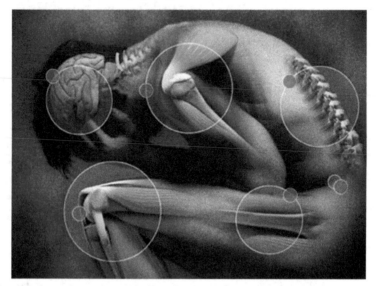

Fig. 1. Acknowledgement to: http://naturalbodyofflorida.webs.com/pain-map_alphachimp_com.jpg for this explicit graphic.

For those dealing with pain it often becomes a fulltime job: monitoring, medicating, resting, exercising, eating, going to bed, take on new meaning when one is in pain. Constantly seeking relief from "the banging drum," as quoted by Dr. Mel Pohl (2), being the top priority for those who suffer. Relief from pain leads to a new quality of life that, in turn, breaks the cycle of chronic pain syndrome.

Cannabis allows new quality of life for many suffering from chronic pain.

Having access to the member's data allows determination of; how much cannabis they're using daily, in what form (smoke able or edible), what strain is preferred, their ailment, etc. This accumulated data is used to take perspective on the cannabis use of the membership of the individual clubs and to track various individuals included in studies.

We have spent five years with our laboratory serving the quality control and standardization needs of one such dispensary, and the past two doing similar duties and research at a second. In all of this time we maintain close association with the members who use cannabis therapeutically for pain, tracking their symptoms with questionnaires, interviews, pain charts, emails, etc.

We have found a psychology that prevails at these dispensaries; they're friendly, non-violent, people whom all seem to be willing to take part in the scientific research that is being carried out. No shortage of volunteers. And many have sustained and continue to deal with disabling injuries that have dramatically affected their lives and families.

Currently we have joined with five medical dispensaries in our local area and are initiating Randomized Controlled Trials (RCT) with roughly one hundred volunteer subjects together taking part in the placebo controlled trial. Our focus will be arthritic pain and we look forward to publication before the end of 2012.

2. The legalities

Cannabis has been legal as a medicine, in Canada, since 2001, when a precedent setting court case ruled that Canadians had a constitutional right to the plant for medical purposes (3). The Medical Marijuana Access Regulations (MMAR) was established in that year allowing qualified individual's licenses to possess and produce their own cannabis for medical reasons.

Only persons who were terminally ill, with severe spinal cord injury, arthritis or multiple sclerosis and unresponsive to routine medical treatment were originally allowed a cannabis license. Often these people were too ill to grow their own, so designated growers were also assigned licenses to specific qualified persons for growing cannabis. An alternative to obtaining an MMAR license was to have a medical doctor fax a letter of acknowledgement of an individuals cannabis use to a local dispensary, releasing the dispensaries from some of the quasi-legal burden of distributing cannabis to members.

Overall the MMAR program has demonstrated itself to be lacking in meeting the needs of it's licensees, with long wait times for initial and renewal licensing and poor supply of government marihuana for those unable to grow for themselves or without a designate. Because of these shortcomings and yet another court case the program is about to be revamped once again to tighter government and industry control.

Nevertheless, most persons in Canada, at this time, with a legitimate complaint of chronic pain and a tenacious attitude can access medical marijuana. And most would do this with their own licensed grows or through dispensaries.

3. The endocannabinoids

As it turns out the receptor that binds THC is one of the most abundant binding sites in the human brain. Expressed at high levels in the hippocampus, cortex, cerebellum, and basal ganglia (4–6), the receptor, is virtually everywhere. An unusual receptor type in that binding occurs at the pre-synapse (upstream) side of the cleft, a type of receptor mechanism, called retrograde signaling. Different, in that depolarization at the post-synapse opens voltage-dependent Ca^{2+} channels, that in turn, activates enzymes that produce endocannabinoids from lipid precursors, in the cell membrane. See Figure 2, courtesy of Dr. Roger Nicoll (7), that illustrates retrograde signaling.

In the Hippocampus, for example, these highly fat-soluble compounds migrate back across the synapse to the pre-synaptic CB1 receptors where binding slows release of the inhibitory neurotransmitter, GABA. G-protein activation liberates Gbg (a receptor subunit), which then directly inhibits presynaptic Ca^{2+} influx, thus preventing release of neurotransmitter vesicles from the presynapse.

Until just a few years ago this type of receptor signaling was unheard of but today characterizes the endocannabinoid mechanism of neuromodulation, protection and plasticity.

In their review, Hohmann and Suplita state that: "Cannabinoid receptors are localized in neuroanatomical regions subserving transmission and modulation of pain signals, such as the periaqueductal gray (PAG), the rostral ventromedial medulla (RVM), (8,9) and the dorsal horn of the spinal cord.(9) These findings suggest that endocannabinoids play a key role in central nervous system modulation of pain signaling.

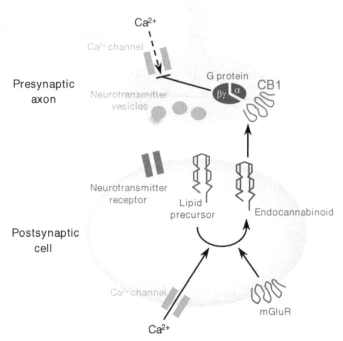

Fig. 2. Retrograde signaling by endocannabionids. Postsynaptic depolarization opens voltage-dependent Ca^{2+} channels; postynaptic Ca^{2+} then activates enzymes that synthesize endocannabinoids from lipid precursors. Activation of postsynaptic mGluRs can also generate endocannabinoids possibly by activation of phospholipase C, generating diacylglycerol, , which is then cleaved by diacylglycerol lipase to yield 2-arachidonylglycerol. Endocannabinoids then leave the postsynaptic cell and activate presynaptic CB1 receptors. G-protein activation liberates $G_{\beta\gamma}$ which then directly inhibits presynaptic Ca^{2+} influx. This decreases the probability of release of a vesicle of neurotransmitter.

Significantly, immunocytochemical studies have demonstrated FAAH expression in the ventral posterior lateral nucleus of the thalamus,(10-12) which is the termination zone of the spinothalamic tract. This pathway is the major source of ascending nociceptive information to the brain. Furthermore, FAAH has been identified in Lissauer's tract and in neurons of the superficial spinal cord dorsal horn (i.e., in close proximity to the termination zone of nociceptive primary afferents). These observations confirm that a mechanism for endocannabinoid deactivation is present in regions of the central nervous system implicated in nociceptive processing and further support the notion that endocannabinoids play a role in pain modulation."

Since the endocannabinoid system includes the G-protein receptors and subunits, the ligands that bind the receptors and the enzymes that make or breakdown the ligands, attention has been paid to all these components in relation to pain.

Mice bred with no CB1 receptors tend to hide in corners, die young and show high incidence of cataplexy and hypoalgesia, or decreased sensitivity to painful stimuli. It was experiments such as these that indicated the role of the endocannabinoid system in the modulation of nociception and pain. And, indeed, the tremendous abundance of the neuromodulatory CB1 receptor in the human central nervous suggests a regulatory role of neurotransmission, far greater than that commanded by the opiate system.

Research carried out between 2005 and 2010 indicates that synthetic cannabinoids and inhaled cannabis are effective treatments for a range of neuropathic disorders.[13] Smoked cannabis has been found to provide relief from HIV-associated sensory neuropathy.[14] This form of cannabis was also found to relieve neuropathy associated with CRPS type I, spinal cord injury, peripheral neuropathy, and nerve injury.[15]

3.1 CB2 receptor

Changes in endocannabinoid levels and/or CB2 receptor expressions have been reported in almost all diseases affecting humans [16]. CB2 receptors are found mostly in peripheral immune tissues such as the spleen, tonsils and thymus glands where they're primarily localized on immune cells such as monocytes, macrophages, B-cells, and T-cells.[17-20] Reducing intracellular levels of cyclic adenosine monophosphate (cAMP), leads to a series of down-regulatory events ultimately resulting in lowered immunity. Other types of cannabinoid receptors (CB3) are proposed and will undoubtedly more will emerge as research continues.

Several putative endocannabinoids have been isolated in the brain, including anandamide, 2-AG, noladin ether, virodhamine, and N-arachidonoyldopamine (NADA), the latter neurotransmitter decidedly involved with the vanilloid receptor and nociception.

4. Dosage

The first step in pain relief is accessing cannabis, once obtained...relief begins.

4.1 Oral vs. smoking

Often the initial use of cannabis for a person in chronic pain is the blessing they have been waiting for. Normally smoked the first time, the instant relief and general well being brought about from cannabis are greatly appreciated. But with smoking relief is short, roughly an hour or two before another dose is needed. With smoking the member of a dispensary or compassion club will cycle through their day with relief one hour, but not the next, for those with severe chronic pain, eating cannabis becomes a better solution. With oral ingestion the effects are often stronger and felt more "in the body than the mind" and pain relief is maintained for four to six hours in a plateau-like fashion rather the cyclical.

Indeed, oral ingestion of cannabis is most often indicated for those with chronic pain. But one cannot just pick a bud off the plant and eat it, since raw cannabis does not contain activated cannabinoids that bind a receptor. In nature the cannabinoids, such as Tetrahydrocannabinol (THC) and Cannabidiol (CBD) are present as acids with carboxyl groups at the 3' or 5' position on the aromatic ring of the molecule, (by the terpene numbering system) . With the carboxyl group in place the cannabinoid does not interact with the receptor; once decarboxylated, normally through heat, the carboxyl group is lost and THC, for example, can now bind. (see section 4.3 on smoking)

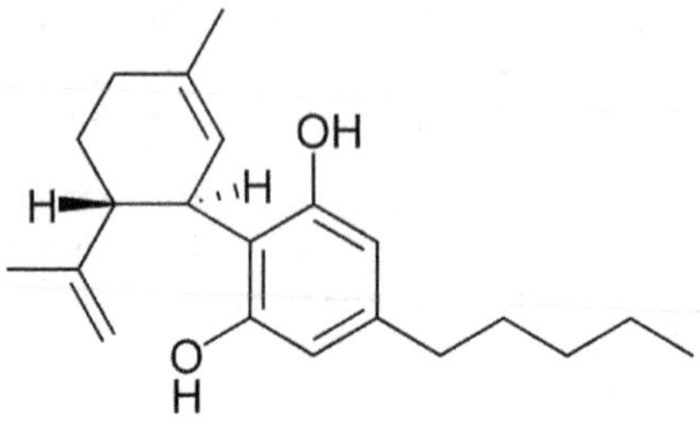

CBD

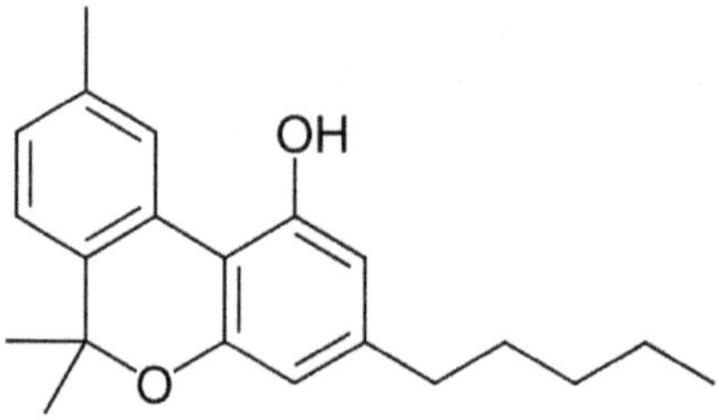

THC

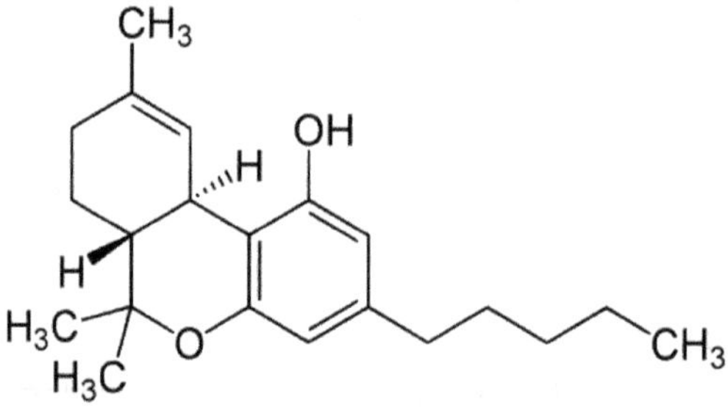

CBN

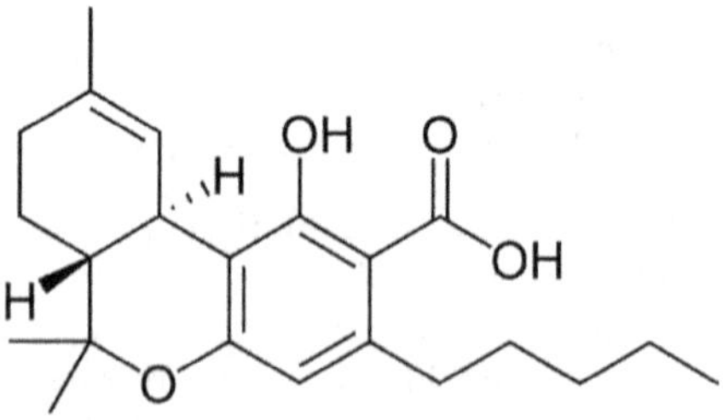

THC-acid

Note that both CBD and CBN also have carboxyl groups as does THC-acid and most other cannabinoids at room temperature.

4.2 Decarboxylation

Decarboxylation of the major cannabinoids, tetrahydocannbinolic acid (THC-A), cannabidiolic acid (CBD-A) and cannabinolic acid (CBN-A), is important to understand particularly with oral administration of cannabis. With smoking de-carboxylation occurs by default with the high heat delivered through burning. With oral preparations the cannabinoids must be decarboxylated to produce an efficacious medicine. Most commonly baking the cannabis into a Brownie not only allows decarboxylation of the primary cannabinoids but also supplies a fatty medium, aiding in absorption of the medicine.

Since decarboxylation requires heating a particular strain of cannabis for a specified time at a specific temperature to achieve optimal release of the carboxyl group, often oral preparations of cannabis have incomplete decarboxylation, yielding only a percentage of the tetrahydorcannabinolic acid (for example) as THC and thus not allowing maximum utilization of the active compound.

Upon realizing the multitude of inefficient decarboxylation methods employed by many dispensary members preparing their own oral cannabis preparations, our research group set about standardizing cannabis into capsules, with known concentrations of the major actives (THC, CBD and CBN), for research purposes.

We also subjected the standardized oral capsules to routine quality control procedures such as screening for heavy metals, pesticides and pathogenic bacteria, yeasts and molds. It is with these standardized capsules that most of our research into the efficacy and safety of cannabis as a medicine as been studied.

4.3 Standardization

By standardizing cannabis into orally administered capsules that we are able to better determine dosage and efficacy and members were able to develop regimens for treating pain. The standardization process involves testing by High Pressure Liquid Chromatography (HPLC) the raw material prior to heating to determine the amounts of the various acids; currently in the heating step we are mostly concerned about the concentration of CBD-A in the raw material, since we consider CBD an extremely important medicinal cannabinoid and indeed it is the last of the three, to decarboxylate with heat.

To clarify, decarboxylation of THC-A occurs at a lower temperature than for CBD-A and since it is our quest to optimize the CBD concentration in a standardized prep, we must heat for long enough at a high enough temperature to fully decarboxylate the CBD-A. Once the heating step is finished the cannabis is re-ground to a fine powder and tested again by HPLC and encapsulated.

In each capsule the concentration of THC, CBD and CBN, is known and of course the ratios of these individual cannabinoids will change depending on the strain of cannabis used (strain specificity, discussed below), therefore there is no generic time or temperature that will optimally decarboxylate every cannabis strain …they're all different. An educated guess for most strains available here in BC and in California would be 160°C (325 °F) for 45 to 60 minutes in a sealed environment. However it is only by pre-analysis of the raw material, and experimentation, that we are able to set a time and temperature for optimal decarboxylation of a specific strain.

The ratios of the three most abundant cannabinoids (excluding CBG), is a good indicator of the observed effects in an individual. For example, a ratio of roughly 1:10 CBD:THC proves useful for pain relief with sedation. Whereas increasing the CBN concentration relative to THC will bring about less pain relief and a more stimulatory effect. Point being, that the ratios of the individual cannabinoids one to t'other are an excellent indicator of efficacy for a given strain.

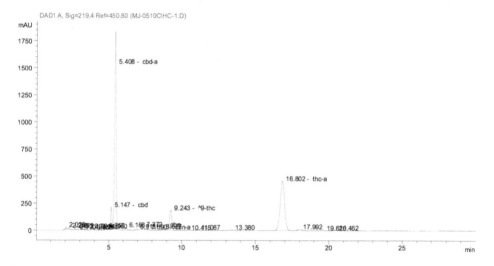

Fig. 3. HPLC (Cannabinoid) profile of a high Cannabidiol (CBD) Strain. Note the undecarboxylated THC-A and CBD-A, before heating.

In terms of dosing an individual there are some important considerations. The first being the individual's genealogy. It is our experience with roughly four thousand people over five years is that body weight is irrelevant to the effects experienced by a person using cannabis. Much more important is the individuals heritage or genetic background. Time and time again in working with persons using cannabis therapeutically it is the British Celtic (Irish, Scottish, Welsh) races that require more cannabis to relieve pain symptoms. Often three to five times more than middle Europeans, Asians or Africans, the latter, often not following theory as well as the former two.

Nevertheless, it is a common observation amongst cannabis users that different races have different tolerances with the Celts being the most tolerant. This phenomenon is important to recognize in sparing many from overdose, particularly with oral preparations and persons with lowered tolerance to cannabis.

Our first question in counseling an individual on cannabis use (particularly with oral administration) is what is their genealogy? Celts will frequently start with 50 to 100 mg of

THC without experiencing any of the effects of overdose, whereas Europeans will start with 20 to 40 mg of THC. We have recently reported two case studies (21,22) where the members being studied were both of Celtic origin, both dealing with pain issues and each required up to 500mg of THC as cannabis per day, to relieve their symptoms.

Now how does one determine THC concentrations in cannabis buds that are to be smoked or even prepped into an oral dose? We will present averages taken here in British Columbia that correlate with other areas of the world were cannabis is being used under medical license. Averages of BC cannabis that was provided to the members of one BC Compassion club is indicative of the concentrations of three cannabinoids found in most commercial cannabis available here and elsewhere.

THC + THC-A (total THC) 172 (± 26) mg/gram

CBD + CBD-A (total CBD) 3.1 (± 0.5) mg/gram

CBN + CBN-A (total CBN) 2.7 (± 0.5) mg/gram

n = 30

Table 1.

Review of the literature on smoked cannabis provides an average ingestion of THC consumed when smoking. A good rule of thumb is that 20% of the available THC is ingested during smoking; the other 80% is lost to atmosphere or pyrolysis. Therefore, of the average 170-mg/gram of THC available, the patient would ingest roughly 34 mg from 1 gram of smoked cannabis, but since most cannabis cigarettes are normally in the 0.5-gram range, this would be approximately 17 mg per dose.

One will note that the concentration of total THC is far greater than CBD or CBN, since breeding, lighting and fertilizer regimens have all been designed to increase THC levels in commercial cannabis. We feel that this is unfortunate considering the growing evidence of the medical benefits of CBD. It is extremely rare to find strains that have anything above these averages for CBD or CBN.

Incidentally, dividing the mg/gram value by 10 provides the percent value.

And, since decarboxylation is a one to one conversion of the acid to the alcohol moiety, with complete loss of the carboxyl group it is possible to administer virtually 100% of the available THC, CBD and CBN, in an oral preparation.

For persons suffering from chronic pain, oral administration of cannabis is greatly preferred over smoking. By oral ingestion, dosing is normally every four to six hours, with the average in the range of 50 to 100 mg of THC, depending on genealogy, cannabis experience and term of use.

4.4 Overdose

An overdose on THC can be a terribly frightening experience. Feelings of fear, paranoia, confusion and vivid death thoughts can occur to a person with low tolerance and unfamiliar with cannabis, who has overdosed on THC. Having done so, it is rare that an individual will want to repeat the event.

Therefore, overdose is to be avoided since a member may miss out on significant pain relief from correct dosing, because of fear of another overdose. This is one of the important aspects of standardized capsules, such that a member can start small and work up, to where relief is found. Important to people with chronic pain, is that low doses won't work, high doses can sometimes make the pain worse and medium doses are best. A medium dose being 50 mg for most, and 150 mg for a Scot. Sorry folks, the phenomenon of Celtic tolerance repeats itself too often to be ignored.

The good thing about overdose is that no one dies. There are no recorded deaths resulting from cannabis use (23). One estimate of THC's LD50 for humans indicates that about 1,500 pounds (680 kg) of cannabis would have to be smoked within 14 minutes.[24], to achieve toxic levels of THC. Cannabis can be considered an anti-toxin with constituents that offer neuroprotection, anti-oxidant activity and reduced stress.

Robert Kampia, Founder and Executive Director of the Marijuana Policy Project. House Subcommittee on Criminal Justice, Drug Policy, and Human Resources. Apr. 1, 2004: Stated that: "Regarding the claim that marijuana is too dangerous to be a medicine, it is interesting to note that there has never been a death attributed to an overdose of marijuana. Clearly, most prescription drugs are far more dangerous than marijuana."[25]

In summary, overdose can easily happen, particularly, when a person orally ingests unstandardized product and is not tolerant to the herb, often resulting in a feeling that one will die...but none do.

4.5 Strain specificity

Important too, when considering dosage is the strain of cannabis in question. There are two subspecies of cannabis, *Indica* and *Sativa*, and since they're the same species they interbreed creating thousands of strains of cannabis each with its own unique pharmacology. It is this latter understanding that holds many of us to it as an extremely useful herbal medicine with a very broad efficacy.

Firstly, correct strain selection is paramount for relief of chronic pain. In general the *Indicas* known as Kushs are widely used for pain relief, as are the Indicas as opposed to *Sativas*. The latter tend to be stimulatory and not as effective for pain. Indeed, Indica's tend to have higher levels of Cannabidiol (CBD), a cannabinoid with demonstrated powerful anti-inflammatory action (26). Our studies using HPLC to quantify cannabinoid concentrations in standardized capsules finds that a ratio roughly 1:10 CBD:THC, works well for pain relief in an oral preparation at doses of 20 to 100 mg (depending on tolerance) THC, every four to six hours (21,22).

Often members at dispensaries will use the term "different strains for different pains", to describe the effects of cannabis on their symptoms. Since high cannabidiol strains are rare, it has been difficult to study the effects of CBD on pain. Touted in the literature as being non-psychoactive we observe markedly different effects with cannabis both smoked and in oral preparations when high CBD levels are found in a strain. CBD brings about sedation at moderate concentrations and shows efficacy with seizure disorder, tremor and neuropathic pain.

We have only discovered one re-producible strain in British Columbia that has a CBD count greater than 50 mg/gram dry, ground, flower weight and, indeed, this strain that has proven most useful in treating persons with chronic pain (patent app). The rarity of high CBD concentrations in B.C. cannabis and other parts of the world where cannabis is grown commercially is a result of selective breeding of high THC strains, over many years, such that cannabidiol has essentially been bred out of commercially available cannabis.

Cannabidiol is useful for a number of reasons…importantly its anti-inflammatory action (26). This property is fully utilized in treating rheumatoid arthritis, irritable bowel syndrome, and bacterial injury, to name a few. Also important is the anti-psychotic effects of CBD, when administered in conjunction with THC. CBD appears to 'buffer' the action of THC at the receptor, allowing less chance of overdose, further permitting higher THC doses, necessary for chronic pain management.

What this means is that CBD can be used to modulate and enhance the effects of THC, in pain management. We have previously discussed the differences in tolerance dependent on genealogy that many persons using cannabis therapeutically can easily overdose particularly on oral preparations. To avoid this we have provided members who are sensitive to cannabis, with high CBD capsules to take along with relatively high THC concentrations and thus prevent the fear and paranoia of overdose and ultimately allowing better pain relief.

5. Cross reaction and allergy

In all of our years studying cannabis effects on members of dispensaries or persons with an MMAR licenses, we have not observed cross-reaction with any other medications, including opiates (synergy observed, discussed below), anti-depressants, NSAIDS or steroids. The apparent neuroprotective, anti-oxidant and homeostatic properties of cannabis, no doubt, playing a role in the non-toxic events arising from combined drug interaction. What is observed occasionally is allergic response to cannabis. Although few in number, on rare occasions a member will present with hives, irritation of the nose, sneezing, itching, and redness of the eyes, symptoms of allergy.

6. Opiate reduction

Although we do not yet have hard data to present on the subject, repeated observation, plus a number of case studies demonstrate the phenomenon of significant reduction in opiate consumption when an individual begins using cannabis therapeutically, particularly by the oral route. In the case study on chronic pain (21) our subject, over the course of one year was able to set aside the following medications and is currently only using cannabis for pain management: Arthrotec, Flexeril, ketorolac, Tylenol 3 with codeine, Naprosyn, Percocet, gabapentin, Marinol, Lyrica, Supradol, oxycodin and Oxycontin for pain. Doxepin, Imovane, Cipralex, Trazadone, Elavil, Effexor XR for depression and HCTZ, Lipitor and ranitidine for a secondary hypercholesterolemia. Even the latter hypercholesterolemia has subsided since using cannabis.

Furthermore, other researchers have noted the same occurrence of opiate reduction or cessation with subsequent use of marijuana (27). And, others have found synergy with opiates, to which we fully agree. Pain relief is better realized when cannabis is used concurrently with opiate medications than with either, alone (28). Dr. Donald Abrams', Chief of Hematology-Oncology at San Francisco General Hospital research team found that plasma levels of opiates did not increase with concurrent use of cannabis, but surprisingly decreased in amounts, yet showed an increase in pain relief. This seemingly paradoxical effect was described as being pharmacodynamic rather than pharmacokinetic...the mechanism remains unexplained, but the finding is significant in that persons using opiates for pain relief could actually use less for equal or better pain relief if cannabis is included in the regimen (28).

The observed reduction in opiate consumption, plus dispensary's, repeatedly using cannabis to significantly reduce or eliminate other addictions suggests its role as a powerful harm reduction agent. Claims of the ability to de-rail crack cocaine and crystal meth addictions, plus reduce or eliminate heroin and methadone were frequently made by dispensary staff members. We believe this to be, once again, the ability of cannabis to lend homeostasis to the human CNS, allowing easier withdrawal and maintenance.

7. Natural supplements

As mentioned earlier in this document chronic pain often cycles with mood disorder. Anxiety and depression are close relatives to pain and although cannabis can help with the symptoms (provided the correct strain and dosage is selected), there are other natural supplements we have found useful for pain management. Taking the lead in popularity with our chronic pain population are free amino acids such as Tyrosine and DL-Phenylalanine, indeed GABA is found to be useful in treating pain as well as anxiety. Other mood enhancing natural products commonly used in pain management are phosphatidylserine (PS) and phosphatidylcholine (PC), S-adenosyl methionine and, of course, B-complex.

Frequently people using cannabis therapeutically, in time, want to eliminate synthetic pharmaceutical drugs from the repertoire entirely and therefore natural supplements fare well, and effectively, in their treatment.

8. Terpenes

It seems appropriate, at this time, to enter another realm of cannabis effects...the terpenes and aromatics contained in the flowers of the plant that are often misunderstood and not realized for medicinal importance. We've conducted experiments creating oral preparations for members that had equal amounts of THC. One, called the "bald" prep, had only THC, the other, termed the "hairy" prep, had an equal amount of THC as the "bald" prep, but also contained the sixty-odd other cannabinoids, plus the terpenes and other essential oils of marijuana. Members reported that the bald prep was boring...indeed it did help with pain, but not to the extent of the "hairy" prep, that provided euphoria and the full cannabis experience. Conclusions from this experiment, that the effects of cannabis are certainly not all about THC, as earlier literature tended to suggest. We have often stated that there is a whole medicinal science called aroma therapy, that incidentally, has not had the use of cannabis essential oils, since they have been banned as long as the plant.

We believe the terpenes, as a result of their chemistry, to be brain active molecules, acting more like anesthetics than receptor binding agonists, playing their role by interacting with nerve cell membranes and modulating subsequent neurotransmission. Failure to include terpenes in cannabis medicine will leave much out of cannabis effects and, furthermore, we do not agree with ozonating cannabis medicine, for sterilization purposes, since we fear the formation of free radicals and reactive acid species (29).

And we do not believe euphoria should be left out of pain management, considering the therapy of laughter and smiles and the mood disorder that often cycles with chronic pain. Euphoria is medically recognized as a mental and emotional state defined as a profound sense of well-being. Technically, euphoria is an affect, but the term is often colloquially used to define emotion as an intense state of transcendent happiness combined with an overwhelming sense of contentment. The word derives from Greek, "power of enduring easily" (30). For those in chronic pain euphoria is welcomed as a break from "the banging drum" and although transient with cannabis it can lead to the preferred psychological state of a better quality of life.

Euphoria is more common to smoked cannabis than oral, since the terpenes enter the blood stream via the lung and are not metabolized first by the liver, as with oral ingestion.

9. Neuroimaging

The inverse agonist MK-9470 makes it possible to produce in vivo images of the distribution of CB1 receptors in the human brain with positron emission tomography.[31] This work, graphically illustrates the abundance of the receptor and its locations.

10. Conclusions

Since discovery of the cannabinoid receptor by Raphael Merchoulam of the Hebrew University in Jerusalem in the early 1990's there has been an absolute explosion in research on what is now called the endocannabinoid system. The system, that is ubiquitous in human physiology is so prolific that it has been said that the human body is "wired for cannabis". Indeed the most common G-protein receptor site in the human brain binds THC. Given the magnitude of this system and its influence of human biochemistry, it is certainly not "of no medical value", yet remains as a Schedule 1 drug in the United States.

As stated a number of times in this Chapter we treat cannabis as a whole plant herbal medicine; we analyze it that way, standardize and quality control it, using the same QC parameters as set out by Health Canada for any other herbal medicine in the country. And we have studied its effects in humans for more than a decade.

Having, in this time observed thousands of persons, most of them in chronic pain, using cannabis therapeutically, in retrospect, we are also impressed by the apparent lack of adverse effects and events seen. We know that panic and anxiety attacks following cannabis use can often be avoided with correct strain selection and dosage. And all of these adverse effects are transient.

After repeated observation, time and time again of desired effects in pain management with persons using cannabis we can only conclude it to be and extremely important and useful herbal medicine. Indeed, a witch's brew of phenolics, flavanoids, vitamins, terpenes, cannabinoids, and many other compounds of medical and human interest, we have always maintained that with sufficient instrumentation and resources, we could complete the story on the efficacy and safety of cannabis, *the whole plant herbal medicine.*

The fact that cannabis is illegal for most people often forces them to use synthetic painkillers that may prove harmful to liver, kidney and heart, with extended use. We have always promoted standardized, quality controlled, herbal cannabis medicine, and, as stated we do not highly purify or synthesize any of its components.

We have not observed any toxic events with any human subjects…not once. Noted on rare occasions are allergic responses to cannabis smoke or oral ingestion that may prevent a person from further use, but never more adverse or toxic reactions to the plant.

Having repeated this exhaustively, our team has concluded that marijuana is a safe and profoundly effective herbal medicine. So effective, in fact, that it has been banned across most of the world for almost 100 years. This is a tragedy, for those who suffer and could gain a new, extended quality of life, for those who do not know of the miracle of cannabis and for those who do.

Research has always been difficult with no government grants or similar resources to support labor or required equipment cost, we have essentially funded the work ourselves, with the help of the dispensaries and their members.

Apart from the occasional overdose, to which full recovery is made, we have only observed benefit in quality of life for those using cannabis therapeutically. Sometimes these benefits are alarming with members setting aside walkers and dancing in waiting rooms, after using marijuana. We have worked with members with crushed, metal impregnated and amputated limbs, addicted to pharmaceutical and street drugs, suffering from bipolar, ADHD, anxiety and depression…all find apparent benefit.

Seems astounding, maybe troubling, why this plant is illegal throughout most of the world, or maybe you've just figured it out too.

11. Acknowledgements

To all of the people of courage we've met at dispensaries, which take their well being into their own hands and make a difference. Thank you for your unwavering support in studies and diligence in cooperation and reporting.

A very special thanks to John Berfelo who's courage in treating his chronic pain with cannabis inspired and lent to our first case study (21) and much of the research referred to in this text.

To Marco Renda for his inspiration and innovation with the Treating Yourself Expo and and Magazine and their support of the Chapter.

12. References

[1] Americans for Safe Access: Cannabis and Chronic Pain Brochure
www.safeaccessnow.org/downloads/pain_brochure.pdf

[2] Mel Pohl MD 2008 in "A Day Without Pain" Central Recovery Press, Las Vegas NV 89129

[3] Hitzig v. Canada, 2003 CanLII 30796 (ON C.A.)

[4] M. Herkenham et al., J. Neurosci. 11, 563 (1991).

[5] L. A. Matsuda, T. I. Bonner, S. J. Lolait, J. Comp.Neurol. 327, 535 (1993).

[6] K. Tsou, S. Brown, M. C. San÷udo-Pen÷a, K. Mackie, J. M. Walker, Neuroscience 83, 393 (1998).

[7] RI Wilson and RA Nicoll Endocannabinoid Signaling in the Brain, Science 296, 678 (2002)

[8] Herkenham M, Lynn AB, Johnson MR, Melvin LS, de Costa BR, Rice KC. Characterization and localization of cannabinoid receptors in rat brain: a quantitative in vitro autoradiographic study. J Neurosci. 1991;11:563-583.

[9] Tsou K, Brown S, Sanudo-Peña MC, Mackie K, Walker JM. Immunohistochemical distribution of cannabinoid CB1 receptors in the rat central nervous system. Neuroscience. 1997;83:393-411.

[10] Egertová M, Cravatt BF, Elphick MR. Comparative analysis of fatty acid amide hydrolase and cb(1) cannabinoid receptor expression in the mouse brain: evidence of a widespread role for fatty acid amide of endocannabinoid signaling. Neuroscience. 2003;119:481-496.

[11] Egertov M, Giang DK, Cravatt BF, Elphick MR. A new perspective on cannabinoid signalling: complementary localization of fatty acid amide hydrolase and the CB1 receptor in rat brain. Proc R Soc Lond B Biol Sci. 1998;265:2081-2085.

[12] Tsou K, Nogueron MI, Muthian S, et al. Fatty acid amide hydrolase is located preferentially in large neurons in the rat central nervous system as revealed by immunohistochemistry. Neurosci Lett. 1998;254:137-140.

[13] http://www.cannabis-med.org/data/pdf/en_2010_01_special.pdf

[14] Abrams DI, Jay CA, Shade SB, Vizozo H, Reda H, Press S, Kelly ME, Rowbotham Mc, Petersen KL (2007). "Cannabis in painful HIV-associated sensory neuropathy: a randomized placebo-controlled trail". J. Neurology 68 (7): 515-21.

[15] Wilsey B, Marcotte T, Tsodikov A, Millman J, Bentley H, Gouaux B, Fishman S (2008). "A randomized, placebo-controlled, crossover trail of cannabis cigarettes in neuropathic pain". J. Pain 9 (6): 506-21.

[16] Pacher P, Mechoulam R (2011). "Is lipid signaling through cannabinoid 2 receptors part of a protective system?". Prog Lipid Res. 50 (2): 193-211.

[17] Sylvaine G, Sophie M, Marchand J, Dussossoy D, Carriere D, Carayon P, Monsif B, Shire D, LE Fur G, Casellas P (1995). "Expression of Central and Peripheral Cannabinoid Receptors in Human Immune Tissues and Leukocyte Subpopulations". Eur J Biochem. 232 (1): 54-61.

[18] Griffin G, Tao Q, Abood ME (2000). "Cloning and pharmacological characterization of the rat CB(2) cannabinoid receptor". J Pharmacol Exp Ther. 292 (3): 886-894.

[19] Tuccinardi T, Ferrarini PL, Manera C, Ortore G, Saccomanni G, Martinelli A. (2006). "Cannabinoid CB2/CB1 selectivity. Receptor modeling and automated docking analysis". J Med Chem 49 (3): 984-994.

[20] Centonze D, Battistini L, Maccarrone M (2008). "The endocannabinoid system in peripheral lymphocytes as a mirror of neuroinflammatory diseases". Curr. Pharm. Des. 14 (23): 2370–42.

[21] Hornby et al.Cases Journal 2009, 2:7487

[22] Hornby, et al. Cases Journal 2010, 3:7

[23] Union movie. Business behind getting high. Quote from Dr. Lester Grinspoon MD | Professor Emeritus, Harvard Medical School.

[24] Annas, George J. (1997). "Reefer Madness — The Federal Response to California's Medical-Marijuana Law". New England Journal of Medicine 337 (6): 435–9.

[25] John A. Benson, Jr., MD, Janet E. Joy, PhD, and Stanley J. Watson, Jr., MD, PhD, co-writers of the Mar. 1999 Institute of Medicine report titled "Marijuana and Medicine: Assessing the Science Base," wrote the following in their Mar. 22, 1999 article titled "From Marijuana to Medicine," published in Issues in Science and Technology:

[26] Scuderi C, Filippis DD, Iuvone T, Blasio A, Steardo A, Esposito G Cannabidiol in medicine: a review of its therapeutic potential in CNS disorders. Phytother Res 2008 Oct 9.

[27] Morel LJ, Giros B, Daugé V (2009). "Adolescent Exposure to Chronic Delta-9-Tetrahydrocannabinol Blocks Opiate Dependence in Maternally Deprived Rats". Neuropsychopharmacology 34 (11): 2469–76.

[28] Dr. Donald Abrams Compares Cannabis To Opiate-based Medicines
http://www.youtube.com/watch?v=cGPtirNqGlM

[29] M. Springs1,J. R. Wells2,G. C. Reaction rates of ozone and terpenes adsorbed to model indoor surfaces Morrison1Article first published online: 7 FEB 2011DOI: 10.1111/j.1600-0668.2010.00707.x

[30] Memidex/WordNet - euphoria

[31] KP, Glaser ST, Gatley SJ.Handb Exp Pharmacol. 2005;(168):425-43. Imaging of the brain cannabinoid system.Lindsey

3

The Research of Lygodium

Zhang Guo-Gang, He Ying-Cui,
Liu Hong-Xia, Zhu Lin-Xia and Chen Li-Juan
*College of Traditional Chinese Materia Medica,
Shenyang Pharmaceutical University, Shengyang,
China*

1. Introduction

Lygodium is the dry root and rhizome of *Lygodium japonicum* (Thunb.)Sw. which belongs to the family Lygodiaceae. *Lygodium* is the only genus of Lygodiaceae comprises 45 species throughout the world. In China, there are 10 species of *Lygodium* distributed in the southwest and south China, and five species of them had been used for Chinese herbs medicine to treat hepatitis and dysentery[1]. They are named Lygodium, Lygodium of hainan, Crankshaft Lygodium, Angustifolia Lygodium, Pinnately lobed Lygodium, Willow-like leaves Lygodium, Reticulata Lygodium, yunnan Lygodium, Lobular Lygodium, Palm leaf Lygodium.

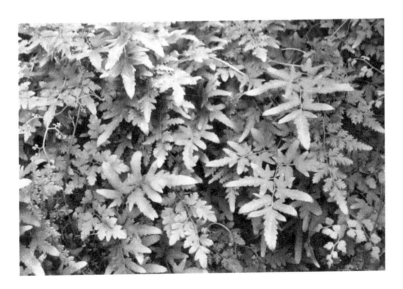

Fig. 1. Leaves and branches of *Lygodium japonicum* (Thunb.)Sw.

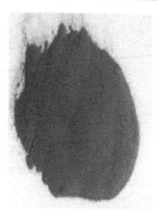

Fig. 2. Dried powder of *Lygodium japonicum* (Thunb.)Sw.

2. Chemical composition

Currently, the research on the active components in the Lygodium were done on the underground parts. We summarize the structure and classification of these compounds from *lygodium*.

2.1 The main components of the Lygodium root[3]

2.1.1 Ecdysteroside

Capitasterone-3-O-β-D-glucopyranoside

Lygodiumsteroside A*

Lygodiumsteroside B*

Makisterone C

2.1.2 Triterpenes

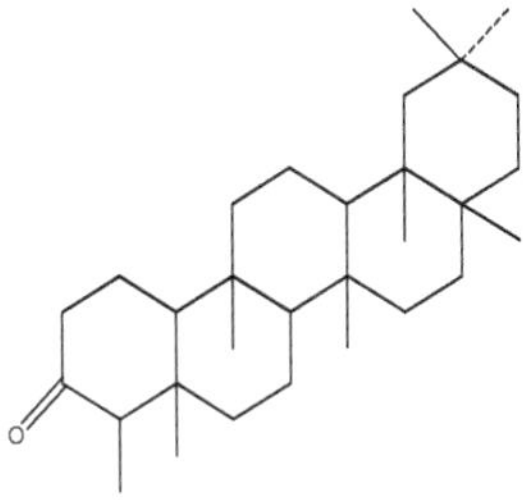

Friedelin

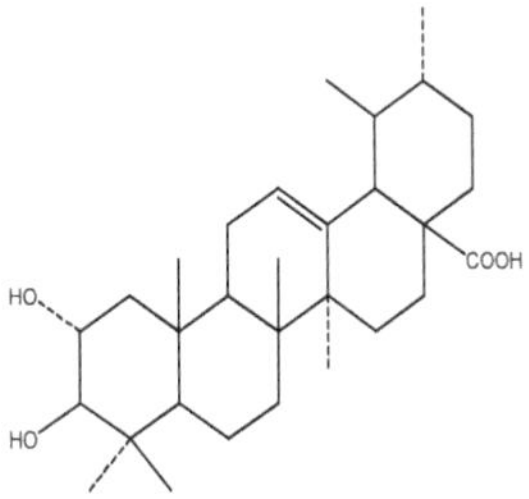

2α-hydroxyursolic acid

2.1.3 Flavonoids

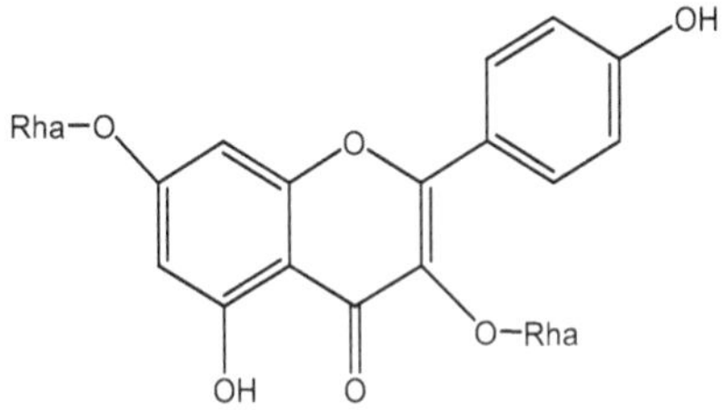

Kaempferol-3-O-α-L- rhamnopyranoside-7-O-α- L-rhamnopyranoside

2.1.4 Phytosterols

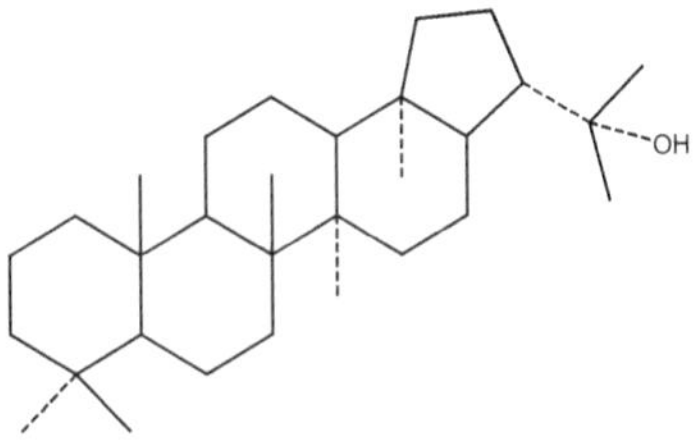

22-hydroxyhopane

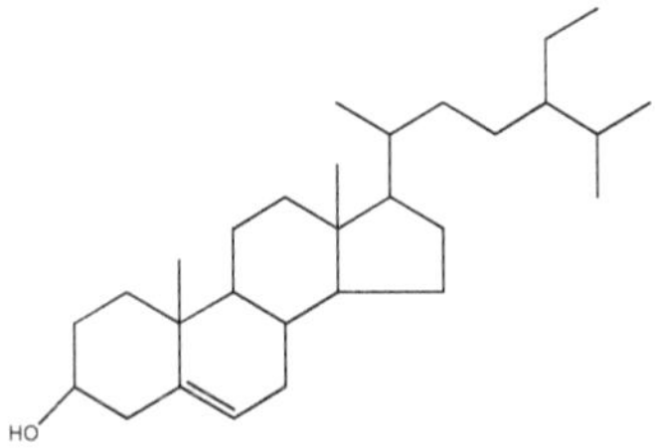

β-phytosterol

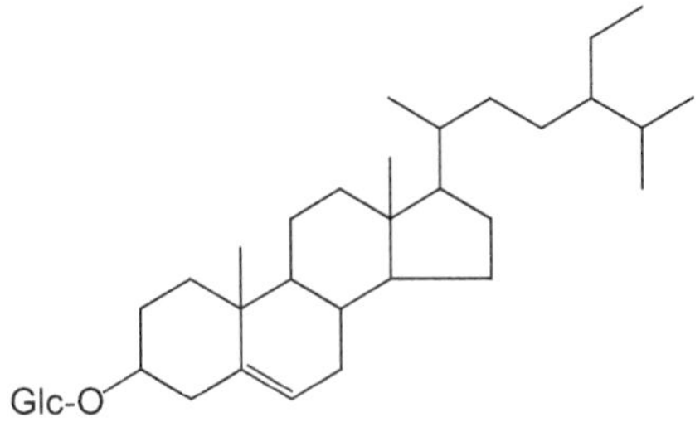

Daucosterol

2.1.5 Glycosides

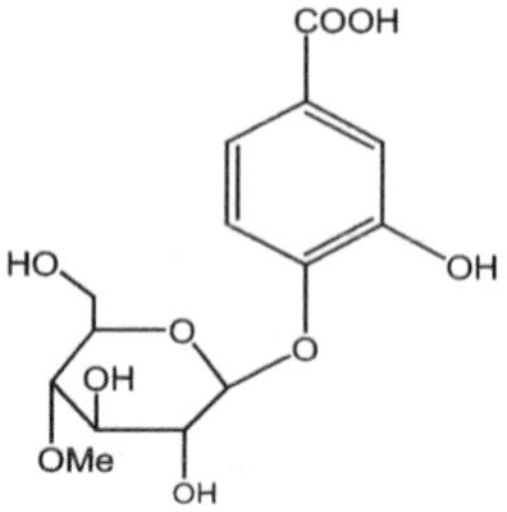

3,4-dihydroxybenzoic acid 4-O- (4'-O-methyl)-β-D-glucopyranoside

2.1.6 Organic acids

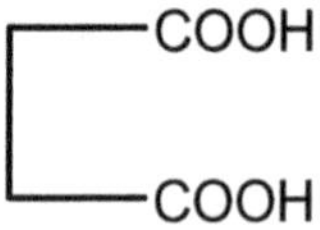

Succinic acid

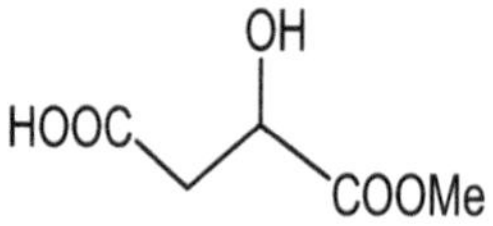

Methylmalic acid

2.1.7 Naphthoquinone

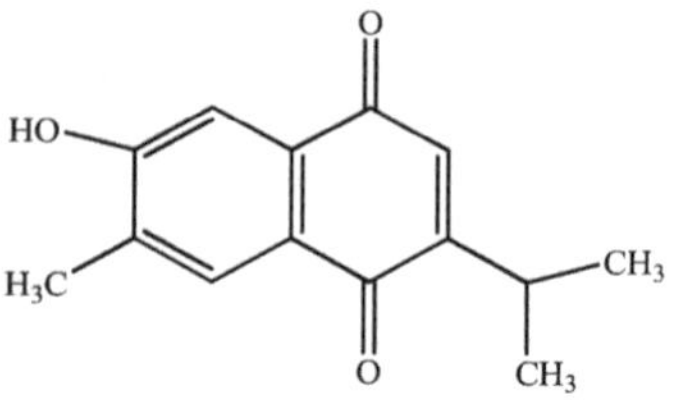

2-isopropyl-7-methly-6-hydroxy-α-(1,4) naphthoquinone∗

2.2 The main components of the root of Lygodium from n-butanol layer[2][3]

2.2.1 flavonoids

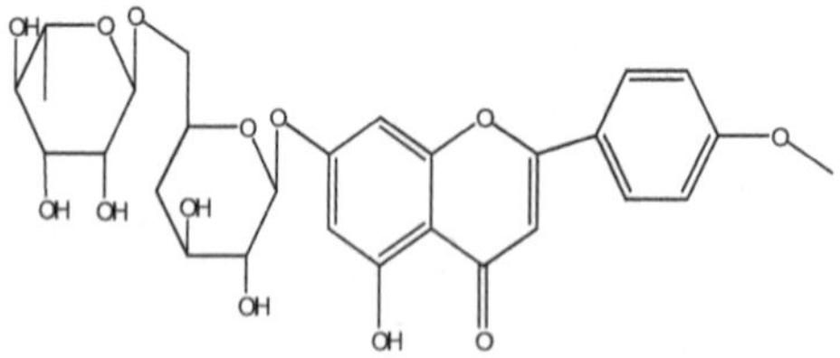

Linaribn

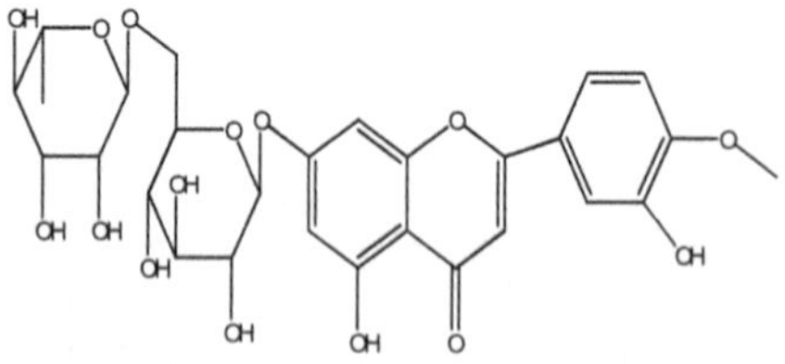

Dosinin

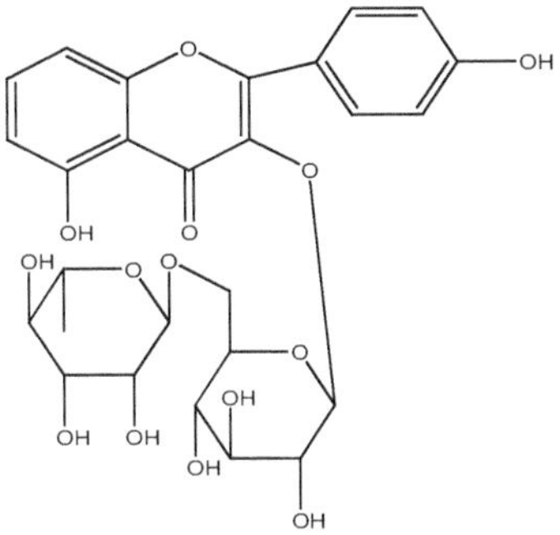

Nicotflorin

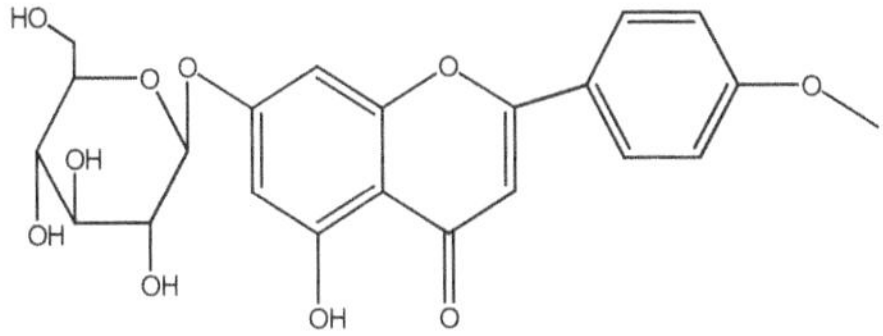

Tilianine

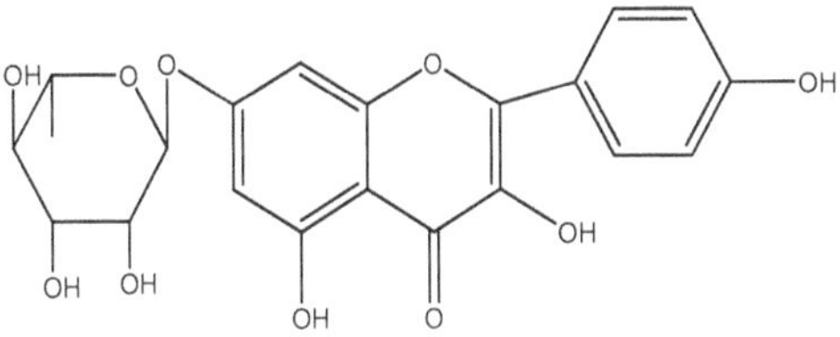

Kaempferol- α

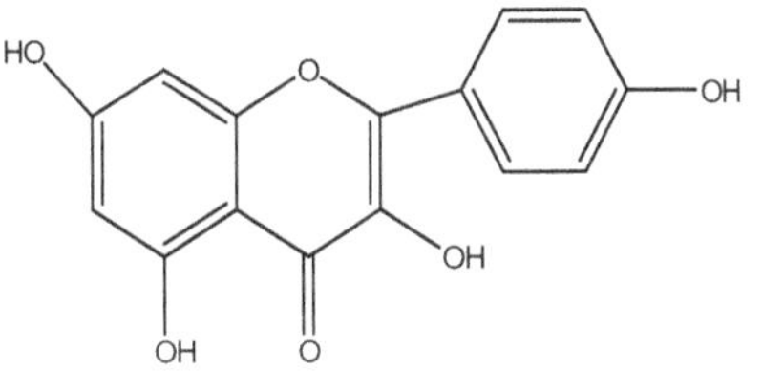

Kaempferol-1-rhamnopyranoside

2.2.2 Phenylpropanoids

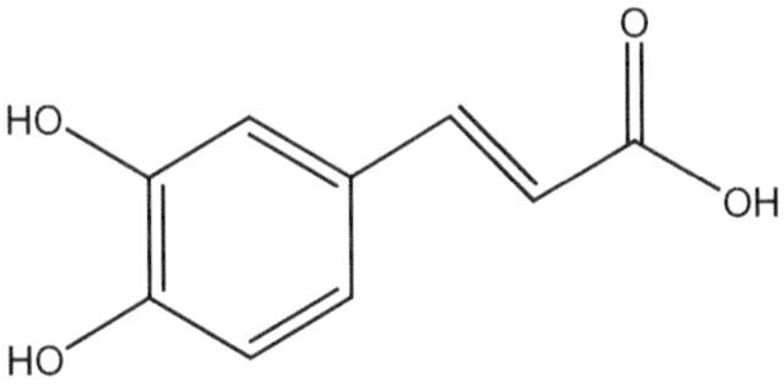

Caffeic acid

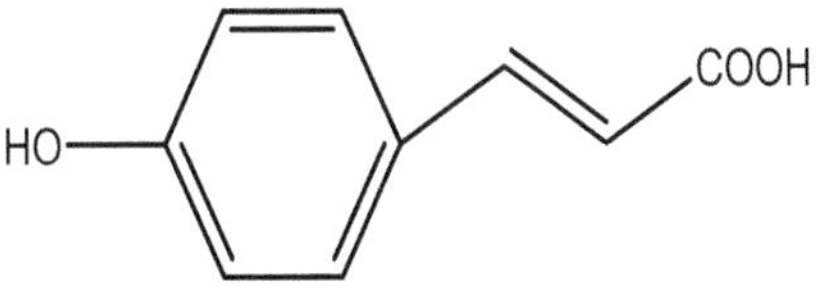

P-coumaric acid

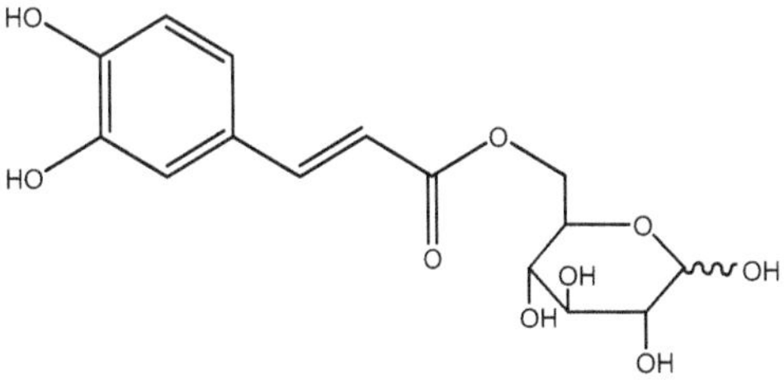

6-O-p-coumaroyl-D-glucopyranose

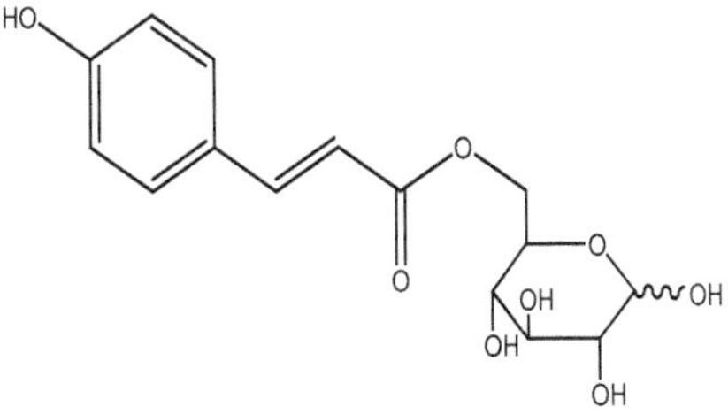

6-O-caffeoyl-D-glucopyranose

2.2.3 Phenolic acids[4]

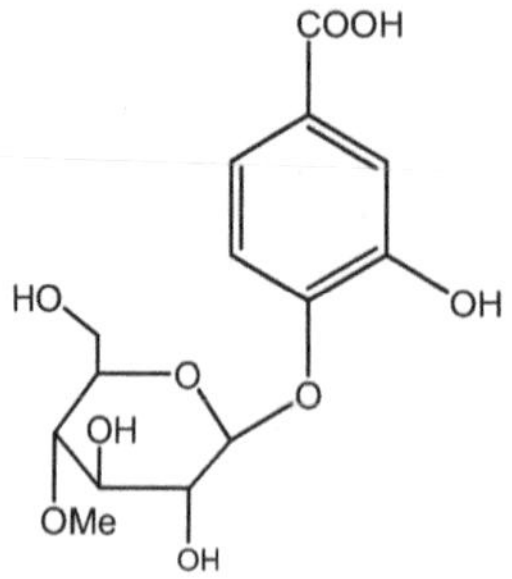

3,4-Dihydroxybenzoic acid 4-O-
(4'-O-methyl)-β-D-glucopyranoside

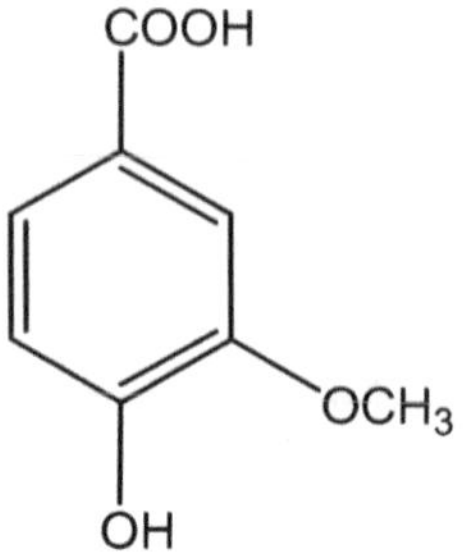

Vanillic acid

2.2.4 Sterols

A new steroidal saponins was Isolated from the root of Lygodium, which is (24- R)-stigmastan-3β, 5a,6β-triol-3-O-β-D-glucopyranoside, in addition to daucosterol and β-sitosterol.

2.2.5 Others

Hexadecanoic acid 2, 3-dihydroxy, propyl ester, hexacosanoic acid, 1-hentriacontanol, pentacosanoic acid, palmitic acid, linoleic acid, (6S, 9R) -6 - hydroxy -3- ketone - Violet alcohol-D-β-9-O-glucoside (roseoside) and so on.

2.2.6 Diterpenoids

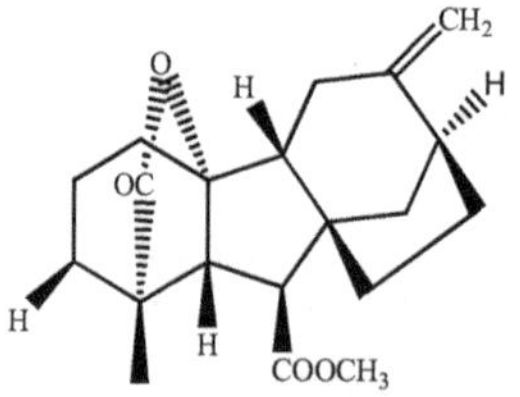

Gibberellin A$_9$ methyl ester

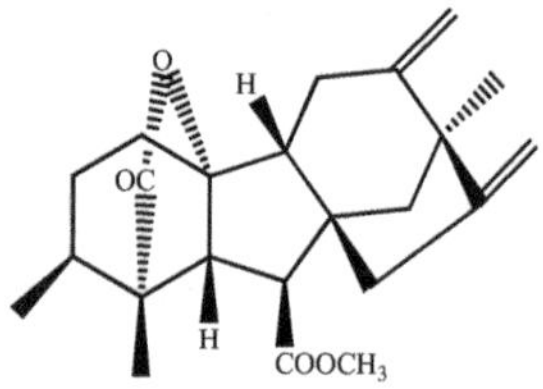

Gibberellin A$_{73}$ methyl ester

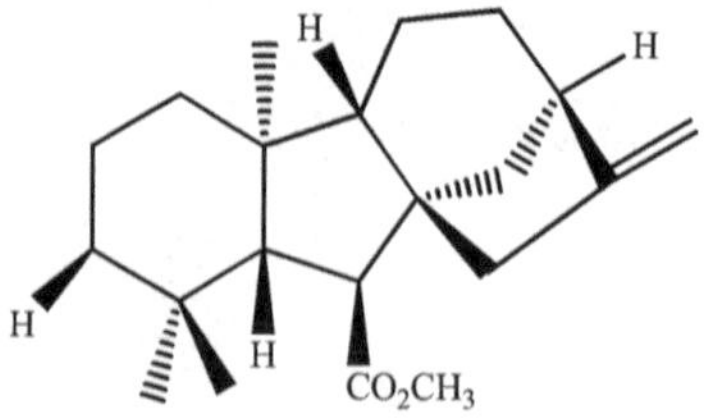

Gibberellin A$_{12}$ methylester

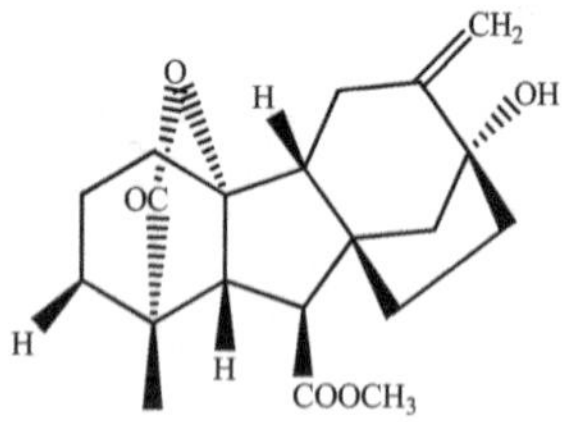

GA$_{20}$-Me

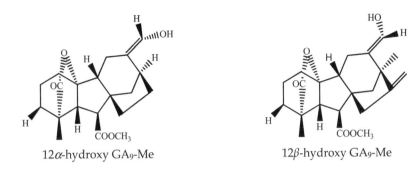

12α-hydroxy GA₉-Me   12β-hydroxy GA₉-Me

3. New compounds from *Lygodium japonicum*

3.1 New naphthalene ketone from the root of *Lygodium japonicum*[5]

3.1.1 Extraction and isolation

Air-dried roots of *L. japonicum* (Thunb.) Sw.(4 kg) were crushed and extracted twice under reflux with 70% EtOH. Evaporation of the solvent under reduced pressure delivered the 70% EtOH extract (around 280 g). The extract was partitioned successively with CHCl₃, AcOEt and n-BuOH. The n-BuOH-soluble fraction(50.0 g) was further eluted on a silica gel column using gradient elution with CHCl₃–MeOH (100:1–1:1) to give ten fractions. Fraction 2 (2.3 g) was subjected to another silica gel column chromatography eluted with petroleum ether (PE)–EtOAc (20:1–1:1) to afford a further five fractions (frs. 2-1 to 2-5). Fraction 2-2 was purified twice by Sephadex LH-20 eluted with MeOH to give the new compound 1(9mg).

3.1.2 Apparatus

Melting points were determined on an X4-A micro-melting point apparatus and were uncorrected. ESI–MS spectra were measured on an Agilent 1100 LC-MSD-Trap-SL, and HR–ESI–MS spectra were measured on an Bruker Dal- tonics MicroTOFQ. NMR spectra were measured on a Bruker ARX-600 and 300 NMR spectrometer with tetra-methylsilane (TMS) as the internal reference and chemical shifts are expressed with δ (ppm). UV spectra were recorded on a Shimadzu UV-2201 spectrometer. IR spectra were recorded on a Bruker IFS-55 spectrophotometer. TLC was performed on silica gel GF254 (10–40 lm; Qingdao,China). Separations were performed by Semiprep-HPLC named Shimadzu SPD-10A apparatus equipped with UV detector under ODS column (i.d. 10 mm 9 200 mm).

3.1.3 Physical data of the new compound 1

The new compound,yellow powder, melting point:193–194℃. The molecular formula was determined as $C_{14}H_{14}O_3$ by HR–ESI–TOF–MS (m/z 231.1004[M + H]⁺, calcd. 231.1016), along with ¹H-NMR and ¹³C-NMR data. The UV spectrum displayed absorption bands at 207, 267 and 347 nm, closely resembling that of 1,4-naphthoquinones. The ¹³C-NMR spectrum revealed 14 carbon resonances; in the low field area of it, two were assigned as carbonyl carbons, eight were assigned as aromatic carbons. However, in the high field area of ¹³C-NMR spectrum, there were four carbon resonances all that assigned as sp3 carbons. By observing these data of

^{13}C-NMR spectrum, nucleus of naphthoquinone was revealed. All protonated carbons were assigned by analysis of the HSQC spectrum (Table 1).The ^{1}H-NMR spectrum showed signals of two aromatic protons at δ 7.30 (1H, s, H-5), 7.77 (1H, s, H-8) and one aromatic methyl proton at d 2.24 (3H, s, 7-CH3) that were assigned by analyzing HMBC spectrum (Table 1; Fig. 1). Additionally, δ 1.12 (6H, d, J = 6.8 Hz,H-12, H-13) and 6.68 (1H, s, H-3) correlated, respectively, with d: δ 26.6 (C-11), δ 156.6 (C-2) in the HMBC spectrum and δ 3.09 (1H, m, H-11) correlated with δ 21.4(C-12 and 13), 156.6 (C-2), 131.6 (C-3), 183.4 (C-1) all that revealed the presence of isopropyl and it connected C-2 of quinone ring. Other detailed correlations in the HMBC spectrum see Table 1. All these spectroscopic data discussed above showed compound 1 as 6-hydroxy-2-isopropyl-7-methyl-1,4- naphthoquinone.

C No.	HSQC		HMBC
	δ_C	δ_H, mult	
1	183.5		
2	156.6		
3	131.6	6.68 (1H, s)	C2/C11
4	185.2		
5	110.3	7. 30 (1H, s)	C6/C9/C4
6	160.9		
7	131.8		
8	129.5	7. 77 (1H, s)	C1/C10/C7 (CH3)/C6
9	124.1		
10	131.7		
CH3-7	16.2	2.24 (3H, s)	C6/C8
11-CH-	26.6	3.09 (1H, m)	C12/ C13/C2
12-CH3	21.4	1.13 (6H, d, J=6.8 Hz)	C11/C2
13-CH3	21.4	1.11 (6H, d, J=6.8 Hz)	C11/C2

Table 1. [1]H and ^{13}C data for New naphthalene ketone (300and 75MHz,in DMSO- d_6).

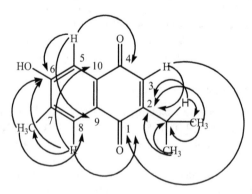

Fig. 3. The key HMBC correlations of the new compound 1.

3.2 The new compound 2 from the roots of *Lygodium japonicum*[6]

lygodiumsteroside B

3.2.1 Extraction and isolation

The air-dried roots of *L. japonicum* (Thunb.) Sw were crushed and extracted twice using reflux with 70% ethanol; the solution was concentrated under reduced pressure to obtain the residue, and then the residue was extracted with MeOH. The MeOH-soluble fraction (100 g) was isolated by column chromatography on silica gel and gradient elution with CHCl$_3$:MeOH (50 : 1 to 1 : 1) gave 14 fractions. Fraction 8 was isolated by semipreparative ODS column using MeOH:H$_2$O (65 : 35) as eluent to afford the new compound 2 (13mg).

3.2.2 Apparatus

Melting point: X-4 micro melting point determination apparatus (uncorrected). ESI–MS spectra: LC-MSD-Trap-SL. HR–ESI–MS spectra: Bruker MicroTOFQ.^{1}H NMR(600MHz) and ^{13} C NMR (150MHz): Bruker ARX-600. UV: Shimadzu UV$_1$ 260 UV–Vis. Semiprep-HPLC: Shimadzu SPD-10A apparatus equipped with UV detector under ODS column (i.d. 10mm*200mm).

3.2.3 The spectrum of new compound

1. ^{1}H-NMR and ^{13}C-NMR data for the new compound 2

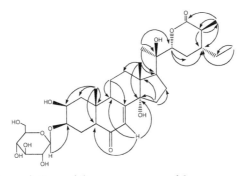

Fig. 4. The key HMBC correlations of the new compound 2.

C	HMQC		HMBC
	δ_C(ppm)	δ_H(ppm)	
1	38.7	1.74(brd, J=12.6Hz), 2.02(m)	C-2,C-3,C-9,C-10,C-19
2	67.5	4.07(br.dt, J=10.8 Hz),	
3	77.7	4.28(brs)	
4	30.6	1.65, 2.20(each m)	
5	51.4	2.93(m)	C-4,C-9
6	203.0	—	
7	121.7	6.23(brs)	C-5,C-9,C-14
8	166.3	—	
9	34.3	3.53(t, J=8.4 Hz)	
10	39.1	—	
11	21.1	1.67, 1.80(each m)	C-8,C-9,C-12,C-13
12	32.0	2.02(m),2.58(dt, J=4.2 and 12.6 Hz)	C-9,C-11,C-18
13	48.1	—	
14	84.2	—	
15	31.9	1.92, 2.17(each m)	C-13,C-16
16	21.4	2.08, 2.45(each m)	C-17
17	50.0	2.89(m)	C-13,C-15,C-16,C-18
18	18.0	1.20(s)	C-12,C-13,C-14,C-17
19	24.1	0.88(s)	C-1,C-2,C-5,C-10
20	76.9	—	
21	21.6	1.58(s)	C-17, C-20, C-22
22	74.2	3.90(m)	C-20
23	36.9	1.45, 1.63(each m)	C-21,C-24,C-28
24	35.6	1.93(m)	
25	33.7	1.46(m)	C-23,C-26,C-27
26	20.3	0.80(d, J=6.6 Hz)	C-24,C-25,C-27
27	18.7	0.76(d, J=6.6 Hz)	C-24,C-25,C-26
28	15.2	0.83(d, J=6.6 Hz)	C-23,C-24,C-25,C-27
C-1'	104.2	4.92(d, J=7.8 Hz)	C-3
C-2'	74.7	4.03(overlap)	C-3'
C-3'	78.7	4.20(overlap)	C-2', C-4'
C-4'	71.6	4.21(m)	C-5', C-6'
C-5'	78.5	3.92(m)	C-4', C-5'
C-6'	62.6	4.32(m),4.52(brd, J=10.8 Hz)	C-4', C-5'

Table 2. ^{1}H and ^{13}C NMR data for lygodiumsteroside B (600 and 150 MHz, in C_5D_5N).

2.   Other spectrum data for the new compound 2

The new compound 2(lygodiumsteroside B): white powder, m.p. 294–295°C,UV⎢max (MeOH): 243 nm; ESI–MS:m/z 675.5 [M+Cl]-, m/z 639.7 [M+H]+; HR–ESI–MS: m/z 639.3701 [M+H]+(Calcd for$C_{34}H_{55}O_{11}$ 639.3750);^{1}H-NMR (600MHz, in C_5D_5N) and ^{13}C-NMR (150MHz, inC_5D_5N), see table 2 .

3.   NMR Analysis of the new compound 2

Lygodiumsteroside B, white powder, m.p. 294–295℃, gave positive responses to Liebermann–Burchard and Molish reactions, which suggested a steroid glycoside structure. The sugar was identified as glucose by co-TLC with authentic sample after acid hydrolysis. The molecular formula was established to be $C_{34}H_{56}O_{11}$ based on HR–ESI–MS([M+H]+,m/z 639.3701, Calcd for $C_{34}H_{55}O_{11}$ 639.3750). Additionally, the UV spectrum showed a maximum at243 nm[Check this typing] for an α, β-unsaturated carbonyl group.The^{1}H NMR(600MHz,C_5D_5N) spectrum showed an olefinic proton at δ 6.23 (1H,brs) and six methyl signals at δ 1.58 (3H, s), 1.20 (3H, s), 0.88 (3H, s), 0.83(3H, d, J¼6.6Hz), 0.80 (3H, d, J¼6.6Hz), 0.76 (3H, d, J¼6.6Hz). The^{13}C –NMR (150MHz,C_5D_5N) spectrum showed six methyl signals and a typical α, β-unsaturated carbonyl group signals at δ 203.0 (C-6), 166.3 (C-8) and 121.7 (C-7). The HMBC spectrum, showed the long-range correlations between δ 6.23 (1H, brs, H-7) and δ 34.3(C-9), 51.4 (C-5), 84.2 (C-14), the correlations between methyl proton signal at δ 0.88 (3H, s,H-19) and the carbon signals at δ 38.7 (C-1), 39.1 (C-10), 51.4 (C-5) and 67.5 (C-2) could also be observed. In addition, the correlations between methyl proton signal at δ 1.20 (3H, s,H-18) and the carbon signals at δ 32.0 (C-12), 48.1 (C-13), 50.0 (C-17) and 84.1(C-14) could also be found. Thus, the ecdysteroid-type skeleton was identified. In the HSQC spectrum, δ 4.07 (1H, brd, H-2) had the correlation with δ 67.5 (C-2) and δ 4.28(1H, brs, H-3) had the correlation with (1H, brs, H-3) had the correlation with (1H, brs, H-3) had the correlation with(1H, brs, H-3) had the correlation withδ77.7 (C-3). δ 1.58 (3H, s,H-21) showed the correlation with δ 50.0 (C-17), δ 74.2 (C-22 and δ 76.9 (C-20) in the HMBC. So the signals of the five hydroxyl carbons C-2, C-3, C-14, C-20, C-22 were evident. Additionally, δ 0.83 (3H, d,H-28) showed correlation with δ 1.93 (1H,m,H-24) in the^{1}H–^{1}H COSY, and the HMBC spectrum showed the correlations between δ 0.83 (3H, s,H-28) and δ 18.7 (C-27),33.7 (C-25), 35.6 (C-24), 36.9 (C-23). These facts indicated that a methyl group (C-28) was attached to C-24.

Compared with polyporusterone A (Ishida et al., 1999; Ohsawa, Yukama, Takao,Murayama, & Bando, 1992), the chemical shifts of C5–C22 were very similar; this fact suggested that the positions of the substituents on the steroid rings and side-chain of the new compound were identical with polyporusterone A except for C24, and the configuration of hydroxyls were 14 α ,20R,22R. Since the signals at 33.7 (C-25), 20.3 (C-26), 18.7 (C-27) were different from the corresponding values of polyporusterone A, the configuration of C-24 could be different. Compared with the compound schizaeasterone A (Fuchino et al., 1997), which has 24R configuration, the chemical shifts of C20–C28 were very similar to those of schizaeasterone A. Moreover, in the NOESY spectrum, a cross peak was observed between δ 3.91 (1H, overlap, H-22) and δ 0.83 (3H, d,H-28). So all these facts indicated that the configuration of C-24 of compound 1 was R (Figure 2). The NOESY spectrum also showed the correlation between the proton signal at δ 4.07 (1H, brd, H-2) and δ 4.28 (1H, brs, H-3), δ 1.65 (1H,m,H α -4), so the relative configuration was confirmed to be2 β ,3 β .

Since the signal at δ 77.7, which could assignable to C-3, was downfield shifted by 9 ppm, and the signal at δ 30.6 (C-4) was upfield shifted, glycosylation was present atC-3. The chemical shifts of the sugar moiety in ^{13}C -NMR (δ 104.2, 74.7, 78.7, 71.6, 78.5,62.6) also confirmed the presence of glucose. The HMBC correlation was observed between the anomeric proton signal at δ 4.92 (1H, d,H-10) and the carbon signal at δ 77.7due to C-3 of the aglycone moiety. The anomeric configurations of glucose were determined to be on the basis of the JH–H values (J¼7.8Hz).Therefore, the structure of 2 was elucidated as 2β ,3β ,14α ,   20R,   22R   -   pentahydroxy-24R-methly-5-cholest-7-en-6-one-3-O- β -D-glucopyranoside, and named lygodiumsteroside B

C No.	HMQC		HMBC
	δ_C(ppm)	δ_H(ppm)	
1	38.7	1.76(m), 2.10(m)	C-2,C-3,C-9,C-10,C-19
2	67.5	4.10(br.dt, J=11.4 Hz),	
3	76.8	4.30(overlap)	
4	30.3	1.73, 2.20(each m)	C-1,C-5,C-9,C-19
5	51.4	2.93(m)	C-1,C-4,C-6,C-9
6	203.1	—	
7	121.7	6.23(d, J=1.8 Hz)	C-5,C-9,C-14
8	166.4	—	
9	34.3	3.55(t, J=8.4 Hz)	C-1,C-11,C-19
10	39.0	—	
11	21.1	1.65, 1.83(each m)	C-8,C-9,C-13
12	32.0	2.02(m),2.58(dt, J=4.2 and 12.6 Hz)	C-11,C-13,C-17,C-18
13	48.1	—	
14	84.2	—	
15	31.8	1.92, 2.15(each m)	C-13,C-16
16	21.5	2.08, 2.44(each m)	C-17
17	50.1	2.91(m)	C-11,C-13,C-15,C-18,C-22
18	17.9	1.19(s)	C-12,C-13,C-14,C-17
19	24.1	0.87(s)	C-1,C-2,C-5,C-9
20	77.7	—	
21	21.6	1.58(s)	C-17,C-22,C-23
22	76.8	3.81(brd, J=10.8 Hz)	C-21,C-24
23	28.2	1.47(m)	C-21,C-24,C-25,C-26,C-27
24	37.2	1.40, 1.70(each m)	C-23,C-26,C-27
25	30.6	1.54(m)	
26	23.4	0.81(d, J=6.0 Hz)	C-23,C-24,C-27
27	22.4	0.82(d, J=6.0 Hz)	C-23,C-24,C-26
C-1'	104.2	4.90(d, J=7.8 Hz)	C-3
C-2'	74.7	4.03(m)	C-3'
C-3'	78.7	4.20(m)	C-2', C-4'
C-4'	71.6	4.18(m)	C-5', C-6'
C-5'	78.5	3.93(m)	C-4', C-5'
C-6'	62.6	4.32(m),4.53(brd, J=10.2 Hz)	C-4', C-5'

Table 3. ^{1}H and ^{13}C NMR data for polyporusterone A (600 and 150 MHz, in C_5D_5N).

4. Attached figure:

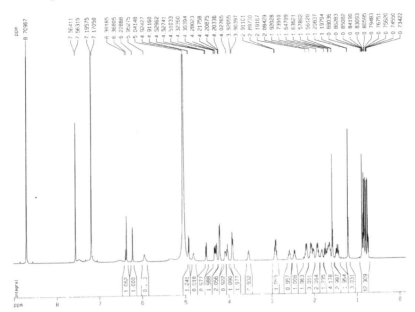

Fig. 5. Lygosteroside B (^{1}H-NMR).

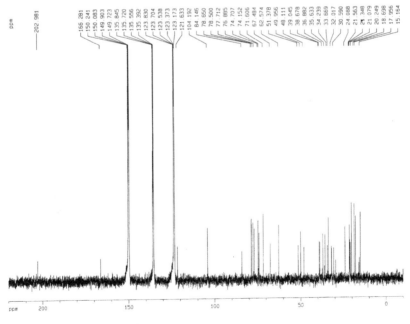

Fig. 6. Lygosteroside B (^{1}H-NMR).

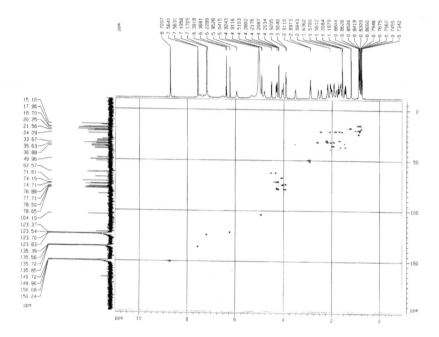

Fig. 7. Lygosteroside B (HSQC).

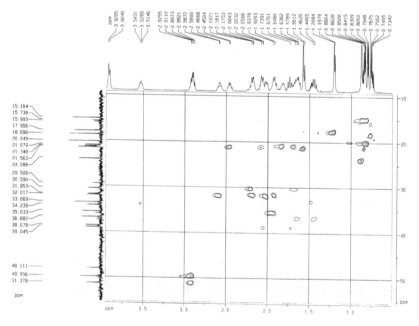

Fig. 8. Lygosteroside B (HSQC).

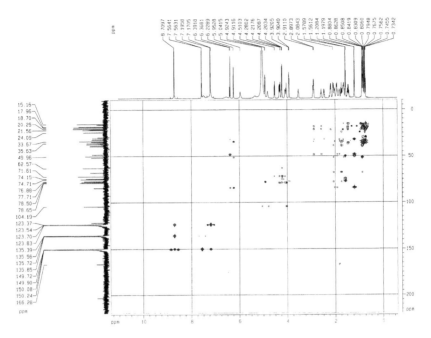

Fig. 9. Lygosteroside B (HMBC).

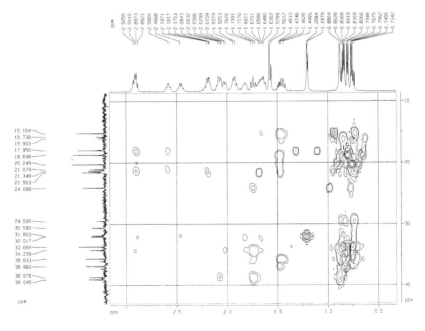

Fig. 10. Lygosteroside B (HMBC).

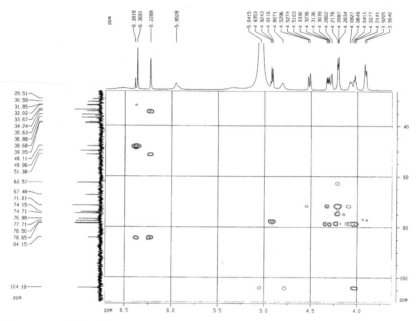

Fig. 11. Lygosteroside B (HMBC).

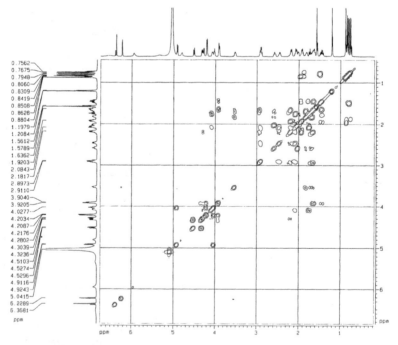

Fig. 12. Lygosteroside B (¹H-¹H COSY).

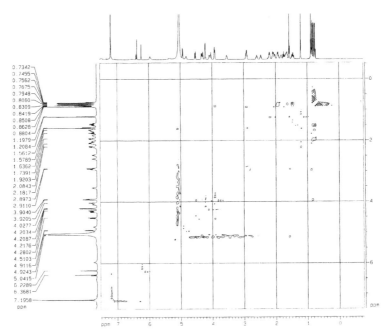

Fig. 13. Lygosteroside B (NOESY).

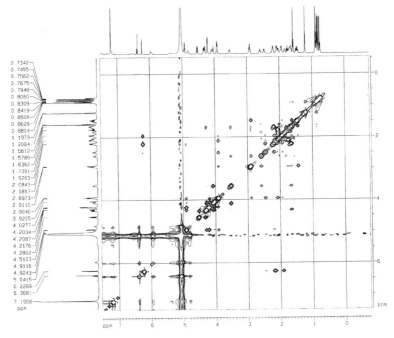

Fig. 14. Lygosteroside B (NOESY).

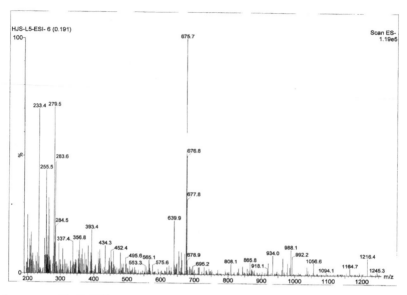

Fig. 15. Lygosteroside B (ESI).

3.3 The new compound 3 from *Lygodium* [7]

lygodiumsteroside A

3.3.1 Extraction and isolation

The air-dried roots of *L. japonicum* (Thunb.) Sw. (4 kg) were crushed and extracted twice under reflux with 70% EtOH. The solution was concentrated under reduced pressure to obtain the residue, and then the residue was extracted with MeOH. The MeOH-soluble fraction (100 g) was isolated by column chromatography on silica gel using gradient elution with $CHCl_3$–MeOH (50:1 to 1:1), which gave 14 fractions. Fraction 9 (10 g) was subjected to silica gel column chromatography using $CHCL_3$–MeOH(40:1 to1:1) in gradient to give fractions 1-4. Fraction 4 (3.7 g) was chromatographed on an ODS column eluting with

MeOH–H$_2$O system, giving two fractions. Fraction 2 (1.3 g) was isolated by a semi-preparative ODS column using MeOH–H$_2$O (65:35) as the eluent to afford lygodium A (9 mg) and a kown compound ponastteroside A(30 mg), respectively.

3.3.2 Apparatus

Melting points were determined on an X4-A micro-melting point apparatus and were uncorrected. ESI-MS spectra were measured on an Agilent1100 LC-MSD-Trap-SL, and HR-ESI-MS spectra were measured on a Bruker Daltonics MicroTOFQ. NMR spectra were measured on a Bruker ARX-600 NMR spectrometer with tetramethylsilane (TMS) as the internal reference and chemical shifts are expressed with δ (ppm). UV spectra were recorded on a Shimadzu UV-2201 spectrometer. IR spectra were recorded on a Bruker IFS-55 spectrophotometer. TLC was performed on silica gel GF254 (10–40 l; Qingdao, China).Separation was performed by semiprep HPLC using Shimadzu SPD-10A apparatus equipped with a UV detector under an ODS column (i.d. 10 mm * 200 mm).

3.3.3 The spectrum of new compound

1. NMR data (nuclear magnetic resonance) of lygodiumsteroside A

C No.	HMQC		HMBC
	δ_C(ppm) DEPT	δ_H(ppm)	
1	38.0 (t)	1.72(t, J=12.6 Hz), 2.05(m)	C-2,C-3,C-9,C-10,C-19
2	66.8 (d)	4.06(br.dt, J=11.4 Hz),	
3	77.1 (d)	4.29(brs)	
4	29.9 (t)	1.66, 2.16(each m)	
5	50.7 (d)	2.90(m)	C-4,C-9
6	202.3 (s)	—	
7	121.1 (d)	6.18(brs)	C-5,C-9,C-14
8	165.4 (s)	—	
9	33.5 (d)	3.50(brt)	
10	38.4 (s)	—	
11	20.3 (t)	1.64, 1.77(each m)	C-8,C-9,C-10,C-12
12	31.2 (t)	1.86, 2.57(each m)	C-9,C-11,C-13,C-18
13	47.2 (d)	—	
14	83.4 (s)	—	
15	31.1 (t)	1.86, 2.12(each m)	C-14,C-16,C-17
16	20.7 (t)	2.05, 2.39(each m)	C-17
17	49.2 (d)	2.93(m)	C-13,C-16,C-18
18	17.3 (q)	1.09(s)	C-12,C-13,C-14,C-17
19	23.4 (q)	0.86(s)	C-2,C-5,C-9,C-10
20	75.1 (s)	—	
21	20.7 (q)	1.44(s)	C-17, C-20, C-22
22	85.3 (d)	4.44(dd, J=11.5Hz and 2.5Hz)	C-23,C-24

C No.	HMQC		HMBC
	δ$_C$(ppm) DEPT	δ$_H$(ppm)	
23	29.0 (t)	1.41, 2.05(each m)	C-24,C-25,C-28
24	39.5 (d)	1.41(m)	
25	40.7 (d)	2.17(m)	C-24,C-27,C-28
26	173.9 (s)	—	
27	15.2 (q)	1.28(d, J=7.2Hz)	C-24,C-25,C-26
28	25.9 (t)	1.01,1.37(each m)	C-23,C-24,C-29
29	9.6 (q)	0.67(t, J=7.2Hz)	C-24,C-28
C-1'	103.5 (d)	4.89(d, J=7.8Hz)	C-3
C-2'	74.0 (d)	4.01(t-like)	C-3'
C-3'	78.0 (d)	4.18(overlap)	C-2', C-4'
C-4'	70.9 (d)	4.06(overlap)	C-5', C-6'
C-5'	77.8 (d)	3.90(t-like)	C-4', C-5'
C-6'	61.9 (t)	4.31(m), 4.49(brd, J=11.5Hz)	C-4', C-5'

Table 4. ^{1}H and ^{13}C NMR data for lygodiumsteroside A (600 and 150 MHz, in C$_5$D$_5$N).

2.   Correlative spectrum data:

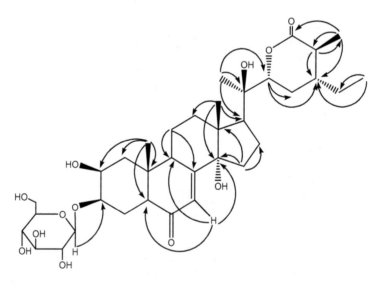

Fig. 16. The key correlations of the new compound 3.

3.   Analysis and conclusions of the new compound 3:

The new compound 3,white powder, mp.245–246℃, gave positive response to Liebermann–Burchard reaction and Molish reaction, suggesting a steroid glycoside structure. The sugar was identified as glucose by co-TLC with authentic sample after acid hydrolysis.

The molecular formula was determined as $C_{35}H_{54}O_{12}$ by HR-ESI-MS (m/z 701.3309 [M+CL]$^-$, calcd. 701.3309), along with ^{1}H-NMR and ^{13}C-NMR data. Additionally, the UV spectrum of compound 1 showed a maximum at λ = 243 nm and the IR spectrum exhibited absorption at 1,730 cm^{-1}for an a, b-unsaturated carbonyl group. The ^{1}H-NMR (600 MHz, C_5D_5N) spectrum showed an olefinic proton at δ 6.18 (1H, brs, H-7) and five methyl signals at δ 1.44 (3H, s, H-21), 1.28 (3H, d, J = 7.2 Hz,H-27), 1.09 (3H, s, H-18), 0.86 (3H, s, H-19), 0.67 (3H, t,J = 7.2 Hz,H-29). The ^{13}C-NMR (150 MHz, C_5D_5N) showed five methyl signals and a typical a, β-unsaturated carbonyl group signals at δ 202.3 (C-6), 165.4 (C-8), and 121.1 (C-7), which revealed an ecdysteroid-type nucleus. It was also confirmed by the HMBC correlations of the new compound 3 . In the HSQC spectrum, δ 4.06 (1H, brd,J = 11.4 Hz, H-2) and δ 4.29 (1H, brs, H-3) had direct correlation with δ 66.8 (C-2) and δ 77.1 (C-3), respectively, which combined with the information of long correlation in the HMBC spectrum — d 1.44 (3H, s, H-21) correlated with d 49.2 (C-17), d 85.2 (C-22), and δ 75.1 (C-20), respectively — all of these signals elucidated the presence of five hydroxyl carbons C-2, C-3, C-14, C-20, and C-22. Additionally, δ 1.09 (3H, s, H-18) and δ 1.44(3H, s, H-21), d 2.17 (1H, m, H-25) and δ 1.28 (3H, d,J = 7.2 Hz, H-27), δ 2.93 (1H, m, H-17) and δ 2.05, 2.39(2H, each m, H-16) correlated mutually with each other in the 2D- COSY spectrum. The occurrence of α - β lactone ring in the side chain was evidenced by the carbonyl absorption at 1,730 cm^{-1}in the IR and the δ 173.9 ppm in the^{13}C-NMR. The HMBC spectrum showed the long correlation between the methyl proton signal at δ 1.28 (3H, d,J = 7.2 Hz, H-27) and the carbon signals at δ 39.5 (C-24),40.7 (C-25), and 173.9 (C-26). The correlation between the methyl proton signal at δ 0.67 (3H, t, J = 7.2 Hz, H-29) and the carbon signals at δ 25.9 (C-28), 39.5 (C-24), and the correlation between the methyl proton signal at δ 2.19 (1H, m, H-25) and the carbon signals at δ 15.2 (C-27), 25.9 (C-28), and 39.5 (C-24) could be observed, respectively. Moreover , δ 4.44 (1H, dd, J = 11.5 Hz and 2.5 Hz, H-22)also showed the correlation with δ 29.0 (C-23), 39.5 (C-24)in the HMBC. Taken together, the structure of the side chain was identified. The HMBC correlation was observed between the anomeric proton signal at δ 4.89 (1H, d, H-10) and the carbon signal at d 77.1 due to C-3 of the aglycone moiety. This key long-range cross peak fixed the glycosidation position.The chemical shifts of the sugar moiety in ^{13}C-NMR (δ 103.5, 74.0, 78.0, 70.9, 77.8, 61.9) also confirmed the presence of B-glucopyranose. The anomeric configuration of glucose was determined to be on the basis of the J_{H-H} values (J = 7.8 Hz) and d 4.09 (1H, brs, H-3) correlated with d 4.85 (1H, d, anomeric proton) in the NOE spectrum. (The NOESY spectra mentioned in this text was recorded in CD_3OD because the key proton signals overlapped in C_5D_5N). The relative configuration of the new compound 3 was identified by the NOESY correlation between the proton signal at δ 4.09 (1H, brs, H-3) and δ 3.85 (1H, brd, H-2), δ 1.87 (1H, m, Ha-4). Careful comparison ^{13}C-NMR data of the new compound 3 and a known compound, named capitasterone[8][9], revealed that the B, C, and D rings and the side chain were very similar to that of capitasterone. Furthermore, the stereochemistry of C-20 and C-22 of capitasterone had established R, in the NOE spectrum (in CD_3OD) of he new compound 3, δ 4.25 (1H, dd, J = 11.5 Hz and 2.5 Hz, H-22) had correlated with δ 1.56 (1H, m, H-24);however, d 1.56 (1H, m, H-24) never correlated with d 2.17 (1H, m, H-25). All of these confirmed the stereochemistry of C24 and C25 as R and S, respectively. The ^{1}H-NMR and^{13}C-NMR signals of the aglycone moiety of he new compound 3 were found to be similar to that of capitasterone .Therefore, the structure of he new compound 3 was elucidated safely as Lygodiumsteroside A (Fig. 15).

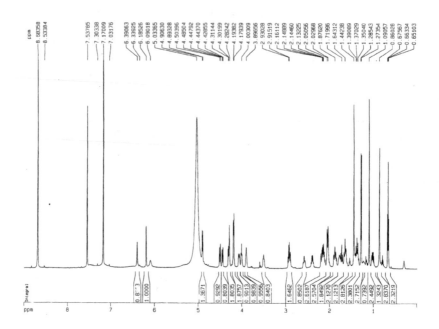

Fig. 17. Lygosteroside A (^{1}H-NMR, in C_5D_5N).

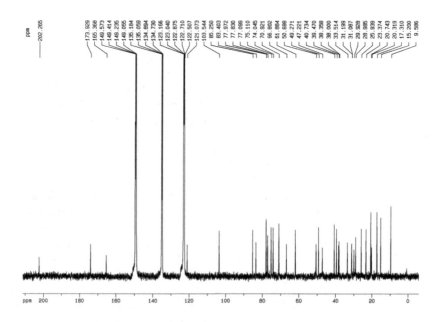

Fig. 18. Lygosteroside A (^{13}C-NMR, in C_5D_5N).

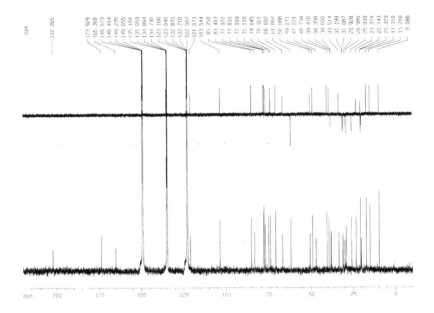

Fig. 19. Lygosteroside A (DEPT).

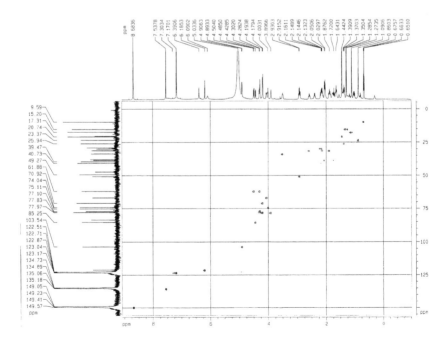

Fig. 20. Lygosteroside A (HSQC, in C₅D₅N).

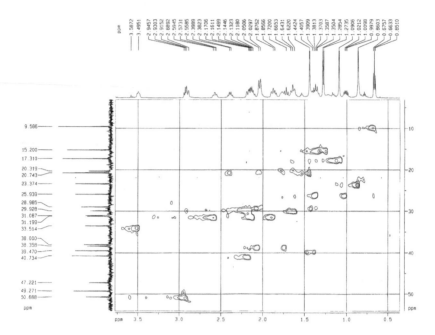

Fig. 21. Lygosteroside A (HSQC, in C_5D_5N).

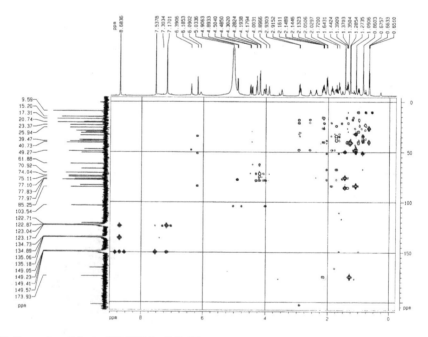

Fig. 22. Lygosteroside A (HMBC, in C_5D_5N).

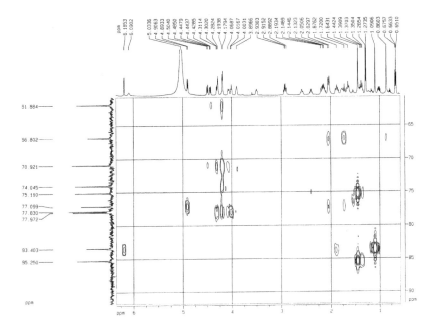

Fig. 23. Lygosteroside A (HMBC, in C₅D₅N).

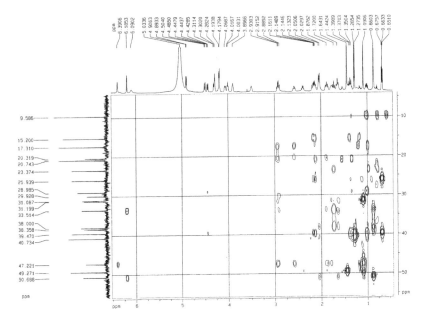

Fig. 24. Lygosteroside A (HMBC, in C₅D₅N).

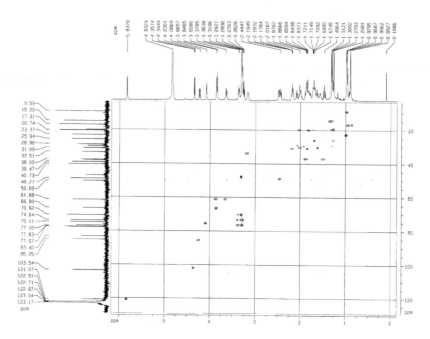

Fig. 25. Lygosteroside A (HSQC, in MeOH).

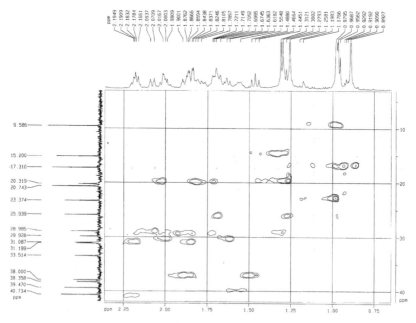

Fig. 26. Lygosteroside A (HSQC, in MeOH).

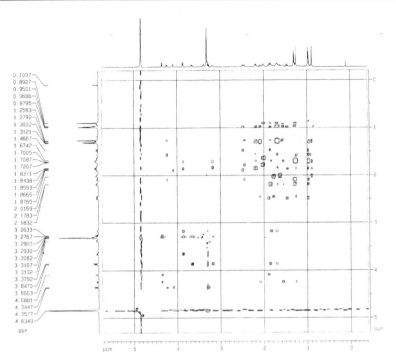

Fig. 27. Lygosteroside A (NOESY, in MeOH).

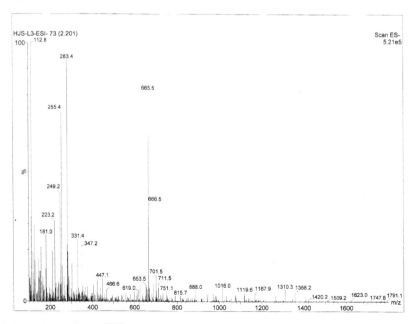

Fig. 28. Lygosteroside A (ESI).

4. Pharmacological actions

4.1 Antibacterial action[10]

Inhibiting *Staphylococcus aureus*, *Pseudomonas aeruginosa*, *Salmonella typhi* and *shigella Flexneri.*

4.2 Antivirus[11]

Water extract and alcohol extract of Lygodium spores both can inhibit HIV-1 virus. The Concertration of water extract above 125ug/ml can wholly inhibit HIV-1 virus.

4.3 Resistance to male hormone and effect on hair growth[12]

50% alcohol extract of Lygodium Spores can inhibit the activity of Testosterone 5-α reductase in vitro and activate hair follicle.

4.4 Normalizing functioning of the gallbladder and dissolving stone[13]

4.5 Liver protection[14]

The water extract of Lygodium (50ug/ml) can significantly reduce the GPT action of liver Cell cultures containing GaIN 5*10~3mol/L,so it has effect on liver protection markably.

4.6 Cure urinary impassability, tumescent feeling below umbilicus,

4.7 Urgent pain:Lygodium powder drinking by licorice soup.

4.8 Have a good effect on urinary tract infection, urinary calculus, nephritis edema, cold with fever ,urine content small and cardial, enteritis diarrhea.

5. Indications[10]

5.1 Stranguria marked by chyluria, stranguria caused by the passage of urinary stone, stranguria from urolithiasis and strangury due to heat. For dribling and painful micturition , there is powder of climbing fern spore from *standards* of *diagnosis* and *treament*: Climbing fern spore 6g,red poria 9g, umbellate pore-fungus 9g, white atractylodes rhizome 9g,peony root 9g, oriental water plantain rhizome 15g, talc 21g, pyrrosia leaf 3g. Grind these herbs into a fine powder. Take 9g each time. For stranguria marked by chyluria ,there is powder of climbing fern spore: Climbing fern spore 30g, talc 30g, licorice root 7.5g. Grind these herbs into a fine powder.Take 6g each time.

5.2 Dampness in the spleen, general edema, distension in the abdomen can be treated with powder of fern spore from *Inventions of medicine:* Morning glory seed 45g, *kansui* root 15g climbing fen spore 15g, grind these herbs into a fine powder. Take 6g each time before meals.

6. Conclusion

Lygodium japonicum (Thunb.)Sw., which belongs to the genus *Lygodium* of the family Lygodiaceae, is the dry root and rhizome of *Lygodium japonicum* (Thunb.)Sw. There are different constituents in different parts of it and distribution of content of these constituents are different.The paper aims at making a systematical research for the root of *Lygodium japonicum* (Thunb.)Sw. that is one specie of medicinal *Lygodium*. According to the existing literature, the main constituents of *Lygodium* are steroidal, flavonoids, organic acids and other substances, but it is no clear whether all these chemical constituents are effective composition or not.

This paper summarize the research on chemical constituents and pharmacological actions of Lygodium, . From our systematic research on Lygodium, we have isolated and identified many kinds of compounds. In this paper, we focus on introduction of three new compounds: lygodiumsteroside A and lygodiumsteroside B and 2-isopropyl-7-methyl-6-hydroxy-α- (1,4) naphthoquinone, as well as the data analysis of UV, IR, ^{1}H-NMR, ^{13}C-NMR、2D-NMR and HR-MS. We also generalize pharmacological actions and clinical applications of Lygodium.

7. References

[1] Ren-chao Zhou,Shu-bin Li,The Rrsearch of Pteridophyta on antibacterial .Hunan newsletter of Traditional Chinese medicine: 1999,5 (1):13-14.

[2] Li-juan Chen , Guo-gang Zhang,Lin-xia Zhu.The research about the components of Lygodium japonicum [D]:2008:3-26.

[3] Li-xia Zhu ,Guo-gang Zhang,Li-juan Chen.The research about the components from N-butanol layer of Lygodium japonicum [D]:2008:3-30.

[4] C Ye, CL Fan, LH Zhang. A new phenolic glycoside from the roots of *Lygodium japonicum*. Fitoperapia, 2007, 78: 600-601.

[5] Lijuan Chen,Guogang Zhang, Jie He.New naphthoquinone from the root of *Lygodium* japonicum(Thunb)Sw.[J] Journal of Natural medicine:2010(64):114-116.

[6] Lixia Zhu,Guogang Zhang,shengchao Wang.A new compound from lygodium japonicum(Thunb)SW[J].Natural product research :2009:1284-1289.

[7] Linxia Zhu,Guogang Zhang,LIjuan Chen.A new ecdysteroside from Lygodium japonicum(Thunb)SW[J].Natural Product Reseach:2009(63):215-219.

[8] Takemoto T, Nomoto K, Hikino Y, Hikino H (1968) Structure of capitasterone, a novel c29 insect-moulting substance from cyathula capitata. Tetrahedron Lett 9:4929–4932.

[9] Huang X-C, Guo Y-W (2003) Ecdysteroids from the stems of Diploclisia glaucescens. Nat Prod Res Dev 15:93–97.

[10] Tieguang tong,Ping Dong.Climbing Fern Spore[M].The practical science of traditional Chinese medicinal herbs:439.

[11] Ma CM, Nakamura N, Miyashiro H, et al. Screening of Chinese and Mongolian herbal drugs for anti-human immunodeficiency virus type 1(HIV-1) activity[J]. Phytotherapy Research, 2002, 16:186-189

[12] Leihong Zhang, Wencai Ye.The research of chemical constituents and biological actions.[J].Natural Product Research and Development2007, (19):552-557:

[13] Jiajun Liu,Jing wang.The experimental study on normalizing functioning of the gallbladder .[J]. Anhui Medical Journal: 1987, 8 (1): 34-35.

[14] Ruiying Fang,Zhongyao Shi.Observing ten kinds of traditional Chinese medicine on the function of resistance to toxic liver in using original generation to cultivate liver cells.[J] Modern pharmaceutical application : 1995, 12 (1): 5-7.

4

Developments in Phytochemistry

Moronkola Dorcas Olufunke
Department of Chemistry,
University of Ibadan,
Nigeria

1. Introduction

Carbohydrates, proteins, fats and oils are utilized as food by man and animals. Other chemical compounds in plants apart from these listed above are phytochemical. Such compounds usually exert peculiar, unique and specific active physiological effects responsible for their therapeutic and pharmacological functions. Activities of such naturally occurring compounds are generally responsible for changes, which are utilized to satisfy man's desires. Phytochemical studies afford revelation and understanding of phytoconstituents, as much as possible conserving their bioactivities, and are on how to standardize them; compared with the crude herbal methods that are not easily standardized. These complex substances of diverse nature occur mostly in plant based foods; they are in very small amounts in grams or mg or µg/Kg of samples. They do not add to body calorie and are numerous in types. These phytochemical are applied mostly for preventive and healing purposes. About 25% of prescribed drugs are obtained from phytochemical in higher plants. Plants are safe means of obtaining drugs. About 250,000 higher plants have promising phytochemical, half of which are located in tropical forests; 60% of these have their biological activities established, while about 15% of them have their phyto-compounds isolated and reported [Hamburger and Hostettman, 1991].

Studies and researches into medicinal constituents of plants, involve qualitative and quantitative analyses. There is rationale behind each experimental work involving definite steps and processes; having in mind properties of compounds analyzed in conjunction with procedures utilized. Also our desired active metabolite to be isolated and studied as interested lead compound, many times is in very complex mixtures of many unwanted and undesired materials [known as contaminants], which have close properties to our desired bioactive molecules.

2. General and specific techniques, procedures and methods in phytochemical analyses, with highlight on recent developments in phytochemistry

Most of the techniques and procedures in phytochemical analyses are cumbersome and tasking, to have detailed understanding of phytoconstituents- [their activities, structures, how to improve on them and standardize them]. If they are carefully followed one achieve the aim of isolations, characterizations and better establish bioactivities of active metabolites.

Phytochemical methods mainly involve EXTRACTIONS, PURIFICATIONS and ISOLATIONS of the active compounds in plants. Procedures are ways of carrying out the methods and techniques. There are numerous methods some specific for interested compounds one is looking for, duly modified to meet the required aim and focus of work. There are daily modifications of techniques and procedures to suit individual purposes of having the phytochemical compound(s) of interest. It is important to say that some natural product may (to variable extent) or may not possess their pharmacological properties and activities when in isolation compared to when among mixture of compounds (synergy) in the natural setting in organism. Recently in genomics whole plant is analyzed which afford easier and truthful analyses of contents in the whole plant as in their natural state.

It is important to first establish proper botanical taxonomic identifications and classification of plant of study. Scientific names must be established, common and local names must be sought. Right choice of study plants or part of plant to study may be from local or traditional surveys i.e. ethno-medicine, ethno-pharmacology or ethno-botanical uses and applications. Geographical location and environmental effects [time and period of plant collection], must be considered also, which may be responsible for variations. Voucher samples of plant of study may be filed in local and national herbaria for accurate authentications. Usually plants are richer in active metabolites during their flowering and fruiting stages [Mendonca-Filho, 2006].

Procedures involve first the analytical stages. Most times our desired active metabolite to be isolated and studied as interested lead compound, is in very complex mixtures of many unwanted and undesired materials [known as contaminants], more so they usually have close properties to our desired bioactive molecules.

Preliminary tests and screenings on plant extracts are faster and easily done following standard procedures and methods in manuals and literature. They detect the presence and amount of basic phytoconstituents like terpenoids, alkaloids, flavonoids, saponin, glycosides, steroids, tannins, phlobatannins and anthraquinones to mention few.

More common and familiar separation and isolation techniques in phytochemical studies are distillation, crystallization, solvent extractions, continuous and liquid-liquid extractions, partitioning using separatory funnels, and chromatography. For accuracy characterizations follow side by side with the above techniques. Bioactivities can also be tested along the above, such as antibacterial, antifungal and antioxidant. The followings are important to consider during choice of procedures for separations and isolation of interested biomolecules of interest:

- Availability of necessary materials, equipments and chemicals. Also economically cheap methods.
- Ease and simplicity of procedures, and risk involved.
- Compatibility of interested solute with phases or solvents such as it distilling out [more volatile phyto-compound], crystallizing and recrystallizing out from phases/ solvents etc.
- Possibility of retrieval methods.

- Selectivity and sensitivity of chosen method(s) and equipments.
- Feasibility of chromatographying out our desired biomolecules from stationary phase using appropriate and suitable solvent or mixture of solvents for elution. Also consider factors like polarity, temperature, agitations etc.
- Provision of rapid online information on activities and structures of the phyto-compound. [Specific methods can be better studied by consulting literature and appropriate textbooks].

3. Isolation, characterization and identification of phytochemical in natural products

Phytochemical are active metabolites that necessarily require extraction and isolation from their natural sources with many unwanted materials. The phytochemical can come singly or as a mixture of important substances to form active principle responsible for its activity (synergy). When singly active, the processes of their separations are of great practical advantages, which in many cases the isolated phytochemical have better and higher activity. We will consider genomics and metabolomics later as more efficient methods of rapid phytochemical screening and characterizations of plant extracts to study their chemical constituents, using NMR-based metabolomics. It utilizes mathematical data; NMR is used directly on extracts before commencing detailed work on plant. It makes it easy to determine which plants are more promising to research into. A large number of variables are collected, then choices on which are important are made, followed by selection procedures.

3.1 More modern spectroscopy utilized in phytochemical studies

Once preliminary separations and detections have confirmed presence of active secondary metabolites, their characterizations as they are separated follows. Chromatographic techniques are utilized in separations and purifications to isolate bioactive constituents based on polarity or other gradient factors. The isolated compound is characterized by spectroscopic methods. The four basic types of spectroscopy are utilized in the characterizations of purified natural product compounds. They are ultraviolet (UV), infra-red (IR), mass-spectroscopy (MS) and nuclear magnetic resonance (NMR) techniques. MS is an instrumental technique, while the other three utilizes different parts of the broad electromagnetic radiation spectrum. UV spectroscopy discovered and utilized in the 1930s gives detailed information on detecting presence of conjugation in molecules and the extents of conjugation. By 1940s the infrared (IR) region of EMR was utilized to detect different vibration frequencies of different chemical bonds present in the molecule. Combination of these two types of spectroscopy [UV & IR] gave information about the functional groups present in the molecule. MS was introduced a decade after by 1950s, involving three important steps: Ionization and vaporization; Separation of ions by m/z; and Detections. The analytical technique provides information which determines the molecular ion. Compounds are ionized for analysis, and also fragments are produced useful for structural characterizations. Almost all compounds can be analyzed by MS, but modes of ionization and type of instruments determine the results. Recent developments have shown the use of others like MALDI[matrix-assisted laser desorption], EI[electron impact], CI[chemical ionization], API[atmospheric pressure ionization], LRMS[low-resolution MS], HRMS[high resolution MS], IT[ion traps], TOF[time of flight] and QQQ[triple quadrupoles]. MS is a destructive technique. In conjunction with UV and IR, and tandem and hyphenations MS is able to give detailed information on molecular formula of the molecule. Recently by 1960s NMR made an easier way of detecting and confirming structures of pure metabolites, and has grown so fast, almost becoming a scientific discipline today.

NMR is a type of absorption chromatography which reveals connectivity of nuclei in the metabolite. Superficially and most common, ^1H and ^{13}C-NMR [1D] techniques [earlier used] are unambiguously and widely utilized in elucidation of structures of naturally occurring metabolites usually isolated and purified from their natural sources. Recently the 2D and 3D-NMR are utilized [as in use of HSCQ, TOCSY, COSY, HMBC and NOESY etc]. Fundamentally NMR reveal (a)information on types of chemical environments in the metabolite from the frequency absorption chemical shift values; (b)number of protons in each type of environment from integral values; (c)details on type of nuclei/ protons on adjacent and neighbouring positions in the metabolite, giving details on the stereochemistry and 3-dimentional structure of metabolites.

The theory of NMR is based on magnetic atomic nuclei with net nuclear spin 'I', capable of having (2I+1) patterns of orientations. Such NMR-active atomic nuclei have odd atomic number and/ or odd mass number. An internal standard, usually TMS [$Si(CH_3)_4$] with equivalent twelve protons and arbitrarily have absorption at δ0, is used in calibrating NMR spectrum for easy interpretations and evaluation of resonances and absorptions. Most used unit is δ (delta), the other unit is τ (tau). Relationship between both is expressed thus: δ=10-τ or τ=10-δ. At high resolutions the splitting patterns (multiplicity) of protons are due to protons on adjacent group of protons; peak is split into (n+1) by n equivalent and adjacent H-atoms in the metabolite.

There are now more rapid strategies for chemical characterizations of phytoconstituents of natural products as well as assessing the bioactivities of the natural products. Coupled or hyphenated methods of separations, isolations, purifications and characterizations are now very appropriate. These include LC/UV, LC/MS, LC-FTIR, LC-NMR, LC/UV-DAD, MS/MS, LC-MS/MS, Q-TOF-MS, CE- capillary electrophoresis, with its added advantage of use of very little solvent consumption, lower costs, short time of analysis and its generally economical; MECC- micellar electrokinetic capillary chromatography, this is when the capillary electrophoresis is in conjunction with electrochemical detections usually along with assay experiments; HSCCC- high speed counter-current chromatography; SPME- solid phase micro extraction; SCFEC- supercritical fluid extraction chromatography; ESI; HPLC-MS/ESI. Introduction of FT [fourier transform] in structural elucidations have increased the enormous power of spectroscopies like IR and NMR.

4. Techniques of establishing phytochemical bio-activities by bio-assay

Bio-assay of extracts or fractions and bioactivity guided fractionations are important and are major steps in phytochemical studies. Bioassay combines biological and chemical screenings to obtain important information on and about plant constituents and chemical compositions. It investigates, establish and estimate biological activities of biomolecules, involving chemical screening techniques. The amount of material to be tested is important determinant of method to be used. There are many methods of in-vitro assays for assessing different activities like antimicrobial or cytotoxic activities. Such have advantages of easy automations with robotics and miniaturized techniques resulting in rapid through-put screening of large numbers of samples. They are more common as their materials are easy to get. Other assays which utilize affected organisms or living cells directly, give more reliable results, though may not be cheap. Such include use of brine shrimps, ants and insects like Drosophila sp., cell lines in different media, tissue culturing, ligand bindings, use of rabbits and rats. Assays may identify promising molecular structures.

Usually many biological activities are screened and tested during a particular bioassay. It is important to note that results of bioassays are not strong enough to establish uses and dosage of compounds found to be bioactive; also they cannot replace pharmacological discovery and establishment of potent drugs in development of lead compounds to consumables and marketed substances. They may be seen as alternatives. Also one must be extremely careful when interpreting in bioassays to get results, especially in cases of clinical studies and investigations. It is best and more reliable for effective results to perform and run bioassays alongside with chemical separations and characterizations. These in modern times are achieved by using hyphenated processes. Particular constituents of extracts or plants as they are separated are characterized as well as assessing their activities side by side. The information obtained from the bioassay and chemical analyses (separations and characterizations) give full description of the bioactive compound, and afford easy and appropriate detection of specific targeted bioactive metabolite(s).

To get pure constituents, modify structures, and carry out toxicological tests bioassay results are very important.

5. General biosynthetic relationships between primary metabolites with interlink precursors and secondary metabolites

The whole plant or organism serves as an active laboratory for the production of natural products from primary metabolites such as proteins, amino acids, carbohydrates, fats and oils, which are mostly obtained from food items. The primary metabolites are basic biological molecules also called biochemist molecules, which are functional compounds found virtually in all plants and organisms. Secondary metabolites are varieties of simple to sophisticated bizarre molecules also called natural products. They are fascinating chemical molecules, very useful and of great importance in nature, as well as highly diversified in structures, properties, uses, chemistry etc. These varied properties and characters emerge from their biological generation, production and formation from basic primary metabolite sources and origin. Natural products are in restricted taxonomic groups and species of organisms. They are from secondary metabolic processes and express individualities of organisms. These are the areas of interest in phytochemistry and pharmacognosy.

We will be examining the underlining principles behind formation, production and generation of natural products syntheses in plants. Primary metabolites are first formed in the first phase (primary metabolism), which is followed by secondary metabolism processes to give the more sophisticated and complicated more specific secondary metabolites.

Successive enzymes which are proteinous organic biocatalysts are utilized in catalyzing specific metabolic reactions and processes, all coded by specific genes in plant's DNA in the nucleus which controls all activities leading to creation of new substances and new organisms. Organelles in cells of the plant carry out specific biochemical functions. Transcriptive processes are involved to get particular enzymes; common reactions in the plant include syntheses, breakdowns, isomerizations, cyclizations, regulations, hydrolysis etc; the key energy molecules in the cell are ATP, ADP, AMP, GRP and derivatives. There are many biosynthetic pathways occurring in plants, initial pathways such as carbon-reduction cycles, pentose phosphate pathways, glycolysis, Krebs cycle, shikimic acid pathway and tricarboxylic acid cycles lead to biosyntheses of primary metabolites, which are precursors of the diverse secondary metabolites. There is need for continuous supply and flow of energy for the ordered transformations of substances in cells. Metabolic activities in specific pathways occur vegetative in cells producing precursors for components of cells to further react and produce simple to complex natural product metabolites. Generally biosynthetic procedures can be viewed as starting (primary metabolism) from biosynthetic activities to produce carbohydrates. From it more complex metabolites are formed. Main metabolites as precursors of specific secondary metabolites include fatty acids and lipids to give the polyketides, amino acids and sulphur containing metabolites to form the peptides and alkaloids, phenyl propanoid and cinnamic acid metabolites, isoprenoids which yield terpenoids, carotenoids, steroids etc. There are now genomic approaches to studies of biosyntheses of natural products, which will be discussed shortly.

6. Importance of the phytochemical to plant producing them and man

Plants are energetic organisms that carry out specific oriented processes to produce useful compounds. They do not waste time to form substances that have no use to the plant. The wide categories of phytochemical produced have their importances to the plant generating them. Some of these are as follows-

1. Starch in plants is hydrolyzed to D-glucose units utilized in syntheses of ATP by aerobic respiration for vigor in growing cells of plants. Starch and sugars are also utilized by plants in development of their storage organs as in rice, tubers of yam and potatoes.
2. Cellulose is the most common naturally synthesized polymer in plants, it is made of glucose units, and it is the main component of plant cell walls, which provides structural supports along with other polysaccharides for the plant.
3. Chlorophyll in plants is photo-receptors which afford the plant important photosynthetic activities to take place.
4. Gums and mucins are hydrophobic acidic residues of hetero-polysaccharides produced by plants. They serve as matrix in cell walls to protect plant against attack of microbes. The gum is also used in sealing up wounds in leaves and stems of plants, and also prevents infections on plants.
5. Lipids are the main constituents of membranes of plasma and cell organelles. Fats and oils are lipid bodies; they are the stored energy forms in fruits and seeds of plants.
6. Proteins are responsible for main cell structures and main constituents of enzymes involved in biochemical reactions and biosynthetic activities.
7. Nucleic acids and nucleotides are for protein coding. They supply metabolic energy molecules like ATP, ADP, AMP, and GRP.

8. Inulins and fructans are soluble polysaccharides made mostly of fructose sugar with some glucose in the chain. Hydrolyses of the stored fructans in plants at spring, provide energy to plant for commencement of its growth in early spring.

9. Lignin are hydrophobic complex polymers in secondary cell walls made of units of aromatics like phenylpropanoids, coumaryl, coniferyl and sinapyl alcohols via shikimic acid pathway. It provides additional supports with rigidity, impermeability to water and prevent water loss from plant, also give compressive strength to cell walls. Ligins resist intrusion of herbivores, but prevent growth and bending of plant tissues.

10. Anthocyanins are flavonoids responsible for colored pigments like blue, red, pink, purple in plant parts like flowers, fruits, stems, leaves, roots, seeds etc. They are flower attractants for birds and insect pollinators, as well as attractants to animals and birds that disperse their fruits and seeds. They also protect plant from UV irradiation.

11. Alkaloids are nitrogen-containing heterocyclic organic bases with complicated structures usually with specific physiological functions. They are biosynthesized and derived from amino acids through mevalonic acid pathways. Most alkaloids are toxic to man and animals, hence prevent herbivores from consuming them; so acts as defensive compounds in plants.

12. Carotenoids are responsible for the bright colours observed in plant pigments like flowers, fruits and seeds such as yellow, orange, red etc. The bright flowers in particular are attractions for pollinators. Carotenoids in fruits and seeds serve to attract animals that disperse them. Usually odoriferous (C10 and C15 terpenoids) are produced along with the carotenoids.

To man, phytochemical have some direct and indirect importance, few are highlighted thus:

a. Cellulose is important industrially in fabrics like cotton. Other plant fibers are used lumber, paper and cardboards. Some are even modified in matrix forms in columns and TLC for chromatographic separation processes.

b. Carotenoids are important in man's diet; they are known to prevent cancer and are important sources of vitamin A.

c. Starch which are stored polysaccharides (of sugar units) in plants serve as primary source of food for man, microbes, insects, birds and other animals. Man consumes it directly and as processed forms like drinks of malt and beers.

d. Anthocyanins are utilized as ornamentals for beautifying man's environment.

e. Fructans and Inulins are beneficial to swine and poultry diets.

f. Alkaloids are generally toxic to man and animals especially in large doses. But in lower doses have been reported to have great medicinal uses e.g. pain relievers, stimulants, antimalaria etc.

7. Aspects of biotechnology in biochemical and molecular regulations in the industrial development of plant phytochemical with the syntheses of metabolites

Biotechnology in phytochemical studies involve bio-reactions and manipulations in plants for producing better and healthier plant growth, developments, protections, expansions and improved potentials of its phytochemical constituents with higher productivity. It applies recent areas of studies like genomics, metabolomics, system-biology and proteomics for producing beneficial natural products. Generally development of plant cells biotechnologically is for economic and industrial purposes. Current methods and techniques utilize high-throughput applications on genomic modifications by homologous and recombinations at specific sites. It applies basic principles of plant and molecular biology, involving recombinant DNA technology modifying functional genes in natural product biosyntheses. The DNA and molecular biomarkers are involved; favourable traits are recognized, identified and isolated, then the selection of the genotype. Results from these assist in appropriate creation of transgenic plants that yield important and economic natural products using plant cells and tissues to get genetically modified plants and natural products. Such results are also utilized in assessments of biodiversities and chemotaxonomy. It is explorative applying foreign genes into plant genomics, so creating improved metabolic biosyntheses with genetic modifications to have faster and better production of active secondary metabolites, than from the conventional ways. But some are opposed to it because of the risk involved, and suggested it should not be applied to food developments. Well it requires first understanding details of genetic information on the plant and its natural product also know and identify the marker genes to be able to successfully transfer its genetic culture, so positively manipulating the plant with beneficial characters which last longer, and so affords better strategies in natural product formation and studies.

Incorporation methods (in-vivo) can be used as well as in-vitro cultivation and regeneration of excised or cultured whole plant provided necessary nutrients and hormones are available. Phytochemical researches in most part of the world utilize wild field cultivated plants or plants in the wilderness. It is more tasking to form plants and natural products from biotechnology, and the yield may even be too low, making it to be more costly and uneconomical. But biotechnology methods are very appropriate for endangered plant species and their natural products. Stereo- and regiospecific bio-transformations and bio-conversions afford in cultured cell suspension cultivations the discovery of new biomolecules which are not in the intact plant, so need to identify the particular enzymes causing this synthesis of new natural products which can be applied on large scale productions.

Molecular farming afford massive production of phytochemical from bioreactor plants to give cheaper and safer ways of forming recombinant proteins of higher values to give more valuable natural products and pharmaceuticals. It is a new area of bioengineering. It has the advantage of expressing gene at specific organs like leaves, fruits, roots or seeds. Gene of the host plant is modified so it forms stable products. These methods are important in fermentation processes, commercial proteins and products, in the generation of therapeutics and vaccines, as well as in diagnostics.

Biotechnology in natural products research afford discovery of bioactive natural products from sources outside the already known conventional plants, so reveals wider diversities of phyto-compounds. This is an important aspect of bio-prospecting.

8. Practical involvements of specific phytochemical in health and treatments as for example antimalaria, antibacterial, anti-fungal, antioxidant, anti-ulcer, anticancer

Active metabolites from natural sources usually have very minimal or no toxic effect on organism using them; hence they are more useful and promising. The great diversity of tropical forest plants are good sources of great number of bioactive substances with many therapeutic uses from which drugs can be discovered and processed. Many lead compounds have been isolated and derived from plants, which are now very useful drugs. [See Table 1]. Optimization follows after identification and establishment of a lead compound.

S/N	Specific use(s)	Active phytochemical	Plant/ Sources
1	Analgesic	Distylin, Rutin flavonoids; Morphine &Papaverine alkaloids.	*Saccharum officinarum, Leersia hexandra, Schrobera arborea,*
2	Antibacteria	Tannins, Saponins	*Nesogordonia papaverifera,*
3	Antifungal	Sterols, Saponins	*Centrosema pubescens, Parinari curatellaefolia, Anthocleista djalonensis, Hygrophila auriculata, Dacryodes edulis,*
4	Antibiotic	Macrolides, Penicillin, Tetracyclines, Cephalosporin, Gentamycins	*Chromolaena odorata, Acalypha wilkesiana/ hispida* & sps., *Mundulea sericera,*
5	Antioxidant	Flavonoids	*Allium sativum,* Apple, Grape, Soyabean,
6	Anti-inflammatory	Flavonoids, Saponins	*Vitex doniana*
7	Antimalaria	Quinines, Pamaquines, Phenacetin Alkaloids, Flavonoids	*Rauwolfia vomitoria, Alstonia boonei, Cinchona officinalis, Polyalthia suaveolens,*
8	Antidepressant	Flavonoids	*Marsderua latifolia,*
9	Anti-tumor	Lignans, Saponins	*Pteris togoensis, Harrisonia abyssinica,*
10	Stimulant	Nicotine & Caffein Alkaloids	*Haemanthus multiflorus, Lagerstroemia speciosa, Vitex cryosocarpa, Leucaena glauca, Cola acuminata,*
11	Antiviral	Ginseng & Saikosaponins	*Hedranthera barteri, Bambusa vulgaris, Dissotis rotundifolia,*
12	Antihypertensive	Reserpine, Flavonoids,	*Voacanga africana, Tapinanthus bangwensis, Adenia cissampeloides,*
13	Tranquilizer	Schizandrins	*Kaempfera nigerica,*
14	Aphrodiasic	Steroids	*Brunfelsia uniflora, Euphorbia deightonii, Prosopis Africana, Rhigiocarya racemifera,*

Table 1. Active phytocompounds from plants and their medicinal uses.

9. Bioinformatics, genomics, and synergies of phytochemical with pathogens

We face challenges on how do plants with its enzymes and regulatory genes biosynthesize specific natural product compounds. It gives deeper and clearer understanding of processes involved in generating our highly interested natural products from perspectives of molecular biology. Studies here are on characterization of functional genes and sequencing of genome because they express and regulate syntheses of natural product which is our main concern in phytochemistry and pharmacognosy. Important areas for molecular biology techniques of studying genomics of natural products in plants include identifying and expressing genes, functional genes and silencing. DNA and RNA isolations and clones with proteins derived from them. The important aspect of phytochemistry is the interest in processes occurring in each plant species for the biosyntheses of the metabolites. Techniques here are very sensitive high-through put plant metabolomics screenings with better separation, purification and structure characterization methods and instruments, as well as very sensitive methods of detections. These will reveal total and detailed natural product constituents in plants, which is our focus, and due to the great importances of natural products in isolated form and as synergies. With great diversities of natural product compounds, this method is highly reliable. The applications of these model plant species to non-model medicinal plants are the new trends in phytochemistry and pharmacognosy. Total genes' content of an organism is its genome, giving understanding of functions of genes proteins on the wide plant genome. The genetic studies are integrated approaches having both experimental and computational sides, later has genomic library with databases called 'bioinformatics'. Experimental work utilizes mutants, gene microarrays in cells and tissues, and spectrometry for analyses to complement the molecular techniques. Very large amount of data is generated from these studies, which are analyzed and interpreted with the computational bioinformatics which are available resources for studying metabolomics pathways from the characterized functional gene, in which a plant can have 20,000 to 50,000 genes responsible for generating its divers metabolites. There are presentations of large size of genome-sequencing projects of great number of plants serving as models with information, maps of genes and molecular markers in known websites. These are mostly on crop plants. Examples are:

www.genome.ad.jp/dbget/ligand.html ; www.p450.kvl.dk; www.stke.org;
www.genome.ad.jp/kegtg; www.arabidopsis.org/tools/aracyc;
www.genome.ad.jp/brite/brite.html; www.signalinggateway.org;

The genes which govern the regulations for the different metabolic pathways and biosynthetic enzymes involved are identified and studied. Understanding families or categories of different biosynthetic genes leading to the production of many specific secondary metabolites is the main focus of natural product metabolomics and its processes. Families of genes function differently and we can even have evolutionary trends where constitution of a group of new genes with same function evolves independently by gene duplications, giving a composite gene evolved from recombination events between two different types. Now combining evolutionary ways of duplications with divergence and domain swapping are most likely the reasons for the very vast diversities of secondary metabolites in plants. Plant metabolomics pathway leadings leading to secondary metabolites have three types of genes which are (1) Glycosyl transferases (2) Acyl transferases and (3) Cytochrome P450s genes.

1. Glycosyl transferases: Here enzymes that cause glycolysation of secondary metabolites see to and ensure sugar moieties are added to organic molecules, so maintains the metabolic homeostasis. The effect causes increase in chemical stability and water

solubility, which may influence or even change the bioactivities. Nucleotide activated sugars are utilized as substrates on many secondary metabolites like flavonoids, carotenoids, steroids, lignin etc.

2. Acyl transferases: They are enzymes which make available the acyl group [RC=O] to other molecules [alcohols, amines, phosphates, carboxylates etc] in different pathways, so controls metabolite levels in biosyntheses of, for examples anthocyanins, alkaloids, cystein and phenylpropanoids.

3. Cytochrome P450 genes: They are heme-thiolate proteins responsible for electron transfers. They cause bio-transformations of xenobiotics and endobiotics in processes like detoxifications, signallings, growth and defenses. They are also important in drugs metabolisms.

Genomics and metabolomics studies will be able to reveal and decipher detail phytochemical in a particular medicinal plant species. Probably in the near future, transgenic methods may also provide good alternative biosynthetic methods of forming new active secondary metabolites not known now. Therefore this will demonstrate biotechnology in natural product studies, and it may even be a potential application in natural product researches, moreso plants are easy organisms to manipulate their genetics so as to obtain diverse natural products. These will also lead to safe nutraceutical natural products.

10. Highlights on thigmonastics, polygraphs, taoism, ancestral aspects of plants with quarantine

'Wellbeing' entails perfect maintenance of man's social, mental, physical and spiritual health. Plants have been highly beneficial to man's health and maintenance. Utilization of herbs for curative applications have been before 2000BC. Some of our ethical believe, behaviour and handlings have effects on plants, and results we get from plants. Man consume plants inform of foods, drinks, fruits and vegetables. The phytochemical in plants determine its smells, flavours, fragrances and colours. It also reduces a lot of risk in man. Man's aggressions and violence are known to decrease with his social interactions with his green environment. Through electromagnetic waves induced by man's activities such as words and music he pronounce in love or show of gratitude, have impact on plants, and vice versa. For examples insectivorous plants trap insects that rest on it; a plant like *Mimosa pudica* re-align its leaflets to a limp up position when touched by man. Likewise, man and animals influence health, pollination and survival of plants (**quarantine**). Experiments on tropisms indicate reactions of plants to factors like applied light, heat, electricity and gravity. Man's physical contact [e.g. applying strokes, rubbings] with plant parts such as flowers, leaves and stems affects its wellness. All described above refers to plant's THIGMONASTICS. Prove of its truthfulness is referred to as **Polygraph**. Emphasis on the natural and simple way of life with the interactions is called **Taoism**. It is believed and proposed that plants have spirits.

11. References

[1] Hamburger M. and Hostettman K., 1991. Bioactivity in plants: The link between phytochemistry and medicine. *Phytochemistry* 30, 3864-3874.

[2] Mendonca-Filho, 2006. Bioactive phytocompounds: New approaches in the Phytosciences. In: Modern phytomedicine- Turning medicinal plants into drugs. I.Ahmad; F.Aqil & M.Owas (Eds). WILEY-VCH Verlag GmbH & Co. KGaA, Weinheim.

[3] B.S. Furniss; A.J. Hannaford; P.W.G. Smith and A.R. Thatchell. 1989. Organic Vogel.Textbook of practical organic chemistry, 5th Edition. ISBN 0-470-21414-7.

[4] Cseke L.J; Kirakosyan A.; Kaufman P.B; Warber S.L; Duke J.A. and Brielmann H.L. 2006. Natural product from plants. 2nd Edition. CRC Taylor & Francis Group. ISBN 0-8493-2976-0.

[5] Odugbemi O. 2008. A textbook of medicinal plants from Nigeria. University of Lagos press. ISBN: 978-978-48712-9-7.

[6] Holton T.A. and Cornish E.C. 1995. Genetics and biochemistry of anthocyanin biosynthesis. *The Plant Cell* 7, 1071–1083.

[7] Nigeria Natural Medicine Development Agency. FMST. Medicinal plants of Nigeria ISBN 978-35642-3-4. (a) North central zone Vol.1. 2006. (b) South west Nigeria. Vol.1. 2005.

[8] Chatwal G.R. 2007. Organic chemistry of natural products. Arora M.(Ed.). Vols 1&2. Himalaya Publishing House. New Delhi-110002.

[9] Xu R.; Ye Y. and Zhao W. 2010. Introduction to natural products chemistry. CRC Press. Taylor & Francis. ISBN 978-1-4398-6076-2.

[10] Dubey R.C. 2009. A Textbook of biotechnology. S. Chand & Co Ltd. ISBN 81-219-2608-4.

[11] Bu'Lock J.D. 1965. The biosynthesis of natural products. An introduction to secondary metabolism. Sykes P. (Ed). McGrw-Hill Publishing Company Ltd.

[12] Can Baser K.H. and Buchbauer G. 2010. Handbook of essential oils. Science, Technology and Applications. CRC Press Taylor & Francis Group. ISBN 978-1-4200-6315-8.

[13] Tringali C.(Ed.). 2011. Bioactive compounds from natural sources. Natural products as lead compounds in drug discovery. CRC Press. Taylor & Francis Group. ISBN: 978-1-4398-2229-6

5

Analytical Evaluation of Herbal Drugs

Anjoo Kamboj

Chandigarh College of Pharmacy, Landran, Mohali
India

1. Introduction

Traditional herbal medicine and their preparations have been widely used for the thousands of years in developing and developed countries owing to its natural origin and lesser side effects or dissatisfaction with the results of synthetic drugs. However, one of the characteristics of oriental herbal medicine preparations is that all the herbal medicines, either presenting as single herbs or as collections of herbs in composite formulae, is extracted with boiling water during the decoction process. This may be the main reason why quality control of oriental herbal drugs is more difficult than that of western drug. As pointed in "General Guidelines for Methodologies on Research and Evaluation of Traditional Medicines (World Health Organization, 2000)", "Despite its existence and continued use over many centuries, and its popularity and extensive use during the last decade, traditional medicine has not been officially recognized in most countries. Consequently, education, training and research in this area have not been accorded due attention and support. The quantity and quality of the safety and efficacy data on traditional medicine are far from sufficient to meet the criteria needed to support its use world-wide. The reasons for the lack of research data are due to not only to health care policies, but also to a lack of adequate or accepted research methodology for evaluating traditional medicine" (WHO, 2000, 2001).

In olden days vaidas used to treat patients on individual basis and prepare drug according to the requirement of the patient but now the scene has changed, herbal medicines are being manufactured on large scale where manufacturers come across many problems such as availability of good quality raw material, authentication of raw material, availability of standards, proper standardization methodology of single drugs and formulation, quality control parameters etc; hence the concept of quality from very first step is paramount factor must get good attention.

The chemistry of plants involves the presence of therapeutically important constituents usually associated with many inert substances (coloring agents, cellulose, lignin etc). The active principles are extracted from the plants and purified for therapeutic utility for their selective pharmacological activity. So quality control of herbal crude drugs and their constituents is of great importance in modern system of medicine. Lack of proper standard parameters for the standardization of herbal preparation and several instances of substandard herbs, adulterated herbs come into existence. To meet new thrust of inquisitiveness, standardization of herbals is mandatory (Chaudhry, 1999; Kokate, 2005; Raina, 2003; Raven, 1999; Yan, 1999).

Hence every single herb needs to be quality checked to ascertain that it confirms to quality requirement and delivers the properties consistently. Standardization assures that products are reliable in terms of quality, efficacy, performance and safety. It is however observed that the drugs in commerce are frequently adulterated and do not comply with the standards prescribed for authentic drug.

2. Drug adulteration

The adulteration and substitution of herbal drugs is the burning problem in herbal industry and it has caused a major effect in the commercial use of natural products. Adulteration in market samples is one of the greatest drawbacks in promotion of herbal products. Adulteration it is a practice of substituting the original crude drug partially or fully with other substances which is either free from or inferior in therapeutic and chemical properties or addition of low grade or spoiled drugs or entirely different drug similar to that of original drug substituted with an intention of enhancement of profits. Or adulteration may be defined as mixing or substituting the original drug material with other spurious, inferior, defective, spoiled, useless other parts of same or different plant or harmful substances or drug which do not confirm with the official standards [Ansari, 2003; Kokate, 2004].

Adulteration may takes place by two ways:

- Direct or intentional adulteration
- Indirect or unintentional adulteration

2.1 Direct or intentional adulteration

Direct or intentional adulteration is done intentionally which usually includes practices in which an herbal drug is substituted partially or fully with other inferior products. Due to morphological resemblance to the authentic herb, many different inferior commercial varieties are used as adulterants. These may or may not have any chemical or therapeutic potential. Substitution by "exhausted" drugs entails adulteration of the plant material with the same plant material devoid of the active constituents. This practice is most common in the case of volatile oil-containing materials, where the dried exhausted material resembles the original drug but is free of the essential oils. Foreign matter such as other parts of the same plant with no active ingredients, sand and stones, manufactured artifacts, and synthetic inferior principles are used as substitutes.

The practice of intentional adulteration is mainly encouraged by traders who are reluctant to pay premium prices for herbs of superior quality, and hence are inclined to purchase only the cheaper products. This encourages producers and traders to sell herbs of inferior quality.

2.1.1 With artificially manufactured materials

Substances artificially manufactured being resemble with original drug are used as substitutes. This practice is generally followed for much costlier drug e.g. nutmeg is adulterated with basswood prepared to the required shape and size, the colored paraffin wax is used in place of beeswax.

2.1.2 With inferior quality materials

Inferior quality material may or may not have same chemical or therapeutic value as that of original natural drug due to their morphological resemblance to authentic drug, they are marketed as adulterants e.g. *Belladonna* leaves are substituted with *Ailanthus* leaves, *papaya* seeds to adulterate *Piper nigrum*, mother cloves and clove stalks are mixed with clove, beeswax is substituted by Japan wax.

2.1.3 With exhausted material

Many drugs extracted on large scale for isolation of active principle, volatile oils etc. the exhausted material may be used entirely or in part as a substituent for the genuine drug e.g. umbelliferous fruits and cloves (without volatile oils) are adulterated with exhausted (without volatile oils) original drugs, exhausted jalap and Indian hemp (without resins) are used as adulterant.

2.1.4 With foreign matter

Sometimes synthetic chemicals are used to enhance the natural character e.g. addition of benzyl benzoate to balsam of Peru, citral to citrus oils like oil of lemon and orange oil etc.

2.1.5 With harmful / Fictitious substances

Sometimes the wastes from market are collected and admixed with authentic drugs particularly for liquids or unorganized drugs e.g. pieces of amber colored glass in colophony, limestone in asafetida, lead shot in opium, white oil in coconut oil, cocoa butter with stearin or paraffin.

2.1.6 Adulteration of powders

Besides entire drug powder form frequently found to be adulterated e.g. powder liquorice or gentian admixed with powder olive stones, under the name of cinchona, *C. calisaya* wedd., *C. officinalis* Linn.f., *C. ledgeriana* and *C. succirubra* are available as mixtures.

2.2 Indirect or unintentional adulteration

Unintentional or undeliberately adulteration which sometimes occurs without bad intention of the manufacturer or supplier. Sometimes in the absence of proper means of evaluation, an authentic drug partially or fully devoid of the active ingredients may enter the market. Factors such as geographical sources, growing conditions, processing, and storage are all factors that influence the quality of the drug [Ansari, 2003; Kokate, 2004].

2.2.1 Faulty collection

Some of the herbal adulteration is due to the carelessness of herbal collectors and suppliers. The correct part of genuine plant should be collected. Other less valuable part of the genuine plant should not be collected. Moreover collection should be carried out at a proper season and time when the active constituents reach maximum. *Datura strumarium* leaves should be collected during flowering stage and wild cherry bark in autumn etc. collection from other plant by ignorance, due to similarity in the appearance, color, lack of knowledge may lead to adulteration. For example in place of *Aconitum napellus*, the other *Aconitum deinorhizum* may be collected or in place of *Rhamnus purshiana* (cascara bark) *Rhamnus colifornica* is generally collected. Confusion existing in the common vernacular name of different plant in various states of india may leads to this type of adulteration. Often in different states the same plant is known by different vernacular names, while quite different drugs are known by same name. This creates confusion which is best illustrated by Punarnava and Brahmi. The Indian pharmacopoeia drugs *Trianthema portulacastrum* L. and *Boerhavia diffusa* L. are both known by the same vernacular name "Punarnava".

2.2.2 Imperfect preparation

Non removal of associated structures eg stems are collected with leaves, flowers, fruits. Non-removal of undesirable parts or structures e.g. cork should be removed from ginger rhizome. Proper drying conditions should be adhered. Improper drying may lead to unintentional adulteration e.g. if digitalis leaves are dried above 65°c decomposition of glycosides by enzymatic hydrolysis. Use of excessive heat in separating the code liver oil from livers, where the proportions of vitamins, odor and color etc are adversely affected.

2.2.3 Incorrect storage

Deterioration especially during storage, leading to the loss of the active ingredients, production of metabolites with no activity and, in extreme cases, the production of toxic metabolites. Physical factors such as air (oxygen), humidity, light, and temperature can bring about deterioration directly or indirectly. These factors, alone or in combination, can lead to the development of organisms such as molds, mites, and bacteria. Oxidation of the constituents of a drug can be brought about by oxygen in the air, causing some products, such as essential oils, to resinify or to become rancid. Moisture or humidity and elevated temperatures can accelerate enzymatic activities, leading to changes in the physical appearance and decomposition of the herb. For example volatile oils should be protected from light and stored in well closed containers in cool place. Belladonna leaf should be stored in moisture free containers, which may cause enzymatic action lead to decomposition of medicinally active constituents. Mites, nematode worms, insects/moths, and beetles can also destroy herbal drugs during storage.

2.2.4 Gross substitution with plant material

Due to morphological resemblance i.e similarity in appearance, colors etc the genuine crude drugs are substituted with others are very often sold in the market e.g. *Podophyllum peltatum* L. is used as a substitute for *P. hexandrum*, *Belladona* leaves are substituted with Ailanthus leaves, saffron is admixed with dried flowers of *Carthamus tinctorius*, mother cloves and clove stalks are mixed with clove.

2.2.5 Substitution with exhausted drugs

In this type, the same drug is admixed but devoid of any medicinally active constituents as they are already extracted out. This practice is more common in case of volatile oil containing drugs like fennel, clove, coriander, caraway etc. sometime, natural characters of exhausted drugs like color and taste are manipulated by adding other additives and then it is substituted eg exhausted gentian made bitter with aloes.

3. Drug evaluation

Evaluation means confirmation of its identity and determination of quality and purity of the herbal drug. Evaluation of crude drug is necessary because of three main reasons: biochemical variations in the drug, deterioration due to treatment and storage, substitution and adulteration as a result of carelessness, ignorance or fraud or variability caused by differences in growth, geographical location, and time of harvesting. For the quality control of a traditional medicine, the traditional methods are procured and studied, and documents and the traditional information about the identity and quality assessment are interpreted in terms of modern assessment or monograph in herbal pharmacopoeia [Ansari, 2003; Kokate, 2004; Gupta, 2007]. The crude drug can be evaluated or identified by five methods:

3.1 Organoleptic evaluation or morphological evaluation

It means evaluation of drug by the organs of sense (skin, eye, tongue, nose and ear) or macroscopic evaluation and it includes evaluation of drugs by color, odor, taste, size, shape and special feature, like touch, texture etc. it is the technique of qualitative evaluation based on the study of morphological and sensory profile of whole drugs. eg. The fractured surfaces in cinchona, quillia and cascara barks and quassia wood are important characteristics. Aromatic odour of umbelliferous fruits and sweet taste of liquorice are the examples of this type of evaluation where odor of drug depends upon the type and quality of odourous principles (volatile oils) present. Shape of drug may be cylindrical (sarsapilla), subcylindrical (podophyllum), conical (aconite), fusiform (jalap) etc, size represent length, breadth, thickness, diameter etc. color means external color which varies from white to brownish black are important diagnostic characters. The general appearance (external marking) of the weight of a crude drug often indicates whether it is likely to comply with prescribed standard like furrows(alternate depression or valleys), wrinkles (fine delicate furrows), annulations (transverse rings), fissures (splits), nodules (rounded outgrowth), scars (spot left after fall of leaves, stems or roots). Taste is specific type of sensation felt by epithelial layer of tongue. It may be acidic (sour), saline (salt like), saccharic (sweetish), bitter or tasteless (possessing no taste).

3.2 Microscopic evaluation

It involves detailed examination of the drug and it can be used to identify the organized drugs by their known histological characters. It is mostly used for qualitative evaluation of organized crude drugs in entire and powder forms with help of microscope [Ansari, 2003; Kokate, 2005; WHO, 1998].

Using microscope detecting various cellular tissues, trichomes, stomata, starch granules, calcium oxalate crystals and aleurone grains are some of important parameters which play important role in identification of certain crude drug. Crude drug can also be identified microscopically by cutting the thin TS (transverse section), LS (Longitudinal section) especially in case of wood and by staining them with proper staining reagents e.g. starch and hemicelluloses is identified by blue color with iodine solution, all lignified tissue give pink stain with phloroglucinol and HCl etc. mucilage is stained pink with ruthenium red can be used to distinguish cellular structure. Microscopic evaluation also includes study of constituents in the powdered drug by the use of chemical reagents.

Quantitative aspects of microscopy includes study of stomatal number and index, palisade ratio, vein-islet number, size of starch grains, length of fibers etc which play important role in the identification of drug.

3.3 Chemical evaluation

Most of drugs have definite chemical constituents to which their biological or pharmacological activity is attributed. Qualitative chemical test are used to identify certain drug or to test their purity. The isolation, purification, identification of active constituents is based on chemical methods of evaluation. Qualitative chemical test such as acid value, saponification value etc. Some of these are useful in evaluation of resins (acid value, sulphated ash), balsams (acid value, saponification value and bester values), volatile oils (acetyl and ester values) and gums (methoxy determination and volatile acidity). Preliminary phytochemical screening is a part of chemical evaluation. These qualitative chemical tests are useful in identification of chemical constituents and detection of adulteration.

3.4 Physical evaluation

Physical constants are sometimes taken into consideration to evaluate certain drugs. These include moisture content, specific gravity, optical *rotation*, refractive, melting point, viscosity and solubility in different solvents. All these physical properties are useful in identification and detection of constituents present in plant.

3.5 Biological evaluation

Some drugs have specific biological and pharmacological activity which is utilized for their evaluation. Actually this activity is due to specific type of constituents present in the plant extract. For evaluation the experiments were carried out on both intact and isolated organs of living animals. With the help of bioassays (testing the drugs on living animals), strength of drug in its preparation can also be evaluated [Ansari, 2003; Kokate, 2005; Williamson, 1996]. Some important biological evaluations are as follow:

3.5.1 Antibiotic activity

Some bacteria such as *Salmonella typhi, styphylococcus aureus* and *E. coli* are used to determine the antiseptic value (the degree of antiseptic activity e.g. phenol co-efficient of certain drugs). The activity of antibiotics is also determined by using *Klebsiella pneumonia, Micrococcus flavus, Sarcira lutea* etc. living bacteria, yeast and molds are used to evaluate certain vitamins. Microbiological assays by cylinder plate method and turbidimetric method are used in evaluation.

3.5.2 Antifertility activity

Antifertility drugs include contraceptives and abortificients. Contraceptive drugs are used to prevent pregnancy and abortificient to terminate pregnancy. Female rats are used for antifertility activity i.e. measure the pregnancy rate (antiovulation and anti-implantation) and male rats are used for antispermatogenic activity (inhibition of spermatogenesis) and spermicidal activity (sperm motility) of herbal drugs.

3.5.3 Hypoglycemic activity

Rabbits, rats or mice are used to test hypoglycemic activity of plant extract. Radio-immuno assay (RIA) or Enzyme linked immunosorbate assay (ELISA) are done for measurement of insulin levels.

3.5.4 Neuropharmacological activity

Testing the herbal drugs with effects on central and autonomic nervous system. CNS acting drugs like cocaine (*Erythroxylum coca*), morphine (*Papaver somniferum*), cannabinol (*Cannabis sativa*) are tested using rodents. For testing the herbal drugs for their effects on ANS guinea pig ileum for antispasmodic activity, rabbit jejunum for adrenergic activity, rat phrenic-nerve-diaphragm for muscle relaxant activity, frog rectus for skeletal muscles activity.

4. Analytical evaluation

In general, quality control is based on three important pharmacopoeias definitions:

Identity: Is the herb the one it should be?
Purity: Are there contaminants, e.g., in the form of other herbs which should not be there?
Content or assay: Is the content of active constituents within the defined limits.

It is obvious that the content is the most difficult one to assess, since in most herbal drugs the active constituents are unknown. Sometimes markers can be used which are, by definition, chemically defined constituents that are of interest for control purposes, independent of whether they have any therapeutic activity or not. To prove identity and purity, criteria such as type of preparation sensory properties, physical constants, adulteration, contaminants, moisture, ash content and solvent residues have to be checked. The correct identity of the crude herbal material, or the botanical quality, is of prime importance in establishing the quality control of herbal drugs [EMEA, 1998; Sharma, 1995; WHO, 1992].

Identity can be achieved by macro- and microscopical examinations. Voucher specimens are reliable reference sources. Outbreaks of diseases among plants may result in changes to the physical appearance of the plant and lead to incorrect identification.

Purity is closely linked with the safe use of drugs and deals with factors such ash values, contaminants (e.g. foreign matter in the form of other herbs), and heavy metals. However, due to the application of improved analytical methods, modern purity evaluation includes microbial contamination, aflatoxins, radioactivity, and pesticide residues. Analytical methods such as photometric analysis (UV, IR, MS, and NMR), thin layer chromatography (TLC), high performance liquid chromatography (HPLC), and gas chromatography (GC) can be employed in order to establish the constant composition of herbal preparations.

Content or assay is the most difficult area of quality control to perform, since in most herbal drugs the active constituents are not known. Sometimes markers can be used. In all other cases, where no active constituent or marker can be defined for the herbal drug, the percentage extractable matter with a solvent may be used as a form of assay, an approach often seen in pharmacopeias. The choice of the extracting solvent depends on the nature of the compounds involved, and might be deduced from the traditional uses.

A special form of assay is the determination of essential oils by steam distillation. When the active constituents (e.g. sennosides in Senna) or markers (e.g. alkydamides in Echinacea) are known, a vast array of modern chemical analytical methods such as ultraviolet/visible spectroscopy (UV/VIS), TLC, HPLC, GC, mass spectrometry (MS), or a combination of GC and MS (GC/MS), can be employed [Booksh, 1994].

5. Chromatography and chemical fingerprints of herbal medicines

Several problems influence the quality of herbal drugs:

- Herbal drugs are usually mixtures of many constituents.
- The active principle(s) is (are), in most cases unknown.
- Selective analytical methods or reference compounds may not be available commercially.
- Plant materials are chemically and naturally variable.
- Chemo-varieties and chemo cultivars exist.
- The source and quality of the raw material are variable.
- The methods of harvesting, drying, storage, transportation, and processing (for example, mode of extraction and polarity of the extracting solvent, instability of constituents, etc.) have an effect.

Strict guidelines have to be followed for the successful production of a quality herbal drug. Among them are proper botanical identification, phytochemical screening, and standardization. Quality control and the standardization of herbal medicines involve several steps. The source and quality of raw materials, good agricultural practices and manufacturing processes are certainly essential steps for the quality control of herbal medicines and play a pivotal role in guaranteeing the quality and stability of herbal preparations [Blumenthal, 1998; EMEA, 2002; Roberts, 1997; WHO, 1992,1998, 2000, 2005, 2004].

The chemical constituents in component herbs in the herbal products may vary depending on stage of collection, parts of the plant collected, harvest seasons, plant origins (regional status), drying processes and other factors. Thus, it seems to be necessary to determine most of the phytochemical constituents of herbal products in order to ensure the reliability and repeatability of pharmacological and clinical research, to understand their bioactivities and possible side effects of active compounds and to enhance product quality control. Thus, several chromatographic techniques, such as high-performance liquid chromatography (HPLC), gas chromatography (GC), capillary electrophoresis (CE) and thin layer chromatography (TLC), can be applied as quality assessment parameters. The concept of phytoequivalence was developed in Germany in order to ensure consistency of herbal products. According to this concept, a chemical profile, such as a chromatographic fingerprint, for an herbal product should be constructed and compared with the profile of a clinically proven reference product.

By definition, a chromatographic fingerprint of an herbal drug is, in practice, a chromatographic pattern of the extract of some common chemical components of pharmacologically active and/or chemically characteristics. This chromatographic profile should be featured by the fundamental attributions of "integrity" and "fuzziness" or "sameness" and "differences" so as to chemically represent the herbal drug investigated. It is suggested that with the help of chromatographic fingerprints obtained, the authentication and identification of herbal medicines can be accurately conducted ("integrity") even if the amount and/or concentration of the chemically characteristic constituents are not exactly the same for different samples of drug (hence, "fuzziness") or, the chromatographic fingerprints could demonstrate both the "sameness" and "differences" between various samples successfully. Thus, we should globally consider multiple constituents in the herbal drug extracts, and not individually consider only one and/or two marker components for evaluating the quality of the herbal products. However, in any herbal drug and its extract, there are hundreds of unknown components and many of them are in low amount. Moreover, there usually exists variability within the same herbal materials. Consequently, to obtain reliable chromatographic fingerprints that represent pharmacologically active and chemically characteristic components is not an easy or trivial work. Fortunately, chromatography offers very powerful separation ability, such that the complex chemical components in herbal extracts can be separated into many relatively simple sub-fractions [Ahirwal, 2006; Brain, 1975; Cheng, 2003; Clarke, 1967; Wanger, 1984].

In general, the methods for quality control of herbal medicines involve sensory inspection (macroscopic and microscopic examinations) and analytical inspection using instrumental techniques such as thin layer chromatography (TLC), HPLC, GC–MS, LC–MS, near infrared (NIR), and spectrophotometer, etc. On the other hand, the methods of extraction and sample preparation are also of great importance in preparing good fingerprints of herbal medicines. As a single herbal medicine may contain a great many natural constituents, and a combination of several herbs might give rise to interactions with hundreds of natural constituents during the preparation of extracts, the fingerprints produced by the chromatographic instruments, which may present a relatively good integral representation of various chemical components of herbal medicines [Bilia, 2002; Choi, 2002; Chuang, 1995; Ebel, 1987; Rozylo, 2002].

5.1 Thin layer chromatography

TLC was the most common, versatile method of choice for herbal analysis before instrumental chromatography methods like GC and HPLC were established. Even nowadays, TLC is still frequently used for the analysis of herbal medicines since various pharmacopoeias such as Indian herbal pharmacopoeia, Ayurvedic pharmacopoeia; American Herbal Pharmacopoeia (AHP), Chinese drug monographs and analysis, Pharmacopoeia of the People's Republic of China, etc. Rather, TLC is used as an easier method of initial screening with a semi quantitative evaluation together with other chromatographic techniques as there is relatively less change in the simple TLC separation of herbal medicines than with instrumental chromatography.

Thin-layer chromatography is a technique in which a solute undergoes distribution between two phases, a stationary phase acting through adsorption and a mobile phase in the form of a liquid. The adsorbent is a relatively thin, uniform layer of dry finely powdered material applied to a glass, plastic or metal sheet or plate. Glass plates are most commonly used. Separation may also be achieved on the basis of partition or a combination of partition and adsorption, depending on the particular type of support, its preparation and its use with different solvent [Herborne ,1928; Stahl, 1969].

Identification can be effected by observation of spots of identical Rf value and about equal magnitude obtained, respectively, with an unknown and a reference sample chromatographed on the same plate. A visual comparison of the size and intensity of the spots usually serves for semi-quantitative estimation.

TLC has the advantages of many-fold possibilities of detection in analyzing herbal medicines. In addition, TLC is rather simple and can be employed for multiple sample analysis. For each plate, more than 30 spots of samples can be studied simultaneously in one time. Thus, the use of TLC to analyze the herbal medicines is still popular. HPTLC is one of the sophisticated instrumental techniques based on the full capabilities of TLC. It is most flexible, reliable and cost efficient separation technique. The advantage of automation, scanning, full optimization, selective detection principle, minimum sample preparation, hypenation, and so on enable it to be powerful analytical tool for chromatographic information of complex mixtures of pharmaceuticals, natural products, clinical samples, food stuffs, and so on. With the help of the CAMAG video store system (CAMAG, Switerland) and TLCQA-UV methods, it is possible to get useful qualitative and quantitative information from the developed TLC plate. For example the four samples of *Cordyceps sinensis* from the joint products of China and Japan cooperation have more valuable medical effect compared to others as they contained the most effective component cordycepin. Moreover, with the help of image analysis and digitized technique developed in computer science, the evaluation of similarity between different samples is also possible.

The advantages of using TLC/HPTLC to construct the fingerprints of herbal medicines are its simplicity, versatility, high velocity, specific sensitivity and simple sample preparation. Thus, TLC is a convenient method of determining the quality and possible adulteration of herbal products. It is worth noting that the new techniques of TLC are also being updated like forced-flow planar chromatography (FFPC), rotation planar chromatography (RPC), over pressured-layer chromatography (OPLC), and electro planar chromatography (EPC). A simple, but powerful preparative forced-flow technique was also reported; in this technique hydrostatic pressure is used to increase mobile-phase velocity. Parallel and serially-coupled layers open up new vistas for the analysis of a large number of samples (up to 216) for high throughput screening and for the analysis of very complex matrices [Funk, 1991;Gong, 2003; Svendsen, 1989; Wanger, 1996].

5.2 Gas chromatography

Gas chromatography (GC), also known as gas liquid chromatography (GLC), is a technique for separation of mixtures into components by a process which depends on the redistribution of the components between a stationary phase or support material in the form of a liquid, solid or combination of both and a gaseous mobile phase.

It is well-known that many pharmacologically active components in herbal medicines are volatile chemical compounds. Thus, the analysis of volatile compounds by gas chromatography is very important in the analysis of herbal medicines. The GC analysis of the volatile oils has a number of advantages. Firstly, the GC of the volatile oil gives a reasonable "fingerprint" which can be used to identify the plant. The composition and relative concentration of the organic compounds in the volatile oil are characteristic of the particular plant and the presence of impurities in the volatile oil can be readily detected. Secondly, the extraction of the volatile oil is relatively straightforward and can be standardized and the components can be readily identified using GC-MS analysis. The relative quantities of the components can be used to monitor or assess certain characteristics of the herbal medicines. Changes in composition of the volatile oil may also be used as indicators of oxidation, enzymatic changes or microbial fermentation. The advantages of GC clearly lie in its high sensitivity of detection for almost all the volatile chemical compounds. This is especially true for the usual FID detection and GC–MS. Furthermore, the high selectivity of capillary columns enables separation of many volatile compounds simultaneously within comparatively short times. Thus, over the past decades, GC is a popular and useful analytical tool in the research field of herbal medicines. Especially, with the use of hyphenated GC–MS instrument, reliable information on the identity of the compounds is available as well. However, the most serious disadvantage of GC is that it is not convenient for its analysis of the samples of polar and non-volatile compounds. For this, it is necessary to use tedious sample work-up which may include derivatization. Therefore, the liquid chromatography becomes another necessary tool for us to apply the comprehensive analysis of the herbal medicines [Nyiredy, 2003].

The first fully automated on-line GC-IR system was developed by Scott et al. Each eluted solute was adsorbed in a cooled packed tube, and then thermally regenerated into an infrared vapor cell. Subsequent to the IR spectrum being obtained, a small sample of the vapor was drawn from the IR cell into a low-resolution mass spectrometer and the mass spectrum was also taken [Gong, 2001; Yan, 2009; Ylinen, 1986].

5.3 High-performance liquid chromatography

High performance liquid chromatography (HPLC), also known as high pressure liquid chromatography, is essentially a form of column chromatography in which the stationary phase consists of small particle (3-50µm) packing contained in a column with a small bore (2-5mm), one end of which is attached to a source of pressurized liquid eluent (mobile phase). The three forms of high performance liquid chromatography most often used are ion exchange, partition and adsorption.

HPLC is a popular method for the analysis of herbal medicines because it is easy to learn and use and is not limited by the volatility or stability of the sample compound. In general, HPLC can be used to analyze almost all the compounds in the herbal medicines. Thus, over the past decades, HPLC has received the most extensive application in the analysis of herbal medicines. Reversed-phase (RP) columns may be the most popular columns used in the analytical separation of herbal medicines.

It is necessary to notice that the optimal separation condition for the HPLC involves many factors, such as the different compositions of the mobile phases, their pH adjustment, pump pressures, etc. Thus, a good experimental design for the optimal separation seems in general necessary. In order to obtain better separation, some new techniques have been recently developed in research field of liquid chromatography. These are micellar electrokinetic capillary chromatography (MECC), high-speed counter-current chromatography (HSCCC), low-pressure size-exclusion chromatography (SEC), reversed-phase ion-pairing HPLC (RP-

IPC-HPLC), and strong anion-exchange HPLC (SAX-HPLC). They will provide new opportunities for good separation for some specific extracts of some herbal medicines. On the other hand, the advantages of HPLC lie in its versatility for the analysis of the chemical compounds in herbal medicines, however, the commonly used detector in HPLC, say single wavelength UV detector, seems to be unable to fulfill the task, since lots of chemical compounds in herbal medicines are non-chromophoric compounds. Consequently, a marked increase in the use of HPLC analysis coupled with evaporative light scattering detection (ELSD) in a recent decade demonstrated that ELSD is an excellent detection method for the analysis of non-chromophoric compounds. This new detector provides a possibility for the direct HPLC analysis of many pharmacologically active components in herbal medicines, since the response of ELSD depends only on the size, shape, and number of eluate particles rather than the analysis structure and/or chromophore of analytes as UV detector do. Especially, this technique is quite suitable for the construction of the fingerprints of the herbal medicines. Moreover, the qualitative analysis or structure elucidation of the chemical components in herbal drug by simple HPLC is not possible, as they rely on the application of techniques using hyphenated HPLC, such as HPLC-IR, HPLC–MS, HPLC-NMR, for the analysis of herbal medicines [Lazarowych, 1998; Li, 1999; Liu, 1999; Li, 2003; Tsai, 2002; Liu, 1993; Zhang, 2004].

5.4 Electrophoretic methods

Capillary electrophoresis was introduced in early 1980s as a powerful analytical and separation technique and has since been developed almost explosively. It allows an efficient way to document the purity/complexity of a sample and can handle virtually every kind of charged sample components ranging from simple inorganic ions to DNA. Thus, there was an obvious increase of electrophoretic methods, especially capillary electrophoresis, used in the analysis of herbal medicines in last decades. The more or less explosive development of capillary electrophoresis since its introduction has to a great extent paralleled that of liquid chromatography. Most of the used techniques are capillary zone electrophoresis (CZE), capillary gel electrophoresis (CGE) and capillary isoelectric focusing (CIEF). CE is promising for the separation and analysis of active ingredients in herbal medicines, since it needs only small amounts of standards and can analyze samples rapidly with very good separation ability. Also, it is a good tool for producing the chemical fingerprints of the herbal medicines, since it has similar technical characteristics of liquid chromatography. Recently, several studies dealing with herbal medicines have been reported and two kinds of medicinal compounds, i.e. alkaloids and flavonoids, have been studied extensively.

In general, CE is a versatile and powerful separation tool with high separation efficiency and selectivity when analyzing mixtures of low-molecular-mass components However, the fast development in capillary electrophoresis causes improvement of resolution and throughput rather than reproducibility and absolute precision. One successful approach to improve the reproducibility of both mobility and integral data has been based on internal standards. But many papers were published unfortunately revealed limited image on the real possibilities of CE in the field of fingerprinting herbal medicines. CE and capillary electrochromatography approaches contribute to be a better understanding of the solution behavior of herbal medicines, especially when additionally combined with the powerful spectrometric detectors [Liu, 1992, 1993; Stuppner ,1992; Yang, 1995].

6. Hyphenation procedures

In the past two decades, combining a chromatographic separation system on-line with a spectroscopic detector in order to obtain structural information on the analytes present in a sample has become the most important approach for the identification and/or confirmation of the identity of target and unknown chemical compounds. For most (trace-level) analytical problems in the research field of herbal medicines, the combination of column liquid chromatography or capillary gas chromatography with a UV-VIS or a mass spectrometer (HPLC-DAD, CE-DAD, GC-MS and LC-MS, respectively) becomes the preferred approach for the analysis of herbal medicines.

The additional and/or complementary information required in number of cases can be provided by, for example, atomic emission, Fourier-transform infrared (FTIR), fluorescence emission (FE), or nuclear magnetic resonance (NMR) spectrometry. It is demonstrated that, from a practical point of view, rewarding results can be obtained, since we need much more information to deal with the most complex analytical systems such as those samples from herbal medicines. Furthermore, the data obtained from such hyphenated instruments are the so-called two-way data; say one way for chromatogram and the other way for spectrum, which could provide much more information than the classic one-way chromatography. With the help of chemo metrics, a rather new discipline developed both in chemistry and statistics in the later part of the 1970s, we will definitely get more chance to deal with the difficult problems in the analysis of herbal medicines and also the problems in quality control of herbal medicines.

6.1 LC-IR, LC-MS, LC-NMR

The hyphenated technique developed from the coupling of liquid chromatography and infrared spectroscopy is known as LC-IR. LC-IR is an important technique as it shows absorption peaks of functional groups in mid IR region which helps in structural identification of compounds present in a sample. The detection technique of IR is comparatively slow than other techniques like MS or NMR. Two approaches used in these techniques are flow cell approach and solvent elimination approach.

Liquid chromatography-mass spectrometry (LC-MS) is an analytical chemistry technique that combines the physical separation capabilities of liquid chromatography with the mass analysis capabilities of mass spectrometry. LC-MS is a powerful technique used for many applications which has very high sensitivity and selectivity. Generally its application is oriented towards the specific detection and potential identification of chemicals in a complex mixture.

There are two common atmospheric pressure ionization (API) LC/MS process: Electrospray Ionization (ESI) & Atmospheric Pressure Chemical Ionization (APCI). Both are soft ionization technique. Both of these processes are compatible with most chromatographic separations.

The combination of liquid chromatography (LC) and nuclear magnetic resonance (NMR) offers the potential of unparalleled chemical information from analytes separated from complex mixtures. Several other hyphenated NMR techniques have been developed to enhance sensitivity of this technique. LC-SPE-NMR increases sensitivity of the instrument by utilizing a solid phase extraction device after LC column. Capillary LC-NMR also practically lowers detection limit to a nanogram range through integration of capillary LC with NMR detection. Further Cryo-LC-probe technology combine the advantage of sample flow and enhanced sensitivity from a cryogenically cooled NMR probe [Wang, 2001].

6.2 GC-MS

Mass spectrometry is the most sensitive and selective method for molecular analysis and can yield information on the molecular weight as well as the structure of the molecule. Combining chromatography with mass spectrometry provides the advantage of both chromatography as a separation method and mass spectrometry as an identification method. In mass spectrometry, there is a range of methods to ionize compounds and then separate the ions. Common methods of ionization used in conjunction with gas chromatography are electron impact (EI) and electron capture ionization (ECI). EI is primarily configured to select positive ions, whereas ECI is usually configured for negative ions (ECNI). EI is particularly useful for routine analysis and provides reproducible mass spectra with structural information which allows library searching. GC–MS was the first successful online combination of chromatography with mass spectrometry, and is widely used in the analysis of essential oil in herbal medicines.

With the GC–MS, not only a chromatographic fingerprint of the essential oil of the herbal medicine can be obtained but also the information related to its most qualitative and relative quantitative composition. Used in the analysis of the herbal medicines, there are at least two significant advantages for GC–MS, that is: (1) with the capillary column, GC–MS has in general very good separation ability, which can produce a chemical fingerprint of high quality; (2) with the coupled mass spectroscopy and the corresponding mass spectral database, the qualitative and relatively quantitative composition information of the herb investigated could be provided by GC–MS, which will be extremely useful for the further research for elucidating the relationship between chemical constituents in herbal medicine and its pharmacology in further research. Thus, GC–MS should be the most preferable tool for the analysis of the volatile chemical compounds in herbal medicines [Gong, 2001, 2003; Li, 1999, 2003,].

6.3 HPLC–DAD, HPLC–MS and others

HPLC-DAD has become a common technique in most analytical laboratories in the world now. With the additional UV spectral information, the qualitative analysis of complex samples in herbal medicines turns out to be much easier than before. For instance, checking peak purity and comparing with the available standard spectrum of the known compound to the one in the investigated sample. Especially, with the introduction of electrospray mass spectrometry, the coupling of liquid chromatography and mass spectrometry has opened the new way to widely and routinely applied to the analysis of herbal medicines. HPLC chromatographic fingerprints can be then applied for documentation of complete herbal extracts with more information and on-line qualitative analysis becomes possible. Several valuable review articles dealing with LC–MS and its application in the analysis of botanical extracts have been published, In last decades, the increasing usage of LC–MS and HPLC-DAD in the analysis of herbal medicines is quite obvious. Several good reviews have been published for the analysis of the bioactive chemical compounds in plants and herbal medicines, in which the technique used most is HPLC, especially the hyphenated

HPLC techniques. Moreover, combined HPLC–DAD–MS techniques take advantage of chromatography as a separation method and both DAD and MS as an identification method. DAD and MS can provide on-line UV and MS information for each individual peak in a chromatogram. With the help of this hyphenation, in most cases, one could identify the chromatographic peaks directly on-line by comparison with literature data or with standard compounds, which made the LC–DAD–MS becomes a powerful approach for the rapid identification of phytochemical constituents in botanical extracts, and it can be used to avoid the time-consuming isolation of all compounds to be identified. Recently, the hyphenation between HPLC and NMR are also available, which might become a vital and an attractive analytical tool for the analysis of drugs in biological fluids and for the analysis of herbal medicines. In fact the tendency of the hyphenation or multi-hyphenation of the chromatography with the common used four spectroscopic detectors, say UV, Fourier transformation infrared spectrum, MS and NMR, for structure elucidation of chemical compounds, is in progress. A "total analysis device" has been recently demonstrated in the case of on-line HPLC–UV (DAD)–FT–IR–NMR–MS analyses. It may be worth noting that the electrode array hyphenated with HPLC is also in progress. As electrochemical detection was described to be superior to UV–Vis and fluorescence spectroscopy for determination of some chemical compound, like polyphenols in trace levels, very sensitive determination was achieved by using a multi channel electrochemical detector (Coul Array). A two-way chromatogram is obtained, since the detector has 12 (or more) electrodes in series set incrementally to different potentials. Thus, similar to the UV–Vis spectra, the hydrodynamic voltammogram can be used for peak purity checking and peak identification [Maillard, 1993; Mellon, 1987; Rajani, 2001; Ravilla, 2001; Sticher, 1992; Wolfender, 1993, 1994, 1995].

6.4 Hyphenation of CE

The situation of the CE analysis in hyphenation development is somewhat like HPLC analysis. The hyphenated CE instruments, such as CE-DAD, CE-MS and CE-NMR, all appeared in the past decades. The techniques have also quickly been used for the analysis of the samples from herbal medicines. On-line coupling of capillary electrophoresis to mass spectrometry and other spectrometry allows both the efficient separation of CE and the specific and sensitive detection to be achieved. Furthermore, the artifacts happened in CE measurements might be overcome with the help of some information handling technique, such as some methods developed in chemometrics, since one could use with the additional information from spectra to correct the artifacts from the chosen separation buffer chemistry or from hidden instrumental constraints. In sum, as the hyphenated techniques in chromatographic and electrophoretic instruments develop, our ability of analysis of herbal medicines, both in qualitative and quantitative respects and our ability of quality control of herbal medicines will become stronger and stronger. We are quite sure that we will have a very prospective future for quality control of herbal medicines [Pusecker, 1998; Stockigt, 2002; Schewitz, 1998].

CE analysis can be driven by electric field performed in narrow tubes which can result in rapid separation of hundreds of compounds. It separates components by applying voltage in between buffer filled capillaries. The components are separated due to production of ions depending on their mass and charge. It is widely used in quantitative determination and the analysis particularly the assay development and trace level determination. When MS is linked to CE then it produces determination of molecular weight of components often termed as CE-MS. Separation is achieved from the etched surface of the capillaries that delivers sample to the ESI MS. This technique runs in full automation and having higher sensitivity and selectivity. The new interface known as coaxial sheath interface has developed which has potential of use of both CE-MS and LC-MS alternatively on same mass spectrometer.

Information features of chromatographic fingerprints of herbal medicines

Hence there are many chromatographic techniques, including the hyphenated chromatographies, available for us to do the instrumental analysis of herbal medicines, and to construct further their fingerprinting. The problem here is that how could we efficiently and reasonably evaluate such-obtained analytical results and/or the fingerprints of the herbal medicines and how could we use the information obtained from chromatographic analysis to address further the problem of quality control for herbal medicines [Liu, 1994, 1993].

7. Phytoequivalence and chromatographic fingerprints of herbal medicines

In general, one could use the chromatographic techniques to obtain a relatively complete picture of an herbal, which is in common called chromatographic fingerprints of herbal medicines to represent the so-called phytoequivalence. The following results show some examples. Fig. 1 shows the total ionic chromatograms (TIC) of essential oils in *Cortex cinnamomi* from four producing areas, say: (a) Zhaoqing, Guangdong province, China; (b) Yulin, Guangxi province, China; (c) Yunnan province, China; and (d) Vietnam, by GC-MS. There are, of course, some differences in the profiles. However, seen from these profiles, phytoequivalence is obvious for *C. cinnamomi*. The other example is shown in Fig. 2a Superimposed HPLC-UV chromatogram of *Ginkgo biloba* in commercial products, Fig 2b in which there are chromatograms of methanol extracts of *Erigeron breviscapus* from 32 different producing places in the same province by HPLC detected at wavelength 280 nm. The integrated feature of the chromatographic fingerprints of herbal medicines can be clearly seen from these examples.

Obtaining a good chromatographic fingerprint representing the phytoequivalence of a herb depends several factors, such as the extracting methods, measurement instruments, measurement conditions, etc. In fact, if we want to obtain an informative fingerprint of a herbal medicine, we need to have a good extracting method, with which we could fortunately obtain almost all the pharmaceutically active compounds to represent the integrity of the herbal medicine.

Furthermore, a chromatogram with good separation and a representative concentration profile of the bioactive components detected by a proper detector are also required. Thus, how to obtain a high quality chromatographic fingerprint of as more as possible information of the herbal medicines is an important task for chemists and pharmacologists. In order to understand bioactivities and possible side effects of active compounds of the herbal medicines and to enhance product quality control, it seems that one needs to determine most of the phytochemical constituents of herbal products so as to ensure the reliability and repeatability of pharmacological and clinical research. Suppose that we have obtained some fingerprints, how to evaluate the information contents of the chromatographic fingerprints of herbal medicines reasonably and efficiently is the second step for the quality control purpose [Beek, 2002; Caoa, 2006; Gong, 2003; Hasler, 1992; Kinghorn, 1998; Liang, 1994; Upton, 2001].

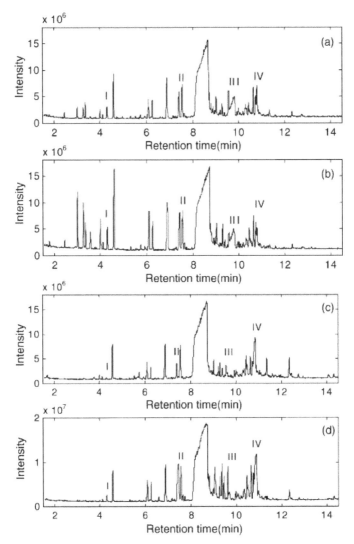

Fig. 1. Total ionic chromatograms of essential oils in C. *cinnamomi* from four different producing areas: (a) Zhaoquing, Guangdong province, china; (b) Yulin, Guangxi province, china; (c) Yunnan province, china; and (d) Vietnam.

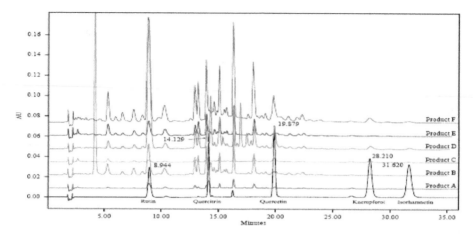

Fig. 2a. Superimposed HPLC-UV chromatogram of *Ginkgo biloba* in commercial products.

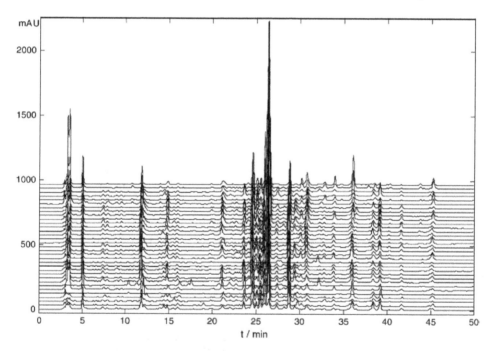

Fig. 2b. Original HPLC chromatograms of 33 herbal samples of *Erigeron breviscapus* at wavelength λ=280nm.

7.1 Information contents of fingerprints of herbal medicines

It is obvious that a chromatographic fingerprint of an herbal medicine is a multivariate system, since in general it embraces most of the phytochemical constituents of herbal products. From a point of view of multivariate, the information content of a chromatogram with lots of peaks might be calculated by means of various approaches. However, as for these methods, the signal intensity, retention time, peak area and/or peak height of each independent peak without overlapping should be all taken into consideration; the calculation burden is also rather heavy. Moreover, if a chromatographic peak is overlapped with its adjacent peak(s), the calculation of the information content will become complex. Vertical splitting is conventionally used for this situation and both peaks on two sides of an overlapping peak cluster are taken as pure ones. Out of question, this approximate treatment on a chromatogram with some overlapping peak clusters will cause some errors on calculation of information content.

In fact, a chromatographic fingerprint, which is a concentration distribution curve of several chromatographic peaks, could be regarded as a continuous signal determined by its chromatographic shape. According to information theory, the information content of a continuous signal might be simply expressed as the following formula:

$$\Phi = -\sum pi \log pi \tag{1}$$

where pi is the positive real numbers of probability property, say $\sum pi = 1$. Based on this idea, we proposed recently a simple method to calculate the information content (Φ) for chromatographic fingerprints of herbal medicines as shown in the following equation, that is

$$\Phi = -\sum \left(\frac{xi}{\sum xi} \log\left(\frac{xi}{\sum xi} \right) \right) \tag{2}$$

where xi is the real chromatographic response of the chemical components involved in the chromatographic fingerprint under study. Here, the normalization of xi divided by their sum is to make the chromatogram investigated be of probability property. In theory, if and only if xi with unchangeable variance is characterized by normal distribution can its information content Φ reach its maximum.

Under an ideal situation, all the chromatographic peaks from a chromatogram can be separated completely and each peak confined to a narrow zone might correspond to a normal distribution profile. A chromatographic fingerprint with all of peaks just completely separated should be featured by maximal information content. Further separation cannot provide any more information and becomes unnecessary. On the contrary, if any of chromatographic peaks is overlapped with its adjacent one(s), this peak will surely show non-Gaussian normal distribution and therefore undoubtedly cause a loss of the information content. There might be, at least, two advantages of the calculation of the information content of complex chromatograms over the available approaches. First, the method uses the whole chromatogram with a simple normalization, thus it is not necessary to identify the retention time, peak intensity, peak width, peak area and/or peak height for all the peaks identified. The calculation burden is reduced significantly. Moreover, the theoretic background of the method is simple and reasonable [Gong, 2003; Hayashi, 1990; Huber, 1993; Matsuda, 1989].

7.2 Correction of retention time shift of fingerprints of herbal medicines

When one deals with several chromatographic fingerprints obtained from the same herbal medicine or from different sources, the first step of our task might be to evaluate their similarity and difference between them. However, correction of retention time shift of the fingerprint of herbal medicines should be taken into consideration first, since some types of variation sources are inevitably encountered from one chromatogram to another. Under this situation, some unacceptable results, one of which is imposed by the retention time shifts, will be produced. Unfortunately, how the retention time shifts are caused by the variation sources is very complex. It might be due to (1) the degradation of the stationary phase, especially, the low stability of silica and silica-based supports at high pH values and the collapse of C- 18 bonded phase because of a highly polar mobile phase; (2) minor changes in mobile phase composition caused by temperature and pressure fluctuations, variations in flow-rate and gradient dispersion; (3) some problems involved in the detectors, for example, a wavelength shift in the UV spectrometer, a spectroscopic intensity variation and the misalignment of the monochromator; (4) the column overloading on account of the great injected amount or some components with high concentration; (5) the possible interaction between analytes; (6) other unknown shifts in the instrument. If these disadvantageous cases are in existence during the chromatographic runs, the retention times will be subsequently shifted. When such retention time shifts occur in chromatographic fingerprints, it is great difficult to conduct data processing, for example, the construction of common chromatographic models of all samples investigated, the similarity comparison between chromatographic fingerprints and pattern recognition based on principal component analysis (PCA) since multivariate analysis with entire chromatographic profiles as input data is very sensitive to even minute variations. As a result, in order to make up a consistent data, it is necessary to detect the retention time shifts of chromatographic fingerprints and then the chromatographic profiles should be adjusted along the retention time direction by means of synchronizing the retention times of the chromatographic peaks from the same components. During the past decades, several kinds of useful approaches have been developed for peak synchronization in chromatographic profiles. Some of them corrected the retention time shifts by making internal standards added or marker peaks coincide in all chromatograms under study. At its first step, chromatographic peaks were identified by setting a retention time window in both of the sample and target chromatograms, and then a list of their retention times was generated. Here, the window meant the maximum shift to be considered. Clearly, the choice of the window size was critical to this technique. However, if the retention time shifts are very serious for complex systems like herbal medicines, the selection of the optimal peak-matching Windows might not be a trivial task. The objective functions on the correlation between the target and sample chromatograms were optimized and then the sample chromatographic profiles were aligned with the target [Bylund, 2002; Hamalainen, 1993; Hayashi, 1990; Huber, 1993; Matsuda, 1989; Pusecker, 1998; Schewitz, 1998].

In general, the methods must be very efficient and elegant if the samples investigated are quite similar in the concentration profiles of the chemical components. However, if the concentration profiles change greatly for the complex samples such as herbal medicines from the different producing places and/or from the various harvest seasons, wrong results might be obtained by simply seeking the optimal correlation coefficient between the chromatograms. It is because that the correlation coefficient is influenced greatly by the big peaks in the chromatographic profiles. In this case, the maximal correlation coefficient does not certainly represent the best correction for the retention time shifts. However, if the data from the hyphenated chromatographic instruments, such as HPLC-DAD, GC–MS, etc. the correction of retention time shift of the fingerprint of herbal medicines will become much clear and easy, which we will discuss later on.

7.3 Evaluation of chemical fingerprints of herbal medicines

In the early chemometric research, chromatographic data were commonly first transformed to retention time–peak area data matrices including only selected peaks, whether the identity of the peaks are known or not. The data such obtained were then used to do the processing, that is, the calculation of similarity or dissimilarity between the fingerprints and the analysis of principal component analysis. However, as pointed by Nielsen, "The quality of the data (including only retention time–peak area data) relies on peak detection (integration) and on how the peaks are selected for the data analysis. It can be very difficult to select an optimal set integration parameters for chromatograms obtained from analysis of complex samples which easily contain more than 100 peaks. Furthermore, the selection and extraction of peaks to include in data analysis is difficult, partly subjective and large amounts of the data in the chromatograms are discarded. The disadvantages of peak detection and integration, and of the introduction of a subjective peak selection can be avoided by using all collected data points in the chemometric analysis." Thus, following the suggestion of Nielsen, the entire chromatographic profiles were utilized to perform direct chemometric analysis. The analysis can be easily done with the help of proper techniques of data compression, such as the technique of wavelet or Fourier transformation, if necessary. Furthermore, another advantage of taking the entire chromatographic profile to perform direct chemometric analysis is that the peak shape can be included in data analysis, which will make the pretreatment of overlapping peaks much easier when one does evaluation of the fingerprints. Of course, the chromatographic profiles should properly aligned to compensate for minor drifts in retention times before one does the fingerprint evaluation and chemometric analysis for the purpose of quality control [Martens, 1991; Sticher, 1992, 1993; Tauler, 1992; Wold, 1987; Zhang, 2003].

7.4 Fingerprints and quality control in herbal medicines

As stated above, one or two markers or pharmacologically active components were currently employed for evaluating the quality and authenticity of an herbal medicine. This kind of the determination, however, does not give a complete picture of an herbal product and therefore it will definitely fail to do the identification of false and true plant extraction. In the following an example will be given to illustrate the situation. Fig. 3 shows 17 fingerprints of *Ginkgo biloba* extractions, which were purchased from several pharmaceutical stores, vendors/companies and collected from various producing areas in the mainland of PR China. All of these samples were supposed to meet the standard measured by UV spectroscopy at wavelength of 318 nm with satisfactory absorbance (old standard method for quality control of *G. biloba* extraction in China), among which standard extract EGb761 from Guangzhou Institute for Drug Control, PR China by a Frenchman from Beaufour-Ipsen Company in France with a satisfactory fingerprint pattern. Analytical grade methanol and phosphoric acid used for mobile phase and all reagents were also of analytical grade. Ultrapure water (18.2M) was obtained by means of a Milli-Q apparatus by Millipore

Corporation (France) and was used for mobile phase preparation. The mobile phase was vacuum filtered through a filter of 0.45 µm pore pore size. From the plot, it is difficult to find some false one. But if we simply do the PCA upon the fingerprints, the results are shown in Fig. 4.

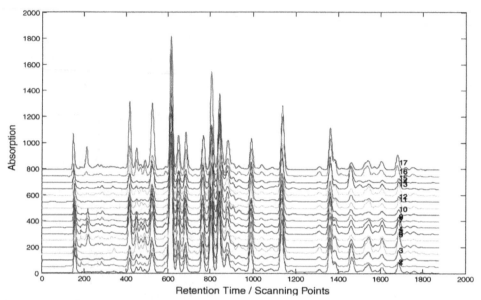

Fig. 3. Chromatograms of 17 extracts of *Ginkgo biloba* meet with the standard measured at wavelength 318nm.

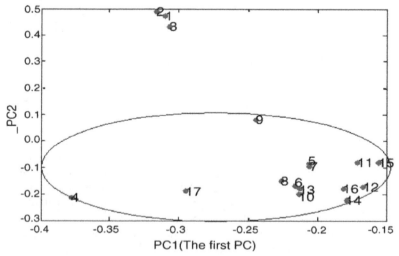

Fig. 4. The score plot obtained by principal components analysis where PC1 means the scores coordinates of principal component 1 and PC2 the ones of principal component 2.

It can be easily seen from the plot that samples marked by numbers 1–3 are clearly outliers. Thus, if we pick up the fingerprints of samples 2 and 3 (see Fig. 5C and D) and comparing them with the fingerprints (see Fig. 5A and B) of the standard extract EGb761 (number 17 in Fig. 4) and the other sample (number 8 in Fig. 4), we can easily find the difference between them. The peak in the fingerprints of samples 2 and 3 around the retention time of 10 min is much higher than the one in the standard extract EGb761 and sample 8. This peak is rutin. In fact, rutin was added in the three outlier samples, say samples 1–3, in order to meet the old standard of enough absorbance. They are quite different from the real *G. biloba* extractions as shown in Fig. 5A. From this example, we can see that the technique of fingerprint could really identify the false herbal products [Chau, 1996].

7.5 Similarity of fingerprints

The construction of chromatographic fingerprints aims at evaluating the quality of herbal medicines. As discussed above, the fundamental reason of quality control of herbal medicines is based on the concept of phytoequivalence of herbs, and then to use this conception to identify the real herbal medicine and the false one, and further to do quality control. Thus, the intuitive evaluation method is to compare the similarities and/or differences of the chromatographic fingerprints' shape. As a result, both the separation degrees and concentration distribution of components involved in a chromatographic fingerprint is also taken into consideration for this evaluation. The most commonly used standards for evaluation of similarity of the multivariate systems are correlation coefficient and congruence coefficient as expressed by the following two formulae correlation coefficient:

$$r_1 = \frac{\sum (xi - \bar{x})(yi - \bar{y})}{(\sum (xi - \bar{x})^2)^2 (\sum (yi - \bar{y})^2)^2} \quad (i = 1, 2, \ldots\ldots.n) \tag{3}$$

congruence coefficient:

$$r_1 = \frac{\sum xiyi}{(\sum (xi^2))^{1/2} (\sum (yi)^2)^{1/2}} \quad (i = 1, 2, \ldots\ldots.n) \tag{4}$$

where xi, yi are the ith elements in two different fingerprints, say x and y, respectively and n is the number of the elements in the fingerprints. $\bar{x}$ and $\bar{y}$ are the mean values of the n elements in fingerprints x and y, respectively, that is,

$$\bar{x} = \frac{\sum xi}{n} \tag{5}$$

$$\bar{y} = \frac{\sum yi}{n} \tag{6}$$

The relationship within a set of chromatographic fingerprints could be currently analyzed through comparison in terms of similarity or dissimilarity of the objects with a certain reference, presented as correlation coefficient or congruence coefficient.

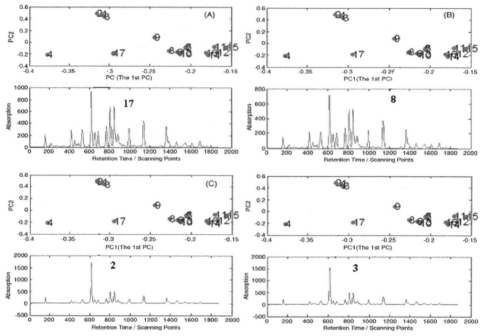

Fig. 5. The relationship between the projection points of score plot of PCA and the corresponding original fingerprints for samples 17, 8, 2 and 3, respectively.

In order to illustrate the situation, the example used in the above subsection is now applied to address such a problem. Table 1 list the correlation coefficients and congruence coefficients of the samples compared with the median spectrum of the whole 17 samples. From the table, we can see that the three false extractions have the smallest similarity values which seem to suggest that the similarity estimation may be used as a standard together with the original fingerprint, even this is very simple.

Sample no.	Correlation coefficients	Congruence coefficients
1	0.8795	0.8939
2	0.8795	0.8899
3	0.8935	0.9051
4	0.9349	0.9474
5	0.9511	0.9604
6	0.9469	0.9574
7	0.9552	0.9637
8	0.9779	0.9821
9	0.9524	0.9568
10	0.9158	0.9269
11	0.9869	0.9895

Sample no.	Correlation coefficients	Congruence coefficients
12	0.9506	0.9593
13	0.9753	0.9801
14	0.9479	0.9581
15	0.9590	0.9640
16	0.8979	0.9187
17	0.9436	0.9547

Table 1. Correlation coefficients and congruence coefficients of the samples compared with the median spectrum of the whole 17 samples.

7.6 Chemical pattern recognition and classification evaluation

As discussed above, the relationship within a set of chromatographic fingerprints could be currently analyzed through comparison in terms of similarity or dissimilarity of the objects with a certain reference, presented as correlation coefficient or congruence coefficient, etc. But, it has been aware that there are two problems for this comparison: how to achieve the reasonable reference (comparing standard) and to what extent the investigated object is similar with the reference. Popularly, the reference may be derived either from standard extract of herbal medicine or proportioned mixture of herbal medicine (e.g. EGb761) or from computation by some mathematical methods (for the example above, the median chromatographic fingerprint of whole samples is taken, since there are three outliers in the samples investigated). However, it is well known that natural products derived from herbal medicines with inherent "uncertainty" feature of its secondary metabolic substances, to define an absolute reference fingerprint by simply calculating their mean or median for one kind of herbal medicine seems somewhat subjective.

From this point of view, the conception of class of one herbal medicine seems to be more reasonable. Thus, the chemical pattern recognition methods, such as K-nearest neighbors (KNN) and soft independent modeling of class analogy (SIMCA), etc. should be taken into consideration for reasonable definition of the class of the herbal medicine. In fact, several researchers in China had worked on the concepts of using chemical analytical and chromatographical fingerprinting to measure the consistency of raw Chinese medicinal herbs and composite formula with the application of fuzzy clustering analysis of HPLC pattern in the early 1990s.

On the other hand, the (dis)similarities of herbal objects with the reference often undertake themselves to a qualified threshold, which is not so easy to define. Although such a comparison attaches importance to the integral relationship of the fingerprints, sometimes masking and swamping effects might occur either explicitly or implicitly. The masking effect is that an unexpected sample is undecided because of high similar value (e.g. the identification of three species of *Coptis chinensis*, *C. teet-Oides* C. Y. Cheng, and *C. deltoidea* C. Y. Cheng et Hsiao from herb *Rhizoma coptidis*). The swamping effect encompasses wrongly discriminating a desirable sample illegal on account of low similarity with the reference influenced by the diversity of chromatographic compositional distribution (e.g. the determination of herb *Houttuynia cordata* Thunb. from different sources). To avoid these effects as much as possible, a method based on PCA after necessary data transformations.

The method has been demonstrated that PCA with standard normal variate transformation of data led to meaningful classification of 33 different *E. breviscapus* herbal samples (see Fig. 2). The result was also colaborated by variance squares discriminant method. The quality of herbal objects was further evaluated, and the causes of this fact have been explained from a chemical point of view. The other method is based on secured principal component regression (sPCR) that was originally developed for detecting and correcting uncalibrated spectral features newly emerging in spectra after the PCR calibration. It can detect and consider unexpected chromatographic features for quality valuation of herbal samples from the point of view of analyzing fingerprint residual [Cheng, 2003; Cheng & Chen, 2003; Collantes, 1997;Vogt, 2003; Welsh, 1996; Wold, 1977; Xie, 2001].

7.7 Qualityfication and validation of two-way data from hyphenated chromatographies by chemometrics

In general, the data generated by the hyphenated instruments are matrices with every row being a spectrum and every column a chromatogram at some wavelength, wave number or m/e unit as illustrated in Fig. 6. The data obtained by such hyphenated instruments in chemistry is generally called two-way or two-dimensional data. In common, the size of the data matrix such-obtained is rather big; sometimes it can be more than 40 megabytes. Thus, this is a really a new challenge for modern analytical chemistry to deal with the chemical information embedded in it.

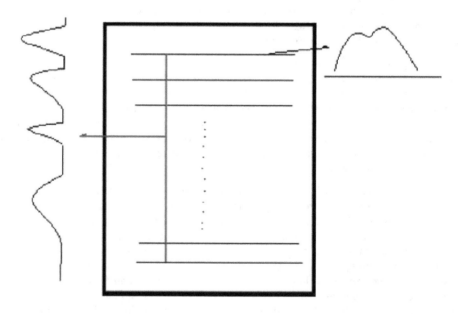

Fig. 6. Illustration of two-dimensional data from hyphenated instruments.

However, data derived from hyphenated analytical techniques have several advantages over the classic one-way chromatograms. Firstly, the two-way data matrix contains both information from spectra and chromatograms, which will make on-line structure identification of some interested compounds possible; secondly, the two-way data has so-called dimension advantages proposed by Booksh and Kowalski, which will make on-line comparison of overlapping chromatographic peaks possible; finally, the hyphenated technique might enhance the chromatographic separation ability by the additional spectral information, since one could easily find some useful component electivity with the help of chemometric local rank analysis methods, which can only be used for two-way chromatographic data but never for one-way chromatographic data. How to use these advantages from the two-way data to address the problems in evaluation of the fingerprints of herbal medicines and the problems in quality control of herbal medicines, which is just the topic we want to discuss in the following subsections. There are still many different kinds of difficult problems unsolved in the research field of herbal medicines. For instance, there may be no big problem for evaluating the fingerprints from the same instruments and/or with the same batch of the herbal products as shown above. However, if we get some fingerprints from different laboratories and/or from the same kind of column, say C-18 for example, but from different companies. Could we still evaluate them reasonably? Moreover, could we do the on-line comparison among the fingerprints of some overlapping chromatographic peaks and/or of big diversity? For instance, if we get some fingerprints from different extraction methods and/or from different herbal medicines, is it possible for us to see whether we have got the same phytochemical constituents or not in order to understand their bioactivities and possible side effects of these herbal products and consequently to enhance product quality control? With the help of the two-way data from the hyphenated chromatographies and chemometric methods recently developed, the answer is positive [Liang, 2001].

7.8 Spectral correlative chromatogram and its applications

As stated above, it is very important for assessment of the quality of various samples to determine the presence or absence of interested components among the different chromatographic fingerprints. They may be obtained either from same herbs or from different ones under the same or similar chromatographic separated conditions. Moreover, another problem is the shift of retention time of some interested peaks of various fingerprints due to inevitable possibility in quality control, such as the fingerprints from different laboratories and the experimental columns from different vendors despite the same type stationary-phase characteristics. This maybe lead to erroneous assess of quality of medical samples. Let us see an example shown in Fig. 6. $x1$ and $x2$ shown in Fig. 7A are the chromatograms of two dimensional data sets of $X1$ (of the G. biloba samples obtained from HPLC–DAD through the column made in Angilent Inc.) and $X2$ (through the column made in Waters Inc.) at wavelength 260 nm, respectively. It can be intuitively seen that the retention time of eluting components of them shift rather seriously, which trouble right identification of them by directly comparing their chromatographic fingerprints.

In order to deal with such a kind of problem a technique named spectral correlative chromatogram (SCC) was developed. The idea of SCC is quite simple, that is, the same chemical component should be of the same spectrum no matter what they are eluted

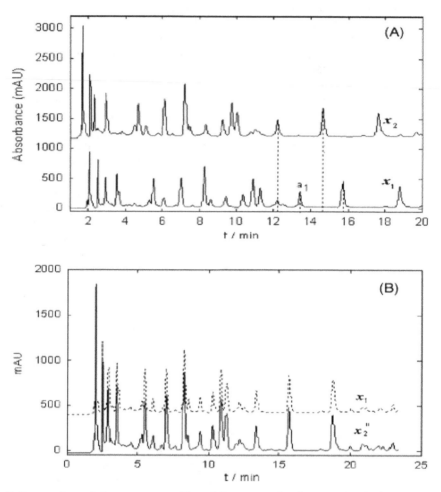

Fig. 7. Comparison of chromatograms X_1 and X_2 measure by the same kind of column but from different companies: X_1 (Angilent Inc.) and X_2 (Waters Inc.). (A) Original chromatograms of samples X_1 and X_2 at wavelength 260nm, respectively. (B) Original chromatograms of samples X_1 and chromatogram X''_2 of sample X_2 after correction of retention time shifting by local least-square technique.

through diverse chromatographic columns. Thus, one could use the spectral information to pick up the interested compound from the other two-way chromatograms. The whole procedure goes in the following steps: (1) assess peak purity of an interested compound and then acquire its spectrum; (2) identify correlative components in the other fingerprint by series correlation coefficients between the spectrum obtained above and the spectra at every scan point for the other two-way chromatogram; (3) get a curve (named SCC) of correlation coefficients at every scan point in the direction of retention time and further validate the result from the second step combining the information of local chromatographic cluster

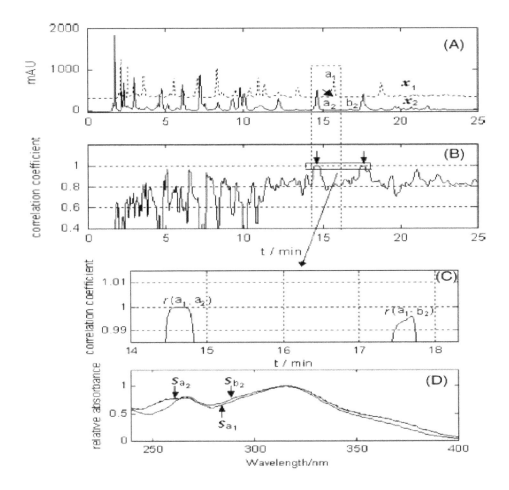

Fig. 8. Illustration of the procedure of spectral correlative chromatogram. (A) Two original samples, say X_1 and X_2, involved in comparison, in which a peak indicated by a1 is the component spectrum to be searched by SCC. (B) The spectral correlative chromatogram obtained for component a1. (C) Enlarged part of spectral correlative chromatogram around retention time range of 14-18.5min. (D) Spectral comparision of spectra s_{a1}, s_{a2} and s_{b2} respectively.

where targets exist; (4) eventually assess the similarity and/or difference of the chromatographic fingerprints after correcting the time shift of correlative components in a piece wise way by using local least squares. Fig. 8 shows an example of this procedure. Pure component $a1$ in $X1$ indicated in Fig. 8 was taken as an example to illustrate this procedure. The obtained SCC is shown in Fig. 8B. As could be seen from Fig. 8, both the correlation coefficients $r(a1, a2)$ and $r(a1, b2)$ corresponding to components $a2$ and $b2$ of $X2$ were larger than others and quite close to 1, say $r(a1, a2)= 0.9998$ and $r(a1, b2)= 0.9940$. Thus, components $a1$ and $a2$ were correlative, even though they were unknown and there were some shift of their retention time. Furthermore, spectrum-dependent principle of identification of substance decided the result. Fig. 7C and D (lower part) exhibits the spectra $sa1$, $sa2$ and $sb2$. It is obvious that $sa1$ and $sa2$ are entirely consistent and factually identical, whereas $sa1$ and $sb2$ are something different. Similarly, other correlative components could also be obtained, as listed in Table 2. With the correlative information available, the retention time shift can be easily corrected by local least squares taking $x1$ as a target reference. The results after shift correction are shown in Fig. 7B. From this plot, we can see that the shift of retention time can be corrected reasonably. Along with this direction, the spectral correlative chromatogram for multi-components' comparing could be also possible and conducted.

7.9 On-line comparison by chemometric methods

In order to understand the bioactivities and possible side effects of some herbal products and consequently to enhance product quality control one might be asked to compare directly some samples to see whether there are same phytochemical constituents in the different samples. For instance, if the extraction method is changed the chemical compositions of the products will also change? **Fig. 9** shows such an example, in which the total ion current chromatograms of the volatile fractions of *Schisandra chinensis* derived from six different extraction methods are presented. It may be observed that the major section (retention time region from 15 to 35 min) is quite similar in each of the six chromatograms. In order to carry out a more detailed analysis, however, it is necessary to compare qualitatively the results from the six methods.

There are three difficulties in comparing such results: (1) it is difficult to conclude if the same compounds are present in overlapping chromatographic peaks; (2) it is difficult to confirm whether a peak with a given retention time represents the same compound in different extractions or whether there is significant chromatographic drift between runs (see top part in Fig. 10 for details); and (3) the chromatographic background makes MS matching difficult. In order to overcome these problems, the mass spectral information together with chemometric methods seems to be necessary to introduced. Sub window factor analysis (SFA) is just such chemometric resolution methods, which focus its attention of comparing the spectra of two overlapping peak clusters to obtain the pure spectrum of the common component in the two overlapping peaks and further to resolve the whole overlapping peak cluster. With the help of SFA, six common components were extracted from the two peak clusters, assigned B1–B6 in the sample from extraction method 1 and b1–b6 in the sample from extraction method II (Fig. 10 (medium part) and (bottom part), respectively [Li, 2003; Liang, 1992, 1994; Karjalainen, 1992; Kvalheim ,1992; Maeder, 1987; Malinowski ,1992; Malinowski, 1991; Windig, 1997; Gemperline, 1984].

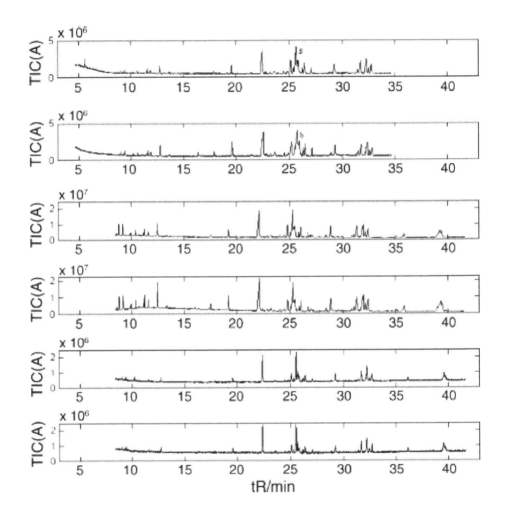

Fig. 9. Total ion current chromatograms of the volatile fractions of *Schisandra chinensis* obtained by the six different extraction methods (1-6, from top to bottom): (1) Use of the Chinese pharmacopoeia committee(1995) method for extracting essential oils from traditional Chinese medicines employing a standard essential oil extractor; (2) Steam distillation; (3) Solvent extraction with petroleum ether using an ultrasonic extractor; (4) Soxhlet extraction with petroleum ether; (5) Solvent extraction with diethyl ether using an ultrasonic extractor; and (6) Soxhlet extraction with diethyl ether.

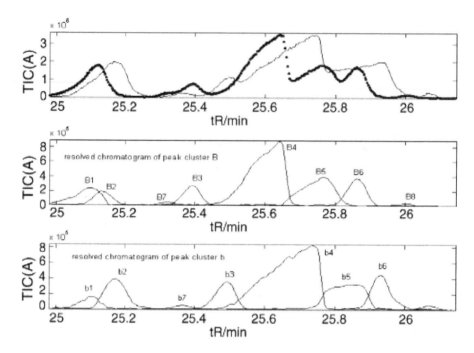

Fig. 10. Total ion current chromatograms of (top part) peak clusters B (bold dotted line) and b (thin continous line) as marked in Fig. 9 and (medium part) and (bottom part) their corresponding resolved chromatograms, respectively.

Correlation component no.	Retention time $(t1,k)$ of $X1$	Retention time $(t2,k)$ of $X2$	$\Delta t = t1,k - t2,k$ (min)
1	2.0820	1.7020	0.3800
2	2.5287	2.1153	0.4134
3	2.9953	2.4753	0.5200
4	5.5287	4.7153	0.8134
5	6.9953	6.1020	0.8933
6	8.2620	7.2087	1.0533
7	9.4220	8.3353	1.0867
8	10.3487	9.2553	1.0934
9	10.8887	9.7287	1.1600
10	11.2820	10.0287	1.2533
11	15.7020	14.6420	1.0600
12	18.7620	17.6020	1.1600

Table 2. Comparison of correlative components and their chromatographic eluting time (min) of *Ginkgo biloba* sample $X1$ with those of $X2$.

7.10 Further comments on quality control of herbal medicines

Western and traditional Chinese medical practices represent totally different philosophies. Thus, this is not a simple exercise of applying modern technologies to quality control of the products that have been in constant use for centuries. The progress on quality control of herbal medicines discussed in this review is just at its beginning stage of a long journey. Of course, the proposal of the use of chromatographic fingerprints of herbal medicines for quality control of herbal medicines is definitely a progress. However, using the chemical fingerprints for the purpose of quality control of herbal medicines can only address to the problem of comparing the integrated sameness and/or difference and controlling their stability of the available herbal products.

The complex relationship between the chromatographic fingerprints and efficacy of the herbal medicines (QRFE) is not taken into account yet, which seems to be the most important aspect for the quality control of herbal medicines. As it is well known that the efficacy of traditional herbal medicines has a characteristic of a complex mixture of chemical compounds present in the herbs, thus how to evaluate reasonably their relationship is obviously not a trivial task. THMs represent a much more daunting challenge due to the natural variability of the individual herbs and the chemical complexity of the formulations. Moreover, the chemical profile by itself is insufficient in determining the efficacy of TCM. This is where biochemistry, molecular biology, and cell biology are invaluable in establishing quantifiable and reproducible assays. Chemical fingerprints might be linked to these biological assays to provide assurance of efficacy and consistency. But the research work on this aspect, to our best knowledge, is far from sufficient to meet the criteria needed. Thus, the researches concerning the relationship between the chromatographic fingerprints and efficacy of the herbal medicines are urgent requirements for the quality control of herbal medicines. On the other hand, the works on possible contaminations in herbal products, such as excessive or banned pesticides, microbial contaminants, heavy metals, chemical toxins, should be also conducted concurrently. In fact, the research field of quality control of herbal medicines is really an interdisciplinary research. It needs crossover of chemistry, pharmacology, medicine and even statistics to provide a platform for the quality control of traditional herbal medicines and further to discover the novel therapeutics composed of multiple chemical compounds.

8. References

Ahirwal B, Ahirwal D and Ram A. 2006. Evaluation of standards and quality control parameters of herbal drugs, *Souvenir, recent trends in herbal therapy,* 25-29.

Ansari SH. 2011. *Essentials of Pharmacognosy,* Birla publications pvt ltd, 10-16.

Beek TAV. 2002. Chemical analysis of Ginkgo biloba leaves and extracts, *J. Chromatogr. A,* 967, 25-55.

Bilia AR, Bergonzi MC, Lazari D, Vincieri FF. 2002. Characterization of commercial Kava-kava herbal drug & herbal drug preparation by means of Nuclear Magnetic Resonance Spectroscopy, *J. Agric. Food Chem.,* 50, 5016.

Blumenthal M, Brusse WR, Goldberg A, Gruenwald J, Hall T, Riggins CW, Rister RS. 1998. *The Complete German Commission E Monographs. Therapeutic Guide to Herbal Medicines,* The American Botanical Council, Austin, TX.

Booksh KS, Kowalski BR. 1994. Theory of analytical chemistry, *Anal. Chem,* 66, 782A-791A.

Brain KR and Turner TD. 1975. *Practical Evaluation of phytopharmaceuticals*. Wright Scientechnica Bristol.

Bylund D, Danielsson R, Malmquist G, Markides KE. 2002. Chromatographic alignment by warping & dynamic programming as a pre-processing tool for PARAFAc modeling of liquid chromatography- mass spectrometry data, *J. Chromatogr.A* , 961, 237-244.

Caoa Y, Wang L, Yu X, Ye J. 2006. Development of the chromatographic fingerprint of herbal preparations Shuang–Huang–Lian oral liquid, *Journal of Pharmaceutical and Biomedical Analysis*, 41, 845–856.

Chau FT, Shih TM, Gao JB, Chan CK. 1996. Application of the Fast Wavelet Transform method to compress Ultraviolet-visible spectra, *Appl. Spectrosc.* 50, 339-348.

Chaudhury RR. 1999. *Herbal medicine for human health*. World Health Organization Geneva, CBS publishers and distributors LTD, New Delhi,

Cheng Y. 2003. An approach to comparative analysis of chromatographic fingerprints for assuring the quality of botanical drugs. *J. Chem. Inf. Comput. Sci*, 43, 1068-1076.

Cheng YY, Chen MJ, Tong WD. 2003. An approach to comparative analysis of chromatographic fingerprints for assuring the quality of botanical drugs, *Chin. J. Chem. Inf. Comput. Sci.*, 43(3): 1068-1070.

Choi DW, Kim JH, Cho SY, Kim DH, Chang SY. 2002. Regulation and quality control of herbal drugs in Korea, *Toxicology*, 181/182, 581-586.

Chuang, W.C., Wu, S.K., Sheu, S.J., Chiou, S.H., Chang, H.C. and Chen, Y.P. (1995). A comparative study on commercial samples of ginseng radix, *Planta Medica*, 61, 459–465.

Clarke ECG. 1967. *Isolation and identification of drugs*, The Pharmaceutical press, London.

Collantes ER, Duta R, Welsh WJ, Zielinski WL, Brower J. 1997. Preprocessing of HPLC trace impurity patterns by wavelet packets for pharmaceutical fingerprinting using artificial neural networks, *Anal Chem*, 69,1392–1397.

Ebel S, Gigalke HJ, Voelkl S. 1987. *AMDHPTLC Analysis of Medicinal Plants*. Proceedings of 4th International Symposium of Instrumental HPTLC, Selvino/Bargamo at Italy, p. 113

EMEA. 1998. Quality of Herbal Medicinal Products. Guidelines. European Agency for the Evaluation of Medicinal Products (EMEA), London.

EMEA. 2002. *Points to Consider on Good Agricultural and Collection Practice for Starting Materials of Herbal Origin*. EMEA/HMPWP/31/99 Review. European Agency for the Evaluation of Medicinal Products (EMEA), London.

Funk W, Droeschel B. 1991. *J. Planar Chromatogr*. Modern TLC 4, 123.

Gemperline PJ. 1984. *J. Chem. Inform. Comput. Sci.*, 24, 206-212.

Gong F, Liang Yi-Z, Xie Pei-S and Chau FT. 2003. Information theory applied to chromatographic fingerprint of herbal medicine for quality control, *Journal of Chromatography A*, 1002, 25 – 30.

Gong F, Liang YZ, Cui H, Chau FT, Chau BTP. 2001. Determination of volatile components in peptic powder by Gas Chromatography- Mass Spectrometry and Chemometric resolution, *J. Chromatogr. A*, 909, 237-247.

Gong F, Liang YZ, Xie PS, Sung AJ. 2003. Information theory applied to chromatographic fingerprint of herbal medicine for quality control, *J. Chromatogr. A*, 1002, 1-2, 25-40.

Gong F, Liang YZ, Xu QS, Chau FT, Leung AKM. 2001. Gas chromatography-Mass spectrometry & Chemometric resolution applied to the determination of essential oils in cortex cinnamomi, *J. Chromatogr. A*, 905, 1-2, 193-205.

Gupta MK and Sharma PK. 2007. *Test Book of Pharmacognosy*, Ayurvedic formulations, Pragati Prakashan Meerut Vol II, Ist edition.

H'am'al'ainen MD, Liang YZ, Kvalheim OM, Andersson R. 1993. *Anal. Chim. Acta*, 271, 101.

Hasler O, Meier SB. 1992. Identification and determination of the flavonoids from Ginkgo biloba by high-performance liquid chromatography. *J. Chromatogr. A*, 605, 41-48.

Hayashi Y, Matsuda R, Nakamura A. 1990. Quantity & Wavelength optimization based on Information Theory of chromatography, *J. Chromatogr. Sci.*, 28, 12, 628-632.

Herbone JB. 1928. *Phytochemical methods*, Chapman and Hall, London, New York, 2nd edition.

Huber JFK, Kenndler E, Reich G, Hack W, Wolf J. 1993. Optimal selection of Gas chromatographic columns for the Analytical control of chemical welfare agents by application of information theory of retention data, *Anal. Chem.* 65, 20, 2903-2906.

Karjalainen EJ, Karjalaien UP. 1991. Component reconstruction in the primary space of spectra and concentrations-alternating regression and related direct methods. Anal. Chim. Acta ,250,169–179.

Kelly L. 2001. International Symposium on Quality of Traditional Chinese medicine with Chromatographic Fingerprint, Guangzhou, i 4-1.

Kinghorn AD, Seo EK. 1998. Chromatographic/chromatographic spectroscopic combination methods for the analysis of botanical drugs. *Drug Info. J.*, 32, 487-495.

Kokate CK, Gokhale SB. 2004. *Pharmacognosy*. Nirali prakashan, Delhi.

Kokate CK, Purohit AP, Gokhale SB. 2005. *Pharmacognosy*, 31st edition Nirali Prakshan, 97-131.

Kvalheim OM, Liang YZ. 1992.Heuristic evolving latent projections: resolving two–way multicomponent data. Part 1. Selectivity, latent projective graph, datascope, local rank and unique resolution. Anal Chem, 64, 936–46.

Lazarowych N.J., Pekos P.1998. Use of fingerprinting and marker compounds for identification and standardization of botanical drugs: Strategies for applying pharmaceutical HPLC analysis to herbal products, *Drug Information Journal*, Vol.32, 497-512.

Li N, Lin G, Kwan YW, Min ZD. 1999. Simultaneous quantification of five major biologically active ingredients of saffron by high-performance liquid chromatography, *J. Chromatogr. A*, 849, 2, 349-355.

Li X N, Cui H, Song Y Q, Liang Y Z, Chau F T. 2003. Analysis of volatile fractions of Schisandra chinensis (Turcz.) Baill. Using GC-MS and chemometric resolution, *Phytochem Anal*, 14(1), 23 - 33.

Liang YZ, Kvalheim OM. 2001. Resolution of two-way data: theoretical background and practical problem-solving. Fresenius *J. Anal. Chem*, 370, 694–704.

Liang YZ, Kvalheim OM, Keller HR, Massart DL, Kiechle P, Erni F.1992. Heuristic evolving latent projections: resolving two–way multicomponent data. Part 2: Detection and resolution of minor constituents. Anal Chem,64, 946–53..

Liang,Yi-Zeng; Kvalheim,Olav M. 1994. Diagnosis and resolution of multiwavelength chromatograms by rank map, orthogonal projections and sequential rank analysis. Anal. Chim. Acta, 292, 5-15.

Liu CL, Zhu PL, Liu MC. 1999. Computer-aided development of a high-performance liquid chromatographic method for the determination of hydroxyanthraquinone derivatives in Chinese herb medicine rhubarb, *J. Chromatogr. A*, 857, 167-174.

Liu YM, Sheu SJ, Chiou H, Chang SH and Chen YP. 1993. A comparative study on commercial samples of ephedrae herba. *Planta Medica*, 59, 376–378.

Liu YM, Sheu SJ, Chiou H, Chang SH and Chen YP. 1994. Capillary electrophoretic analysis of alkaloids in commercial samples of coptidis rhizoma. *Phytochemical Analysis*, 5, 256 –260.

Liu YM, SheuSJ. 1992. Determination of quaternary alkaloids from Coptidis Rhizoma by capillary electrophoresis, *J. Chromatogr.*, 623, 1, 196-199.

Liu YM, SheuSJ. 1993. Determination of coptisine, berberine and palmatine in traditional Chinese medicinal preparations by capillary electrophoresis, *J. Chromatogr.*, 639, 2, 323-328.

Maeder M. 1987. Evolving factor analysis for the resolution of overlapping chromatographic peaks, *Anal. Chem.*, 59, 527-530.

Maillard MP, Wolfender JL, Hostettmann K. 1993. Use of liquid chromatography thermospray mass spectrometry in phytochemical analysis of crude plant extract, *J. Chromatogr.*, 647, 147-154.

Malinowski ER. 1991. Factor Analysis in Chemistry, second ed., Wiley, New York.

Malinowski ER. 1992. 'Window factor-analysis-theoretical derivation and application to flow-injection analysis data, *J. Chemometr.* 6: 29-40 (1992). *J. Chemom.*, 6, 29.

Martens H, Naes T. 1991. *Multivariate Calibration*, second ed., Wiley, New York.

Matsuda R, Hayashi Y, Ishibashi M, Takeda Y. 1989. An information theory of chromatography-II, application of FUMI to the optimization of overlapped chromatograms, *J. Chromatogr.* 462, 13, 23-30.

Mellon FA, Chapman JR, Pratt JAE. 1987. Thermospray liquid chromatography- mass spectrometry in food and agricultural research, *J. Chromatogr.* 394, 209-222.

Nyiredy S. 2003. Progress inforced flow planar chromatography, *J. Chromatogr. A*, 1000, 985-999.

Pusecker K, Schewitz J, Gfrorer P, Tseng LH, Albert K, Bayer E, Wilson ID, Bailey ND, Scarfe GB, Nicholson JK, Lindon JC. 1998. *Anal. Commun.* 35, 3159.

Raina MK. 2003. Quality control of herbal and herbo-mineral formulations, *Indian journal of natural products*, 19, 11-15.

Rajani M, Ravishankara MN, Shrivastava N, Padh H. 2001. A sensitive high performance thin layer chromatography method of estimationof diospyrin, a tumor inhibiting agent from stem bark of Diospyros Montana, *J. Planar Chromatogr.* 14, 34.

Raven PH, Evert RF, Eichhorn SE. 1999. *Biology of Plants*, sixth ed.,Freeman, New York.

Revilla E, Beneytez EG, Cabello F, Ortega GM, Ryan JM. 2001. Value of high performance liquid chromatographic analysis of anthocyanins in the differentiation of red grape cultivars and red wines made from them, *J. Chromatogr. A*, 915, 53-60.

Roberts JE, Tyler VE. 1997. *Tyler's Herbs of Choice. The Therapeutic Use of Phytomedicinals.* The Haworth Press, New York.

Rózylo JK, Zabinska A, Matysiak J, Niewiadomy A. 2002. OPLC and HPTLC methods in physicochemical studies of a new group of antimycotic compounds , *J. Chromatogr. Sci*, 40, 10, 581-4.

Schewitz J, Gfrorer P, Pusecker K, Tseng LH, Albert K, Bayer E, Wilson ID, Bailey NJ, Scarfe GB, Nicholson JK, Lindon JC. 1998. Directly coupled CZE-NMR and CEC-NMR spectroscopy for metabolite analysis: paracetamol metabolites in human urine, *Analyst* ,123, 12, 2835-7

Sharma PP. 1995. How to practice GMPs Vandana publications.

Stahl E. 1969. *Thin layer chromatography*, Springer verlag Berlin Heidel berg, New York, Springer international student edition.

Sticher HO. 1992. *J. Chromatogr.*, 605, 41. Hasler, A., Sticher, O. and Meier, B., Identification and determination of the flavonoids from Ginkgo biloba by high-performance liquid chromatography. J Chromatogr A, 605:41-48, 1992.

Sticher O. 1993. Quality of Ginkgo preparations. Planta Med, 59,2-11.

Stockigt J, Sheludko Y, UngerM, Gerasimenko I, Warzecha H, Stockigt D. 2002. High-performance liquid chromatographic, capillary electrophoretic and capillary electrophoretic-electrospray ionisation mass spectrometric analysis of selected alkaloid groups, *J. Chromatogr. A*, 967, 1, 85-113.

Stuppner H, Sturm S, Konwalinka G. 1992. Capillary electrophoresis analysis of oxindole alkaloids from uncaria tomentosa, *J. Chromatogr.* 609, ½, 375-380.

Svendsen B. 1989. Thin layer chromatography of alkaloids, *J. Planar Chromatogr.* Modern TLC 2, 8.

Tauler R, Izquierdo-Ridorsa A, Casassas E. 1992. Applicayion of factor analysis to speciation in multiequilibria systems, Analysis, 20, 255-268.

Tsai TR, Tseng TY, Chen CF, Tsai TH. 2002. Identification and determination of geniposide contained in *Gardenia jasminoides* and in two preparations of mixed traditional Chinese medicines, *J. Chromatogr. A* . 961, 83-88.

Upton R. 2001. International Symposium on Quality of Traditional Chinese Medicine with Chromatographic Fingerprint, Guangzhou, i 2-1.

Vogt F, Mizaikoff B. 2003. Fault-tolerant spectroscopic data evaluation based on extended principal component regression correcting for spectral drifts and uncalibrated spectral features, *J. Chemom.*, 17, 225-236.

Wagner H, Bladt S, Rickl V. 1996. *Plant Drug Analysis: A Thin LayerChromatography Atlas*, second ed., Springer-Verlag.

Wagner SB and Gainski EMZ. 1984. *Plant drug analysis*, A Thin layer chromatograpy atlas, New Delhi.

Wang Y, Sheng LS, Lou FC. 2001. Analysis and structure identification of trace constituent in the total ginkgolide by using LC/DAD/ESI/MS, *Yao Xue Xue Bao*, 36, 606-608.

Welsh WJ, Lin W, Tersigni SH, Collantes E, Duta R, Carey MS. 1996. Pharmaceutical fingerprinting: evaluation of neural networks and chemometric techniques for distinguishing among same-product manufacturers, *Anal. Chem.* 68 (19), 3473-82.

WHO. 1988. *Quality Control Methods for Medicinal Plant Materials*. World Health Organization, Geneva.

WHO. 1992. *Quality Control Methods for Medicinal Plant Materials*. World Health Organization, Geneva.

WHO. 1998. *Quality Control Methods for Medicinal Plant Materials*, World Health Organization, Geneva.

WHO. 1999. *Quality Control Methods for Medicinal Plant Materials*. World Health Organization, Geneva.

WHO. 2005. General Guidelines for Methodologies on Research and Evaluation of Traditional Medicines, p. 1.

WHO. 2001. General Guidelines for Methodologies on Research and Evaluation of Traditional Medicines, p. 1.

WHO. 2000. *General Guidelines for Methodologies on Research and Evaluation of Traditional Medicine*. World Health Organization, Geneva.

WHO. 2003. *Guidelines on Good Agricultural and Collection Practices* (GACP). World Health Organization Geneva.

WHO. 2004. *Guidelines on Good Agricultural and Collection Practices (GACP) for Medicinal Plants*. World Health Organization, Geneva.

Williamson E, Okpako DT, Evans F J. 1996. *Pharmacological Methods in Phytotherapy Research*, Vol. 1. Selection, Preparation and Pharmacological Evaluation of Plant Material. John Wiley and Sons, Chichester.

Windig W. 1997. *Chem. Intell. Lab. Syst.* 36, 3. W. Windig, Spectral Data Files for Self-Modeling Curve Resolution with Examples Using the SIMPLISMA Approach, Chemometrics and Intelligent Laboratory Systems, 36, 1997, 3-16.

Wold S, Esbensen K, Geladi P. 1987. Principal component analysis. *Chemom. Intell. Lab. Syst.* 2(1-3), 37-52.

Wold S, Sjostrom M. 1977. *Chemometrics:Theory and Applications*, ACS Ser., vol. 52, p. 243.

Wolfender JL, Hostettmann K. 1995. *Phytochemistry of Medicinal Plants, Recent Advances in Phytochemistry*, vol. 29, Plenum Press, New York, p. 189.

Wolfender JL, Maillard MP, Hostettmann K. 1993. Liquid chromatographic thermospray mass spectrometric analysis of crude plant extracts containing phenolic and terpene glycosides, *J. Chromatogr.*, 647, 183-190.

Wolfender JL, Maillard MP, Hostettmann K. 1994. Thermospray liquid chromatography mass spectrometry in phytochemical analysis, *Phytochem. Anal.* 5, 153.

Xie PS. 2001. A feasible strategy for applying chromatography fingerprint to assess quality of Chinese herbal medicine. *Tradit. Chin. Drug Res. Clin. Pharm.* 2001, 12 (3), 141-169.

Yan XJ, Zhou JJ, Xie GR, Milne GWA. 1999. Traditional Chinese Medicines: Molecular Structures, Natural Sources and Applications, Aldershot, Ashgate.

Yan S, Yang Y, Wu Y, Liu R, Zhang W. 2009. Chemical fingerprinting and quantitative analysis of volatiles in *Shexiang Baoxin* Pill by Gas chromatography with flame ionization and Mass spectrometric determination, *J of Analytical Chemistry*, 64, 2, 165-171.

Yang SS, Smetena I. 1995. Evaluation of capillary electrophoresis for the analysis of nicotine and selected minor alkaloids from tobacco *Chromatographia*, 40,7-8, 375-378.

Ylinen M , Naaranlahti T, Lapinjoki S, Huhtikangas A, Salonen ML, Simola LK, Lounasmaa M. 1986. Tropane alkaloids from Atropa belladonna part-I. capillary gas chromatographic analysis, Planta Med. 52, 2, 85-87.

Zhang H. 2004. Identification and determination of the major constituents in traditional Chinese medicine, Si-Wu-Tang by HPLC coupled with DAD and ESI-MS. *J. Pharm. Biomed. Anal*, 34,705,713.

Zhang MH, Xu QS, Massart DL. 2003. Robust principal components regression based on principal sensitivity vectors. *Chemom. Intell. Lab. Syst.* 67(2), 175-185.

6

Natural Alkamides: Pharmacology, Chemistry and Distribution

María Yolanda Rios

Centro de Investigaciones Químicas, Universidad Autónoma del Estado de Morelos,
Col. Chamilpa, Cuernavaca, Morelos,
México

1. Introduction

Alkamides are a broad and expanding group of bioactive natural compounds found in at least 33 plant families. Despite the relatively simple molecular architecture of alkamides (fig. 1), these natural products show broad structural variability and an important range of biological activities, such as immunomodulatory, antimicrobial, antiviral, larvicidal, insecticidal, diuretic, pungent, analgesic, cannabimimetic and antioxidant activities. Additionally, alkamides are involved in the potentiation of antibiotics and the inhibition of prostaglandin biosynthesis, RNA synthesis and the arachidonic acid metabolism, among others.

Many plant species containing alkamides have been used in traditional medicine by different civilizations around the world. Many of the plants containing these natural products have been used in the treatment of toothaches and sore throats (Rios-Chavez et al., 2003). These compounds are present in different organs of the plant, such as roots (*Heliopsis longipes, Echinaceae purpurea, Achillea wilhelmsii, Acmella oppositifolia, Asiasarum heterotropoide, Cissampelos glaberrima,* etc.), leaves and stems (*Aristolochia gehrtii, Phyllanthus fraternus, Amaranthus hypochondriacus, Achyranthes ferruginea,* etc.), the pericarpium (*Zanthoxylum piperitum* and *Piper spp.*), the placenta of *Capsicum spp.*, the fruits of *Piper longum*, the flowers of *Spilanthes acmella*, the seeds of the *Piper* species and tubers of *Lepidium meyenii*. It is believed that alkamides act as plant growth regulators, promoting or inhibiting the growth and formation of roots in a dose-dependent manner and showing a positive effect in plant biomass production (Campos-Cuevas, et al., 2008).

Structurally, natural alkamides commonly have an aliphatic, cyclic or aromatic amine residue, and a C8 to C18 saturated or unsaturated chain (including double or triple bonds, or both) acid, which can also be aromatic. The nature of the acid (carbon chain lengths, unsaturation level, stereochemistry, etc.) and the amine residues are characteristic of each family and genus of plants such that these characteristics serve as chemotaxonomic criteria (fig. 1). Because the nitrogen atom of alkamides is not part of a heterocyclic ring, these compounds are classified as protoalkaloids or pseudoalkaloids.

Alkamides represent a class of lipidic compounds structurally related to animal endocannabinoids. Notably, based on the structural similarity of these compounds to anandamide (N-arachidonoylethanolamine), an endogenous cannabinoid cerebral neurotransmitter, alkamides are highly active in the central nervous system (CNS, fig. 2).

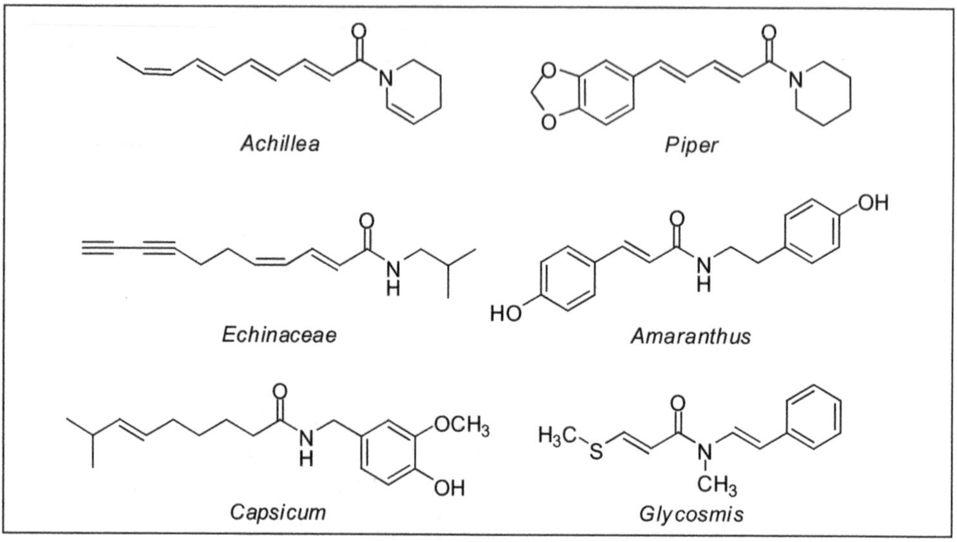

Fig. 1. Characteristic alkamides from different plant genera.

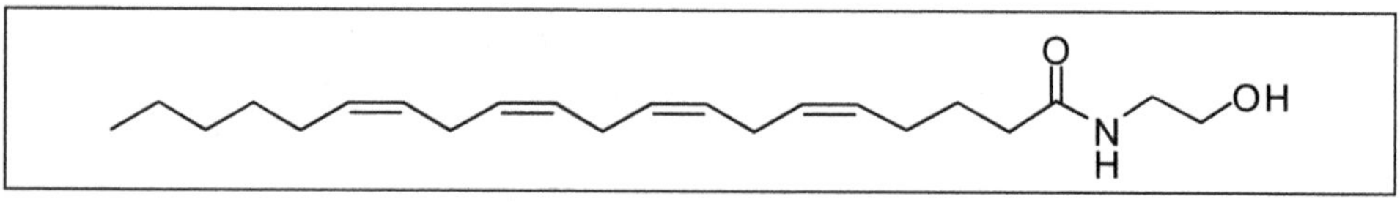

Fig. 2. Anandamide (N-arachidonoylethanolamine) structure.

In general, when alkamide-producing plants are chewed, a pungent taste is released causing itching and salivation. Chloroform is the best solvent for the extraction of alkamides, though both methanol and ethanol have also been used. Pure alkamides are sensitive to oxidation and polymerization of double and triple bonds occur during the drying, handling and storage of these compounds. Notably, alkamides are promising chemical and pharmacological entities that are useful therapeutics for the treatment of several important illnesses. This chapter describes the distribution of alkamides, the chemical aspects used to distinguish these important natural products and the pharmacological properties of the plants from which these compounds are isolated.

2. Aliphatic alkamides

Plants belonging to the Asteraceae, Convolvulaceae, Euphorbiaceae, Menispermaceae and Rutaceae families specialize in the biosynthesis of alkamides with both amine and acid aliphatic residues. Chemical analysis of these species revealed that aliphatic alkamides are the major and most characteristic components of several Asteraceae plants based on the number of isolated compounds from each plant and the yield obtained for each alkamide. In contrast, Convolvulaceae, Euphorbiaceae, Menispermaceae and Rutaceae families produce alkamides along with other types of natural products, resulting in alkamides being the minor components.

2.1 Alkamides from the Asteraceae family

The Asteraceae family is characterized by the accumulation of aliphatic alkamides. *Aaronsohnia, Achilea, Acmella, Anacyclus, Artemisia, Echinaceae, Heliopsis, Spilanthes, Salmea, Sanvitalia* and *Wedelia* are genera that belong to this alkamide-producing family. These genera share the biogenetic capacity to combine C8 to C18 (with exception of C17) olefinic and acetylenic acid residues with the more widespread N-isobutyl, N-2-methylbutyl, N-phenethyl and cyclic amines [piperidinyl (piperidide), 2,3-dehydro-piperidinyl (piperideide), pyrrolidinyl and pyrrolidyl]. However, other minor amides including N-4-methylbutyl, N-tyramidyl and O-methyl-tyramidyl residues have also been found (fig. 3).

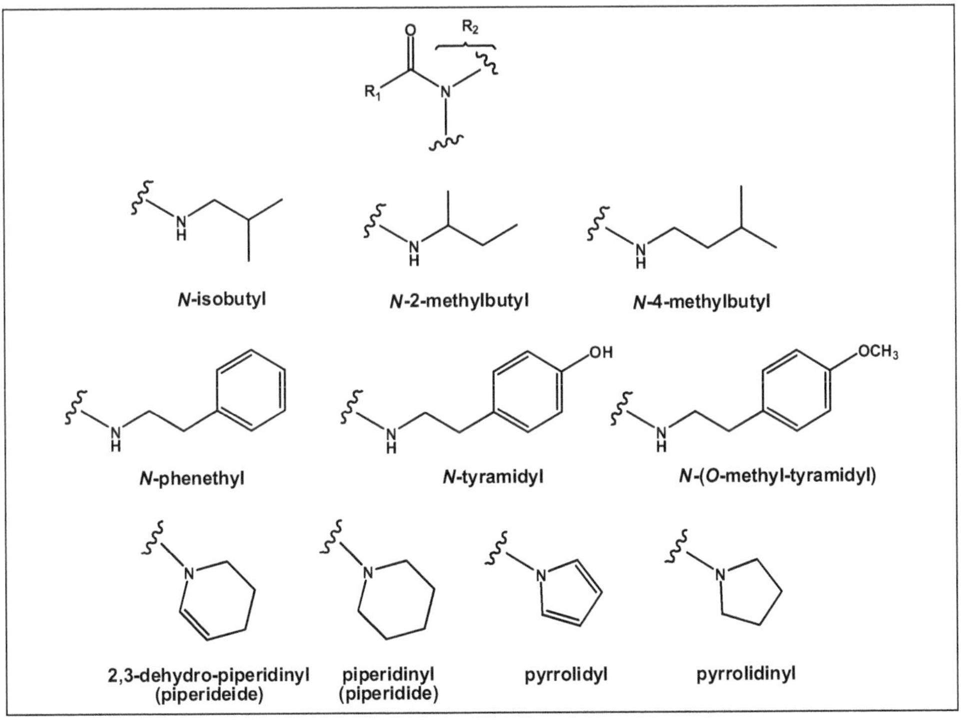

Fig. 3. Amine residues (R₂) of aliphatic alkamides from the Asteraceae family.

Currently, the most commonly found alkamides in the Asteraceae family include a C10, C11 and C12 long chain residue acids, which represent approximately 72% of aliphatic alkamides isolated from this family. The second most important group of these natural products includes C14 and C18 long chain residue acids, constituting approximately 13% of Asteraceae alkamides. Most phytochemical and pharmacological studies have been conducted with *Achillea*, *Acmella*, *Sphilantes*, *Echinaceae* and *Heliopsis* genera, which will be discussed in subsequent sections.

2.1.1 *Achillea* genus

The occurrence of alkamides with cyclic amide moieties is confined to the Anthemideae tribe, being *Achillea* species especially rich in both pyrrolidides and piperidides and their corresponding dehydroderivatives. Apart from the more widespread isobutylamides, this genus is characterized by the frequent occurrence of saturated and unsaturated 5- and 6-ring amides (Greger et al., 1987a, 1987b). The accumulation of amides with characteristic olefinic and acetylenic patterns is characteristic of this genus. These amides are mainly accumulated in the subterranean parts of these plants (table 1).

2.1.2 *Acmella* genus

A name frequently used in folk medicine for species containing alkamides is "the tooth herb". These plants exhibit analgesic properties and are frequently used as odontologic agents. For example, *Acmella decumbens* roots have a pungent taste and when chewed a numbing sensation is felt on the tongue. *Acmella radicans* is another species also used for the treatment of toothache (Rios-Chavez et al., 2003).

Alkamides from the *Acmella* genus consist of an *N*-isobutyl, *N*-2-methylbutyl or *N*-phenethyl amine and C8 to C12 acid residues. Of the seven *Acmella* species that have been chemically analyzed, four species have been observed to produce affinin (spilanthol, *N*-isobutyl-2*E*,6*Z*,8*E*-decatrienamide, **70**), an alkamide with established analgesic properties (Rios et al., 2007). Several affinin analogues are present in extracts from these *Acmella* species (see table 1), which probably contribute to the analgesic sensation induced by these plants.

2.1.3 *Spilanthes* genus

For years *Spilanthes acmella* has been used as traditional folk medicine to treat toothaches, stammering, and stomatitis. Previous studies have demonstrated the diuretic, antibacterial, and anti-inflammatory activities of *Spilanthes acmella*. Spilanthol (**70**), the main alkamide isolated from this plant, exhibits antiseptic activity. Additionally, spilanthol (**70**) is involved in immune stimulation and the attenuation of the inflammatory responses in murine RAW 264.7 macrophages (Wu et al., 2008).

2.1.4 *Echinaceae* genus

Echinacea is a native herb from North America and Europe that is used as an immunostimulant. Extracts from the *Echinacea* species are widely used due to the strong belief that the components of the extract stimulate the immune system and help to prevent infections, colds, respiratory infections and influenza. However, the clinical efficacy of this

Tribe	Genus	Species	Alka-mide	R₁ (including C=O) Chain	R₁ (including C=O) Double and triple bonds	R₂	Reference
Anthe-mideae	Aaronsohnia	pubescens	1	C10	2E,4E-dies-6-(thien-2-yl)	N-isobutyl	(Muller-Jakic et al., 1994)
	Achillea	ageratifolia	2	C12	2,6-epoxy	pyrrolidyl	(Muller-Jakic et al., 1994) (Greger et al., 1987b)
			3	C16	2E,7Z-dienyl	pyrrolidyl	
			4	C16	7Z-en-9-yne	pyrrolidyl	
			5	C16	2E,7Z-dien-10-yne	pyrrolidyl	
			6	C16	2E,6E,8E-trien-10-yne	pyrrolidyl	
			7	C14	2E,4E-dien-8-yne	pyrrolidyl	
			8	C14	2E,4E,7Z,10Z-tetraenyl	pyrrolidinyl	
			9	C16	6E,8E-dien-10-yne	pyrrolidinyl	
			10	C16	4E,7Z-dien-10-yne	pyrrolidinyl	
			11	C16	2E,6E,8E-trien-10-yne	pyrrolidinyl	
		beibersteinii	12	C14	2E,4E,12E-trien-8,10-diyne	piperidinyl	(Muller-Jakic et al., 1994)
		chamaeme-lifolia	13	C18	12-oxo	piperidinyl	(Greger et al., 1987a)
			14	C18	12-oxo	pyrrolidyl	
			15	C18	2E-en-12-oxo	piperidinyl	
			16	C18	2E-en-12-oxo	pyrrolidyl	
			17	C18	2E,4E,9Z-trien-12-yne	N-isobutyl	
			18	C18	2E,8E,10E-trien-12-yne	piperidinyl	
			19	C18	2E,4E,8E,10E-tetraen-12-yne	N-isobutyl	
			20	C18	2E,4E,8E,10Z-tetraen-12-yne	N-isobutyl	
		crithmifolia	21	C11	2E,4E-dien-8,10-diyne	N-isobutyl	(Muller-Jakic et al., 1994)
		distans subsp. distans	22	C10	2E,4E-dienyl	N-isobutyl	(Lazarevic et al., 2010)
			23	C10	2E,4E-dienyl	piperidinyl	
			24	C10	2E,4E-dienyl	2,3-dehydro-piperidinyl	
			25	C10	2E,4E,6Z-trienyl	2,3-dehydro-piperidinyl	
		lycaonica	26	C15	2E,4E-dien-12-oxo	N-isobutyl	(Greger et al., 1987a)
			27	C18	2E-enyl	piperidinyl	

Tribe	Genus	Species	Alka-mide	Chain	R₁ (including C=O) Double and triple bonds	R₂	Reference
			28	C18	2E,9Z-dienyl	piperidinyl	
			29	C18	9Z-en-12-yne	piperidinyl	
			30	C18	2E,9Z-dien-12-yne	piperidinyl	
			31	C18	9Z,14Z-dien-12-yne	piperidinyl	
			32	C18	2E,9Z-dien-12,14-diyne	piperidinyl	
			22	C10	2E,4E-dienyl	N-isobutyl	
			33	C10	2E,4E-dien-8,10-diyne	N-isobutyl	
			34	C10	2E,4E,8Z-trienyl	N-isobutyl	
			35	C14	2E,4E-dien-8,10-diyne	N-isobutyl	(Muller-Jakic et al., 1994)
			36	C14	2E,4E,12E-trien-8,10-diyne	N-isobutyl	(Greger & Hofer, 1989)
			37	C14	2E,4E,12Z-trien-8,10-diyne	N-isobutyl	(Greger & Hofer, 1990)
			38	C15	2E,9Z-dien-12,14-diyne	N-isobutyl	(Greger, H. & Werner, 1990)
			39	C10	2E,4E-dien-8,10-diyne	N-isobutyl	
			40	C10	2E,4E-dienyl	N-tyramidyl	
			41	C10	2E,4E-dienyl	N-(O-methyl-tyramidyl)	
		millefolium	23	C10	2E,4E-dienyl	piperidinyl	
			42	C10	2E,4E,8Z-trienyl	piperidinyl	
			24	C10	2E,4E-dienyl	2,3-dehydro-piperidinyl	
			25	C10	2E,4E,6Z-trienyl	2,3-dehydro-piperidinyl	
			43	C10	2E,4E-dien-8,10-diyne	2,3-dehydro-piperidinyl	
			44	C10	2E,4E,8Z-trienyl	2,3-dehydro-piperidinyl	
			45	C10	2E,4E,6E-trienyl	2,3-dehydro-piperidinyl	
			46	C10	2E,4E,6Z,8Z-tetraenyl	2,3-dehydro-piperidinyl	
			47	C10	2E,4E,6E,8Z-tetraenyl	2,3-dehydro-piperidinyl	
			48	C11	2E,4E,6E,8E-tetraenyl	2,3-dehydro-piperidinyl	
			49	C11	2E,4E-dien-8,10-diyne	piperidinyl	
			50	C11	2E,4E-dien-8,10-diyne	2,3-dehydro-piperidinyl	
		nana	51	C14	2E,4E,10Z-trien-8-yne	pyrrolidinyl	(Muller-Jakic et al., 1994)
		spinulifolia	52	C13	2E,4E-trien-8,10,12-triyne	piperidinyl	(Muller-Jakic et al., 1994)

Tribe	Genus	Species	Alka-mide	Chain	R₁ (including C=O) Double and triple bonds	R₂	Reference
		ptarmica	22	C10	2E,4E-dienyl	N-isobutyl	(Lazarevic et al., 2010)
			53	C10	2E-en-4-yne	N-isobutyl	
		wilhelmsii	54	C10	2E,8Z-dien-4,6-diyne	N-isobutyl	(Muller-Jakic et al., 1994) Greger, 1987c]
			55	C10	2E,4E-dienyl	N-(3-methylbutyl)	
			56	C10	2E,8Z-dien-4,6-diyne	N-(3-methylbutyl)	
			57	C10	2E-en-4,6,8-triyne	N-(3-methylbutyl)	
			58	C10	2E,4E-dienyl	N-phenethyl	
			59	C10	2Z,8E-dien-4,6-diyne	N-phenethyl	
			60	C10	2E-en-4,6,8-triyne	N-phenethyl	
			61	C14	2E,4E,6Z,12Z-tetraen-8,10-diyne	N-isobutyl	
			62	C14	2E,4E,6E,12Z-tetraen-8,10-diyne	N-isobutyl	
			63	C14	2E,4E-dien-8,10-diyne	N-(3-methylbutyl)	
			64	C14	2E,4E,12Z-trien-8,10-diyne	N-(3-methylbutyl)	
			65	C14	2E,4E,6Z,12Z-tetraen-8,10-diyne	N-(3-methylbutyl)	
			66	C14	2E,4E,6E,12Z-tetraen-8,10-diyne	N-(3-methylbutyl)	
	Anacyclus	pyrethrum	40	C10	2E,4E-dienyl	N-tyramidyl	(Muller-Jakic et al., 1994)
	Artemisia	dracunculus	22	C10	2E,4E-dienyl	N-isobutyl	(Saadali et al., 2001)
			67	C11	2E,4E-dien-7,9-diyne	N-isobutyl	
			23	C10	2E,4E-dienyl	piperidinyl	
Berbe-sininae	Salmea	scandens	68	C12	2E,4E,8Z,10E-tetraenyl	N-isobutyl	(Herz & Kulanthaivel, 1985) (Bohlmann et al., 1985)
			69	C12	2E,4E,8Z,10Z-tetraenyl	N-isobutyl	
Ecliptinae Less.	Wedelia	parviceps	70	C10	2E,6Z,8E-trienyl	N-isobutyl	(Johns et al., 1982)
Galin-soginae B. and H	Acmella	alba	68	C12	2E,4E,8Z,10E-tetraenyl	N-isobutyl	(Bohlmann et al., 1980)
		ciliata	71	C8	2E,4Z-dienyl	N-isobutyl	(Martin & Becker,

Tribe	Genus	Species	Alka-mide	Chain	Double and triple bonds	R_2	Reference
					R_1 (including C=O)		
			72	C10	6Z,8E-dienyl	N-isobutyl	1984)
			70	C10	2E,6Z,8E-trienyl	N-isobutyl	(Martin & Becker, 1985)
			68	C12	2E,4E,8Z,10E-tetraenyl	N-isobutyl	
			73	C12	2E,4Z,8Z,10E-tetraenyl	N-isobutyl	
			74	C8	2Z,4E-dienyl	N-2-methylbutyl	
			75	C10	2E,6Z,8E-trienyl	N-2-methylbutyl	
			76	C10	3E,6Z,8E-trienyl	N-phenethyl	
			77	C10	2E,6Z,8E-trienyl	N-phenethyl	
			78	C12	2E,4E,8Z,10E-tetraenyl	N-phenethyl	
		decumbens	79	C9	2Z-en-6,8-diyne	N-phenethyl	(Casado et al., 2009)
			80	C10	2E,4E-dien-9-yne	N-phenethyl	
			81	C11	4E,6E-en-10-yne	N-isobutyl	
		mauritiana	82	C12	2E,4E,8E,10Z-tetraenyl	N-isobutyl	(Casado et al., 2009)
		oloracea	70	C10	2E,6Z,8E-trienyl	N-isobutyl	(Greger et al., 1985)
			75	C10	2E,6Z,8E-trienyl	N-2-methylbutyl	
		oppositifolia	70	C10	2E,6Z,8E-trienyl	N-isobutyl	(Calle et al., 1988)
			75	C10	2E,6Z,8E-trienyl	N-2-methylbutyl	(Molina et al., 1996)
			68	C12	2E,4E,8Z,10E-tetraenyl	N-isobutyl	
		radicans	83	C8	2E-enyl	N-isobutyl	(Rios-Chavez et al., 2003)
			84	C8	2E,4Z-dienyl	N-isobutyl	
			70	C10	2E,6Z,8E-trienyl	N-isobutyl	
			68	C12	2E,4E,8Z,10E-tetraenyl	N-isobutyl	
			21	C11	2E,4E-dien-8,10-diyne	N-isobutyl	
			75	C10	2E,6Z,8E-trienyl	N-2-methylbutyl	
			85	C12	2E,4Z,8E,10E-tetraenyl	N-2-methylbutyl	
			86	C8	2E,4Z-dienyl	N-phenethyl	
			87	C8	2Z,4E-dienyl	N-phenethyl	
			77	C10	2E,6Z,8E-trienyl	N-phenethyl	
			88	C9	2E-en-6,8-diyne	N-phenethyl	

Tribe	Genus	Species	Alka-mide	Chain	R₁ (including C=O) Double and triple bonds	R₂	Reference
Heli-anthinae	Spilanthes	acmella	89	C9	cis-2,3-epoxy-6,8-diyne	N-phenethyl	
			90	3-phe-C3	3-phenyl- 2-propenyl	N-phenethyl	
			91	C9	2E-en-6,8-diyne	N-isobutyl	
			70	C10	2,6,8-trienyl	N-isobutyl	
			92	C10	2E,7Z-dienyl	N-isobutyl	
			70	C10	2E,6Z,8E-trienyl	N-isobutyl	(Pandey et al., 2011)
			93	C10	2,4,6,8-tetraenyl	N-isobutyl	(Boonen et al., 2010)
			94	C12	2E,7Z,9E-trienyl	N-isobutyl	(Ramsewak et al., 1999)
			69	C12	2E,4E,8Z,10Z-tetraenyl	N-isobutyl	
			95	C11	2E-en-8,10-diyne	N-isobutyl	
			96	C11	2E,6Z-dien-8,10-diyne	N-isobutyl	
			97	C11	2E,7Z,9E-trienyl	N-isobutyl	
			98	C13	2E,7Z-dien-10,12-diyne	N-isobutyl	
			99	C13	7Z-en-10,12-diyne	N-isobutyl	
			75	C10	2E,6Z,8E-trienyl	N-isobutyl	
			100	C11	2E-en-8,10-diyne	N-2-methylbutyl	
			101	C11	2E,4Z-dien-8,10-diyne	N-2-methylbutyl	
			89	C9	2-epoxy-6,8-diyne	N-2-methylbutyl	
						N-phenethyl	
		ocymifolia	102	C9	cinnamamidyl	N-2-phenylethyl	(Ramsewak et al., 1999)
	Echinaceae	angustifolia	95	C11	2E-en-8,10-diyne	N-isobutyl	(Bauer et al., 1989)
			103	C11	2Z-en-8,10-diyne	N-isobutyl	(Bauer & Reminger, 1989)
			104	C11	2E,4Z-dien-8,10-diyne	N-isobutyl	
			105	C11	2Z,4E-dien-8,10-diyne	N-isobutyl	(Woelkar et al., 2005)
			106	C12	2E,4E-dienyl	N-isobutyl	
			107	C12	2E,4E,8Z-trienyl	N-isobutyl	(Muller-Jakic et al., 1994)
			68	C12	2E,4E,8Z,10E-tetraenyl	N-isobutyl	
			69	C12	2E,4E,8Z,10Z-tetraenyl	N-isobutyl	
			108	C12	2E-en-8,10-diyne	N-isobutyl	(Schulthess et al., 1990)
			109	C12	2E,4Z-dien-8,10-diyne	N-isobutyl	
			110	C12	2E,4Z,10Z-trien-8-yne	N-isobutyl	(Chen et al., 2005)

Tribe	Genus	Species	Alkamide	R₁ (including C=O)		R₂	Reference
				Chain	Double and triple bonds		
			111	C12	2Z,4E,10Z-trien-8-yne	N-isobutyl	
			112	C14	2E-en-10,12-diyne	N-isobutyl	
			38	C15	2E,9Z-dien-12,14-diyne	N-isobutyl	
			113	C16	2E,9Z-dien-12,14-diyne	N-isobutyl	
			114	C11	2Z-en-8,10-diyne	N-2-methylbutyl	
			115	C12	2E-en-8,10-diyne	N-2-methylbutyl	
			116	C12	2E,4Z-dien-8,10-diyne	N-2-methylbutyl	
		angustifolia var. *strigosa*	95	C11	2E-en-8,10-diyne	N-isobutyl	(Senchina et al., 2006)
			103	C11	2Z-en-8,10-diyne	N-isobutyl	
			105	C11	2Z,4E-dien-8,10-diyne	N-isobutyl	
			106	C12	2E,4E-dienyl	N-isobutyl	
			107	C12	2E,4E,8Z-trienyl	N-isobutyl	
			68	C12	2E,4E,8Z,10E-tetraenyl	N-isobutyl	
			69	C12	2E,4E,8Z,10Z-tetraenyl	N-isobutyl	
			108	C12	2E-en-8,10-diyne	N-isobutyl	
			117	C12	2E,4E,10E-trien-8-yne	N-isobutyl	
			118	C12	2E,4Z-dien-8,10-diyne	N-isobutyl	
			101	C11	2E,4Z-dien-8,10-diyne	N-2-methylbutyl	
		pallida	104	C11	2E,4Z-dien-8,10-diyne	N-isobutyl	(Bauer & Reminger, 1989) (Senchina et al., 2006) (Schulthess et al., 1990) (Chen et al., 2005)
			105	C11	2Z,4E-dien-8,10-diyne	N- isobutyl	
			106	C12	2E,4E-dienyl	N-isobutyl	
			107	C12	2E,4E,8Z-trienyl	N-isobutyl	
			68	C12	2E,4E,8Z,10E-tetraenyl	N-isobutyl	
			69	C12	2E,4E,8Z,10Z-tetraenyl	N-isobutyl	
			118	C12	2E,4Z-dien-8,10-diyne	N-isobutyl	
			119	C12	2Z,4E-dien-8,10-diyne	N-isobutyl	
		pallida var. *pallida*	38	C15	2E,9Z-dien-12,14-diyne	N-isobutyl	(Binns et al, 2002)
		pallida var. *angustifolia*	95	C11	2E-en-8,10-diyne	N-isobutyl	(Binns et al, 2002)
			103	C11	2Z-en-8,10-diyne	N-isobutyl	
			68	C12	2E,4E,8Z,10E-tetraenyl	N-isobutyl	

Tribe	Genus	Species	Alka-mide	Chain	R_1 (including C=O) Double and triple bonds	R_2	Reference
			69	C12	2E,4E,8Z,10Z-tetraenyl	N-isobutyl	
			38	C15	2E,9Z-dien-12,14-diyne	N-isobutyl	
		pallida var. tennesseensis	95	C11	2E-en-8,10-diyne	N-isobutyl	[(Binns et al, 2002)
			103	C11	2Z-en-8,10-diyne	N-isobutyl	
			38	C15	2E,9Z-dien-12,14-diyne	N-isobutyl	
		pallida var. sanguinea	95	C11	2E-en-8,10-diyne	N-isobutyl	(Binns et al, 2002)
			103	C12	2Z-en-8,10-diyne	N-isobutyl	
			38	C15	2E,9Z-dien-12,14-diyne	N-isobutyl	
		purpurea	95	C11	2E-en-8,10-diyne	N-isobutyl	(Bauer & Reminger, 1989) (Senchina et al., 2006) (Schulthess et al., 1990) (Chen et al., 2005) (Cech et al., 2006) (Binns et al., 2002) (Perry et al., 1997)
			103	C11	2Z-en-8,10-diyne	N-isobutyl	
			104	C11	2E,4Z-dien-8,10-diyne	N-isobutyl	
			105	C11	2Z,4E-dien-8,10-diyne	N-isobutyl	
			106	C12	2E,4E-dienyl	N-isobutyl	
			107	C12	2E,4E,8Z-trienyl	N-isobutyl	
			68	C12	2E,4E,8Z,10E-tetraenyl	N-isobutyl	
			69	C12	2E,4E,8Z,10Z-tetraenyl	N-isobutyl	
			108	C12	2E-en-8,10-diyne	N-isobutyl	
			117	C12	2E,4E,10E-trien-8-yne	N-isobutyl	
			118	C12	2E,4Z-dien-8,10-diyne	N-isobutyl	
			119	C12	2Z,4E-dien-8,10-diyne	N-isobutyl	
			120	C12	2E,4Z,10E-trien-8-yne	N-isobutyl	
			98	C13	2E,7Z-dien-10,12-diyne	N-isobutyl	
			38	C15	2E,9Z-dien-12,14-diyne	N-isobutyl	
			121	C16	2E,9Z-12Z,14E-tetraenenyl	N-isobutyl	
			101	C11	2E,4Z-dien-8,10-diyne	N-2-methylbutyl	
			122	C12	2E,4E-dien-8,10-diyne	N-2-methylbutyl	
			116	C12	2E,4Z-dien-8,10-diyne	N-2-methylbutyl	
		sanguinea	95	C11	2E-en-8,10-diyne	N-isobutyl	(Senchina et al., 2006)
			103	C11	2Z-en-8,10-diyne	N-isobutyl	
			104	C11	2E,4Z-dien-8,10-diyne	N-isobutyl	
			105	C11	2Z,4E-dien-8,10-diyne	N-isobutyl	

Tribe	Genus	Species	Alkamide	Chain	R$_1$ (including C=O) Double and triple bonds	R$_2$	Reference
Zinniinae B. and H.		simulata	106	C12	2E,4E-dienyl	N-isobutyl	
			107	C12	2E,4E,8Z-trienyl	N-isobutyl	
			68	C12	2E,4E,8Z,10E-tetraenyl	N-isobutyl	
			69	C12	2E,4E,8Z,10Z-tetraenyl	N-isobutyl	
			108	C12	2E-en-8,10-diyne	N-isobutyl	
			118	C12	2E,4Z-dien-8,10-diyne	N-isobutyl	
			101	C11	2E,4Z-dien-8,10-diyne	N-2-methylbutyl	
			116	C12	2E,4Z-dien-8,10-diyne	N-2-methylbutyl	(Bauer & Foster, 1991)
			95	C11	2E-en-8,10-diyne	N-isobutyl	
			103	C11	2Z-en-8,10-diyne	N-isobutyl	
			68	C12	2E,4E,8Z,10E-tetraenyl	N-isobutyl	
			69	C12	2E,4E,8Z,10Z-tetraenyl	N-isobutyl	
			98	C13	2E,7Z-dien-10,12-diyne	N-isobutyl	
		tennesseensis	95	C11	2E-en-8,10-diyne	N-isobutyl	
			103	C11	2Z-en-8,10-diyne	N-isobutyl	
			106	C12	2E,4E-dienyl	N-isobutyl	(Senchina et al., 2006)
			68	C12	2E,4E,8Z,10E-tetraenyl	N-isobutyl	(Bauer et al, 1990)
			9	C12	2E,4E,8Z,10Z-tetraenyl	N-isobutyl	
			108	C12	2E-en-8,10-diyne	N-isobutyl	
			114	C11	2Z-en-8,10-diyne	N-2-methylbutyl	
			115	C12	2E-en-8,10-diyne	N-2-methylbutyl	
	Heliopsis	longipes	70	C10	2E,6Z,8E-trienyl	N-isobutyl	
			123	C10	2E-enyl	N-isobutyl	
			124	C10	2E,6Z-dienyl	N-isobutyl	(Rios et al., 2007)
			125	C10	2E,6Z-dien-syn-8,9-dihydroxyl	N-isobutyl	(Molina et al., 1996)
			126	C10	2E,7E-dien-syn-6,9-dihydroxyl	N-isobutyl	(Rios et al., 2011)
			127	C11	3Z-en-8,10-diyne	N-isobutyl	
			95	C11	2E-en-8,10-diyne	N-isobutyl	
			104	C11	2E,4Z-dien-8,10-diyne	N-isobutyl	
	Sanvitalia	ocymoides	128	C14	2E,4E,8Z,10E-tetraenyl	N-isobutyl	(Dominguez et al., 1987)
			129	C14	2E,4E,8Z-trienyl	N-isobutyl	

Table 1. Alkamides from the Asteraceae family.

agent has not been proven. *E. angustifolia*, *E. pallida* and *E. purpurea* are three species of *Echinacea* that are used in commercial preparations with reported alkamide profiles. These species contain complex mixtures of alkamides that are good chemotaxonomic characters (table 1). The major alkamides in *E. purpurea* roots are the C12-2,4-diene and C12-2,4-diene-diyne type, while the C11 diene-diynes were highest in vegetative stems (Binns et al., 2002). *E. angustifolia* roots are characterized by the presence of di-, tri- and tetraenes in coexistence with mono- and diynes, all of them with variable insaturation degree at the C2, C4, C9 or C10 position. In *E. pallida*, the major compounds are polienes (also di-, tri- and tetraenes) and diynes (C2 or C2 and C4 unsaturated)

Lipophilic alkamides from *Echinacea* show immunostimulatory activity and have been used for the treatment of cold, flu, respiratory infections and inflammations, making a considerable contribution to the activities attributed to *Echinaceae* plants (Bauer, 1989a, 1989b, 1990, 1991). Studies on the mechanisms of action of the immunomodulatory activity of *Echinacea* have indicated that alkylamides can act as cannabinomimetics. Endogenous ligands for cannabinoid receptors such as anandamide (fig. 2), an animal alkamide that shares structural similarity with the *Echinacea* alkylamides, can bind to CB2 cannabinoid receptors (LaLone et al., 2010). The cannabinoid receptors CB1 and CB2 have been implicated in the modulation of the CNS and the inflammatory response. CB1 receptors are present in neurons from the central and peripheral nervous system and are concentrated in the brain. CB2 receptors are mainly present in immune cells, such as macrophages.

2.1.5 *Heliopsis* genus

Heliopsis longipes is a Mexican plant that was broadly used by the Náhuatl civilization as flavoring in food preparation. The stems of this climber are used in traditional medicine as a condiment, buccal anesthetic, analgesic in pain toothache, antiparasitic, anti-inflammatory and antiulcerative agent and to prepare homemade insecticides that, similar to pyrethrins, are toxic and exhibit paralyzing effects. Chewing of a little piece of the *Heliopsis longipes* stem results in intense salivation and a local analgesic effect (Molina et al., 1996). An ethanolic extract of this plant exhibited antinociceptive effects on acute thermal and chemical inflammation induced nociception in mice with a mechanism partly linked to the lipoxygenase and/or cyclooxygenase systems (Cariño-Cortés et al., 2010). This extract exhibited synergistic interactions with diclofenac in the Hargreaves model of thermal hyperalgesia (Acosta-Madrid et al., 2009). Various unsaturated aliphatic alkamides have also been identified and characterized from the roots of this plant (table 1), such as affinin (**70**), its most abundant and bioactive alkamide. The analgesic activity of affinin was determined by measuring the release of GABA in mice brain slices (Rios et al., 2007). Furthermore, dose-dependent antinociceptive effects have been observed to be a result of the activation of opiodergic, serotoninergic and GABAergic systems (Déciga-Campos et al., 2010).

2.2 Aliphatic alkamides from other plant families

Convolvulaceae, Euphorbiaceae, Menispermaceae and Rutaceae are other plant families that produce aliphatic alkamides. *N*-isobutyl, 2'-hydroxy-*N*-isobutyl, NH_2 and pyrrolidinyl amine residues have been identified in the structures of alkamides isolated from these plants (table 2).

Species	Alka-mide	Name	Chain (inclu-ding C=O)	R₁ saturation, unsaturation		R₂	Reference
Ipomoea quinquefolia (Convolvulaceae)	130	Alkaloid MQ-A₁	C15	$C_{14}H_{29}$	branched	pyrrolidinyl	(Tofern et al., 1999)
	131	Alkaloid MQ-A₂	C16	$C_{15}H_{31}$	branched	pyrrolidinyl	
	132	Alkaloid MQ-B₂	C16	$C_{15}H_{31}$	linear	pyrrolidinyl	
	133	Alkaloid MQ-A₃	C17	$C_{16}H_{33}$	branched	pyrrolidinyl	
	134	Alkaloid MQ-A₄	C18	$C_{17}H_{35}$	branched	pyrrolidinyl	
	135	Alkaloid MQ-B₄	C18	$C_{17}H_{35}$	linear	pyrrolidinyl	
	136	Alkaloid MQ-A₅	C19	$C_{18}H_{37}$	branched	pyrrolidinyl	
Merremia aquatica (Convolvulaceae)	132	Alkaloid MQ-B₂	C16	$C_{15}H_{31}$	linear	pyrrolidinyl	
	133	Alkaloid MQ-A₃	C17	$C_{16}H_{33}$	branched	pyrrolidinyl	
	136	Alkaloid MQ-A₅	C19	$C_{18}H_{37}$	branched	pyrrolidinyl	
Phyllanthus fraternus subsp. togoensis (Euphorbiaceae)	137	E,E-2,4-octadienamide	C8	2E,4E-diene		NH₂	(Sittie et al., 1998) (Sailaja & Setty, 2006)
	138	E,Z-2,4-decadienamide	C10	2E,4Z-diene		NH₂	
Cissampelos glaberrimma (Menispermaceae)	139	octa-2E,4E-dienoic acid isobutylamide	C8	2E,4E-diene		N-isobutyl	(Rosario et al., 1996)
	140	deca-2E,4E-dienoic acid isobutylamide	C10	2E,4E-diene		N-isobutyl	
	141	decden-2-oic acid isobutylamide	C10	2E-ene		N-isobutyl	
	142	decanoic acid isobutylamide	C10	---		N-isobutyl	

Species	Alka-mide	Name	R₁		R₂	Reference
			Chain (inclu-ding C=O)	saturation, unsaturation		
Zanthoxylum integrifoliolum (Rutaceae)	143	lanyuamide I	C14	2E,4E,12-oxo	N-isobutyl	(Chen et al., 1999)
	144	lanyuamide II	C14	2E,4E,8Z-12-oxo	N-isobutyl	
	145	lanyuamide III	C14	2E,4E,8Z-11E-tetraene	N-isobutyl	
	146	tetrahydrobungeanool	C14	2E,4E-diene	2'-hidroxy-N-isobutyl	
	147	γ-sanshool	C14	2E,4E,8Z-10E,12E-pentaene	N-isobutyl	
	148	hydroxy-γ-sanshool	C14	2E,4E,8Z-10E,12E-pentaene	2'-hidroxy-N-isobutyl	
	140	(2E,4E,8Z,11E)-2'-hydroxy-N-isobutyl-tetradecatetraenamide	C14	2E,4E,8Z-11E-tetraene	2'-hidroxy-N-isobutyl	
	150	(2E,4E,8Z,11Z)-2'-hydroxy-N-isobutyl-tetradecatetraenamide	C14	2E,4E,8Z-11Z-tetraene	2'-hidroxy-N-isobutyl	
	151	hazaleamide	C14	2E,4E,8Z-11Z-tetraene	N-isobutyl	

Table 2. Aliphatic alkamides from Convolvulaceae, Euphorbiaceae, Menispermaceae and Rutaceae plant families.

2.2.1 Convolvulaceae alkamides

Convolvulaceae alkamides are also known as alkaloids MQ. These alkamides are characterized by linear or branched saturated acid residues. All Convolvulaceae alkamides have a pyrrolidinyl residue as the amine group and have been isolated from the *Ipomoea* and *Merremia* genera (compounds **130-136**).

2.2.2 Euphorbiaceae alkamides

Phyllanthus fraternus is used by traditional healers and tribes in the northern region of India as a folklore remedy for the treatment of malaria and various liver diseases. An aqueous extract of this plant exhibited antioxidant activity, preventing the oxidation of proteins and lipids. Additionally, aqueous extracts of *Phyllanthus fraternus* protect against allyl alcohol-induced oxidative stress in liver mitochondria (Sailaja & Setty, 2006). Two aliphatic alkamides C_4 isomers , *E,E*-2,4-octadienamide (**137**) and *E,Z*-2,4-decadienamide (**138**), have been isolated from this plant. Both isomers lack an alkyl residue at the amine group, which is typically joined to an acid residue (Sittie et al., 1998). Instead, these compounds possess an $\alpha,\beta,\gamma,\delta$-unsaturated conjugated amide, a feature believed to enhance antiplasmodial activity. Notably, *in vitro* assays of these two isomers demonstrated that these compounds possess moderate antiplasmodial activity.

2.2.3 Menispermaceae alkamides

The roots of some species of the *Cissampelos* genus exhibit significant activity against mechanical, chemical and arthritic pain, increasing the pain threshold and dictating the medicinal value of the plants of this genus. For example, *C. glaberrimma* is a plant whose bioactivity is a reflection of its alkamide content (alkamides **139-142**, Rosario et al., 1996).

2.2.4 Rutaceae alkamides

The fruits of *Zanthoxylum integrifoliolum* possess a pungent taste. Chemical analysis enabled the isolation and identification of nine isobutylamides (**143-151**). These amides have a 2*E*,4*E*-dienamide moiety, including an oxo, diene, tetraene or pentaene acidic fragment (table 2). However, no activity has been reported for these molecules.

Amides have also been isolated from the *Glycosmis* genus (Rutaceae); however, those isolated from this genus are sulfur-containing amides, a rare group of secondary metabolites that have an aromatic amine residue. *Glycosmis* alkamides will be discussed in section 3.3 (*vide infra*).

3. Aromatic alkamides

Alkamides isolated from Solanaceae, Piperaceae, Brassicaceae and Rutaceae plant families either have one aromatic ring at the amine residue, at the acid residue or both. Capsaicinoids, amides from *Lepidium meyenii*, and sulfur derivatives from the *Glycosmis* genus are alkamides with one aromatic ring at the amine residue. Piperine and its analogs are amides with one aromatic residue at the acid fragment. Alkamides that have an aromatic ring at the amine and acid residues are distributed among a large group of plants.

3.1 The alkamides from Solanaceae family: Capsaicinoids

Capsicum (also known as "chile" or "chilli") are species used as vegetables, condiments, and for an important number of medicinal preparations. The fruits of *Capsicum* have been utilized in food preparation, for medicinal applications to tone body muscles after workouts, hot infusions for toothache and muscle pain and aerosols such as *Capsicum* extracts that are used as personal protection. This species are the source of highly pungent capsacinoids that induce a hot or burning sensation. Capsaicinoids are the major chemical constituents from the following five domesticated species of *Capsicum* (peppers) genus: *C. annuum* L., *C. baccatum* L., *C. chinense* Jacq., *C. frutescens* L. and *C. pubescens*. All of these species have *N*-vanillylamides (all contain a 4-hydroxy-3-methoxybenzyl amine group) of C8 to C18 fatty acids (table 3).

Alka-mide	Name	R$_1$ long chain (including C=O)	Chain	Reference
152	caprylic acid vanillylamide	C8	linear	
153	nonivamide	C9	linear	
154	nordihydrocapsaicin	C9	7-CH$_3$	
155	norcapsaicin	C9	5E; 7-CH$_3$	
156	decylic acid vanillylamide	C10	linear	
157	dihydrocapsaicin	C10	8-CH$_3$	(Kozukue
158	capsaicin	C10	6E; 8-CH$_3$	et al., 2005)
159	homocapsaicin-I	C11	6E; 9-CH$_3$	(Kobata
160	homocapsaicin-II	C11	6E; 8-CH$_3$	et al., 2010)
161	homodihydrocapsaicin-I	C11	9-CH$_3$	
162	homodihydrocapsaicin-II	C11	8-CH$_3$	
163	*N*-vanillyl-hexadecanamide (palvanil)	C16	linear	
164	*N*-vanillyl-octadecanamide (stevanil)	C18	linear	
165	*N*-vanillyl-9E-octadecenamide (olvanil)	C18	9E	
166	*N*-vanillyl-9E,12E-octadecadienamide (livanil)	C18	9E,12E	

Table 3. Capsaicinoids from *Capsicum annuum*.

Some capsaicinoids exhibit strong pungent sensory properties when consumed as part of the diet. Additionally, capsaicinoids possess a variety of biological properties that may affect human health (Kozuke et al., 2010), such as antiviral, antibacterial, antifungal, insecticidal, antioxidative, anti-inflammatory and anticancer activities. Furthermore, capsaicinoids influence neuronal structures that contain substances that are associated with pain transmission and neurogenic inflammation. As a result, these compounds are used as topical analgesics for treating pain. The aforementioned properties are the basis for the use of capsaicinoids to prevent or reduce chronic and age-related pain (Kozuke et al., 2005). Capsaicin (**158**) and dihydrocapsaicin (**157**) are notable among natural capsaicinoids because they constitute approximately 90% of the total capsaicinoids in many varieties of peppers. The burning sensation caused by capsaicin is induced by the direct activation of a nonselective cation channel-transient receptor potential, vanilloid 1 (TRPV1), located at the end of sensory nerves. Several physiological activities caused by capsaicin are related to the activation of the TRPV1 receptor. Meghvansi and coworkers have written a review of capsaicinoids in which their ethnopharmacological applications are discussed (Meghvansi et al., 2010). Long acyl chain capsaicinoids exhibiting similar activities to capsaicin, such as anti-inflammatory, antinociceptive and enhanced adrenaline secretion, have been recently reported. The advantages of these compounds are the lack of irritancy or pungency due to the lower accessibility of TRPV1 in the tongue due to higher lipophilicity compared to capsaicin (Kobata et al., 2010).

3.2 The alkamides from *Lepidium meyenii* (Brassicaceae)

The roots from of *L. meyenii* are used to enhance fertility and sexual behavior in men and women. Additionally, *L. meyenii* roots serve as a traditional remedy for menopausal symptoms, the regulation of hormone secretion, immunostimulation, memory improvement, as an antidepressant or anticancer agent, and to prevent anemia. Phytochemical analysis of the roots of this plant led to the identification of *m*-methoxybenzyl and *N*-benzyl amine residues and macamides, linear C16, C18 or C24 alkamides with one or two double bonds and possible oxidation of C_5, C_9 or C_{13} (table 4).

3.3 The alkamides from *Glycosmis* (Rutaceae)

Sulfur-containing amides (phenethyl/styrylamine-derived amides) form a rare group of secondary metabolites in the Rutaceae family. These amides are only present in the leaves of plants that belong to the *Glycosmis* genus. Sulfur-containing amides represent a typical chemical profile of this genus. The acid moieties of these alkamides are probably derived from cysteine, which can be oxidized to sulfones and sulfoxides or shortened by β-oxidation (as in ritigalin). With the exception of simple methylamides, the amine residues are characterized by the presence of phenethyl or styryl groups (derived from phenylalanine) that can be linked to different prenyloxy (dambullins) or geranyloxy groups in *para* position (gerambullins). More recently, a group of similar (methylsulfonyl)propenoic acid amides has been detected in which dopamine is linked to various oxidized geranyl chains (sakerines). Some of these alkamides exhibit pronounced antifungal and/or insecticidal activity (Greger & Zechner, 1996) (table 5).

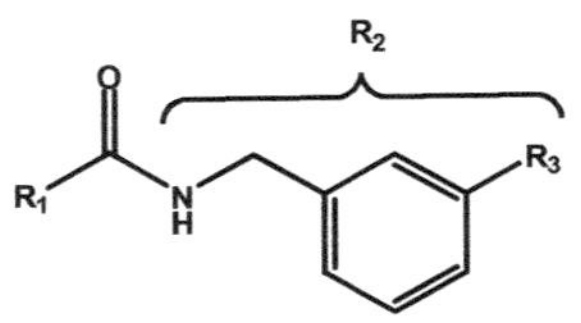

R_2

$R_3 = H$ *N*-benzyl

$R_3 = OCH_3$ *N*-*m*-methoxybenzyl

Alkamide	Name	R_1 long chain (including C=O)	chain	R_2	Reference
167	N-(*m*-methoxybenzyl)hexadecanamide	C16	$C_{15}H_{31}$	*m*-methoxybenzyl	(Zhao et al., 2005) (Muhammad et al, 2002)
168	N-benzylhexadecanamide	C16	$C_{15}H_{31}$	*N*-benzyl	
169	N-benzyl-9-oxo-12Z-octadecenamide	C18	9-oxo-12Z	*N*-benzyl	
170	N-benzyl-9-oxo-12Z,15Z-octadecadienamide	C18	9-oxo-12Z,15Z	*N*-benzyl	
171	N-benzyl-13-oxooctadeca-9E,11E-dienamide	C18	13-oxo-9E,11E	*N*-benzyl	
172	N-benzyl-5-oxo-6E,8E-octadecadienamide	C18	5-oxo-6E,8E	*N*-benzyl	
173	N-benzyl-15Z-tetracosenamide	C24	15Z	*N*-benzyl	

Table 4. Alkamides from *Lepidium meyenii*.

Species	Alk	Name	R1	R2	
G. angustifolia	174	penamide A	E-CH3-S-CH=CH-	R3=CH3; R4=O; R5=R6=R7=H	(Greger et al., 1994)
	175	penamide B	Z-CH3-S-CH=CH-	R3=CH3; R4=O; R5=R6=R7=H	
	176	dambullin	E-CH3-SO2-CH=CH-	R3=H; R4=H,H; R5=R6=H; R7=O-isopentenyl	
	177	methyldambullin	E-CH3-SO2-CH=CH-	R3=CH3; R4=H,H; R5=R6=H; R7=O-isopentenyl	
	178	gerambullin	E-CH3-SO2-CH=CH-	R3=H; R4=H,H; R5=R6=H; R7=O-geranyl	
	179	methylgerambullin	E-CH3-SO2-CH=CH-	R3=CH3; R4=H,H; R5=R6=H; R7=O-geranyl	
	180	gerambulindiol	E-CH3-SO2-CH=CH-	R3=R5=R6=H; R4=H,H; R7=O-6,7-dihydroxy-geranyl	
	181	methylgerambullone	E-CH3-SO2-CH=CH-	R3=CH3; R4=H,H; R5=R6=H; R7=O-5-oxo-geranyl	
	182	methylisogerambullone	E-CH3-SO2-CH=CH-	R3=CH3; R4=H,H; R5=R6=H; R7=O-5-oxo-isogeranyl	
G. chlorosperma	183	penangin	E-CH3-S-CH=CH-	-NH(CH3)	(Greger et al., 1993a)
	184	isopenanangin	Z-CH3-S-CH=CH-	-NH(CH3)	
	185	sinharine	-CH3-S-CH2-CH2-	2,3-*trans*; R3=H; R4=R5=R6=R7=H	
	186	methylsinharine	-CH3-S-CH2-CH2-	2,3-*trans*; R3=CH3; R4=R5=R6=R7=H	
	187	gerambullol	E-CH3-SO2-CH=CH-	R3=R5=R6=H; R4=H,H; R7=O-8-hydroxygeranyl	
	188	β-hydroxy-gerambullin	E-CH3-SO2-CH=CH-	R3=R6=H; R4=H,H; R5=OH; R7=O-geranyl	
	189	β-hydroxy-gerambullol	E-CH3-SO2-CH=CH-	R3=R6=H; R4=H,H; R5=OH; R7=O-8-hydroxy-O-geranyl	
	190	β-hydroxy-gerambullal	E-CH3-SO2-CH=CH-	R3=R6=H; R4=H,H; R5=OH, R7=O-geran-8-al	
	191	sakerinol A	E-CH3-SO2-CH=CH-	R3=R5=H; R4=H,H; R6=OH, R7=O-8-hydroxy-O-geranyl	
	192	O-methyl-sakerinol A	E-CH3-SO2-CH=CH- 176	R3=R5=H; R4=H,H; R6=OCH3, R7=8-hydroxy-O-geranyl	
	193	sakambullin	E-CH3-SO2-CH=CH-	R3=R5=H; R4=H,H; R6=OH; R7=O-isopentenyl	
	194	O-methyl-sakambullin	E-CH3-SO2-CH=CH-	R3=R5=H; R4=H,H; R6=OCH3; R7=O-isopentenyl	
	195	sakerol	E-CH3-SO2-CH=CH-	R3=H; R4=H,H; R5=R6=H; R7=5-hydroxy-O-isopentenyl	

Species	No.	Name	R_1	R_2 (and substituents)	Reference
G. citrifolia	196	glycothiomin A	E-CH_3-SO-CH=CH-	-NH(CH$_3$)	(Wu et al., 1995)
	197	glycothiomin B	Z-CH_3-SO-CH=CH-	-NH(CH$_3$)	
G. cyanocarpa	198	dehydronarinin A	CH_3-S-	2,3-trans; R$_3$=CH$_3$; R$_4$=R$_5$=R$_6$=R$_7$=H	(Greger & Zechner, 1996) (Greger & Hofer, 1993b)
	199	dehydronarinin B	CH_3-S-	2,3-cis; R$_3$=CH$_3$; R$_4$=R$_5$=R$_6$=R$_7$=H	
	200	thalebain B	isobutyl	2,3-cis; R$_3$=CH$_3$; R$_4$=R$_5$=R$_6$=R$_7$=H	
	201	methylillukumbin A	E-CH_3-S-CH=CH-	2,3-trans; R$_3$=CH$_3$; R$_4$=R$_5$=R$_6$=R$_7$=H	
	202	dehydrothalebain A	isobut-2,3-enyl	2,3-trans; R$_3$=CH$_3$; R$_4$=R$_5$=R$_6$=R$_7$=H	
	203	dehydrothalebain B	isobut-2,3-enyl	2,3-cis; R$_3$=CH$_3$; R$_4$=R$_5$=R$_6$=R$_7$=H	
		183, 184, 185, 198, 199, 200, 201, 202, 203			
G. mauritiana	204	ritigalin	CH_3-S-	R$_3$=CH$_3$; R$_4$=O; R$_5$=R$_6$=R$_7$=H	
	205	niranin	CH_3-S-	R$_3$=CH$_3$; R$_4$=H,H; R$_5$=R$_6$=R$_7$=H	
	206	illukumbin A	Z-CH_3-S-CH=CH-	2,3-trans; R$_3$=H; R$_4$=R$_5$=R$_6$=R$_7$=H	
	207	methylillukumbin B	Z-CH_3-S-CH=CH-	2,3-trans; R$_3$=CH$_3$; R$_4$=R$_5$=R$_6$=R$_7$=H	
G. parviflora		204			
G. pentaphylla		183, 184, 185, 201, 207			(Greger & Hofer, 1993b)

Table 5. Sulfur-containing alkamides from the *Glycosmis* species.

3.4 The Piperaceae family. Piperine and its analogs

Alkamides from the Piperaceae family are produced by plants that are classified as being in either the *Piper*, *Ottonia* or *Peperomia* genera. These alkamides are characterized by the presence of *N*-isobutyl, *N*-3-acetoxy-isobutyl, piperidinyl (piperidide), 5,6-dihydro-2(1*H*)pyridinone and pyrrolidinyl groups as amine residues, with *N*-isobutyl and piperidinyl being the most commonly found. The presence of carboxylic acid fragment is also characteristic of the alkamides isolated from plants that belong to the Piperaceae family. These fragments include the 3',4'-methylenedioxyphenyl as the most common terminal group. However, *p*-methoxyphenyl, 3',4',5'-trimethoxyphenyl and 4'-hydroxy-3'-methoxyphenyl groups can also be joined to a chain of 2, 4, 5, 6, 8, 9, 10, 11, 12 or 14 carbons, with one, two or three unsaturations at the even-numbered carbons (with the exception of C_{12}, fig. 4).

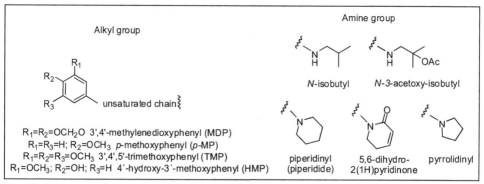

Fig. 4. The most common alkyl and amide residues of alkamides from the Piperaceae family.

Dimeric alkamides have been found in *P. chaba* and *P. nigrum*. *P. chaba* dimers are [4+2] adducts obtained from the combination of piperlonguminine and piperine [chabamide H (**208**) and I (**209**)], two molecules of pellitorine [chabamide J (**210**), and K (**211**)], two molecules of piperine [chabamide (**212**)], or two molecules of piperamine [chabamide F (**213**) and G (**214**)] (fig. 5). Notably, these dimeric alkamides exhibited potent cytotoxic activity against the COLO-205 cell line (Rao et al., 2011).

In contrast, *P. nigrum* dimers constituting [2+2] adducts are the combination of either two molecules of piperine [pipercyclobutanamide A (**215**) and nigramide R (**216**)] or from the piperine analogue piperrolein A [pipercyclobutanamide C (**217**)] (Rao et al, 2011; Subehan et al., 2006) (fig. 6).

The compounds produced by the Piperaceae family are pharmacologically very important, as several species of these plants are being used in folkloric medicine in different parts of the world. For example, the roots of plants from the *Ottonia* genus have a piquant taste and cause intense salivation when are in contact with the mouth. These roots exhibit local anesthetic and hallucinogenic effects and are used in the treatment of toothaches and sore throats. The toothache-relieving reputation of plants that belong to this genus led to the isolation of piperovatine (**222**), a buccal local anesthesic isobutyl amide isolated from *O.*

corcovadensis. Alkamides isolated from the *Ottonia* genus contain 1-oxo-5-(3',4'-methylenedioxyphenyl)-2E,4E-pentadien-1-yl and 1-oxo-6-(*p*-methoxyphenyl)-2E,4E-hexadien-1-yl residues as acidic fragments with N-isobutyl or N-3-acetoxy-isobutyl fragments as the amide residues (Antunes et al., 2001; Costa & Mors, 1981, table 6).

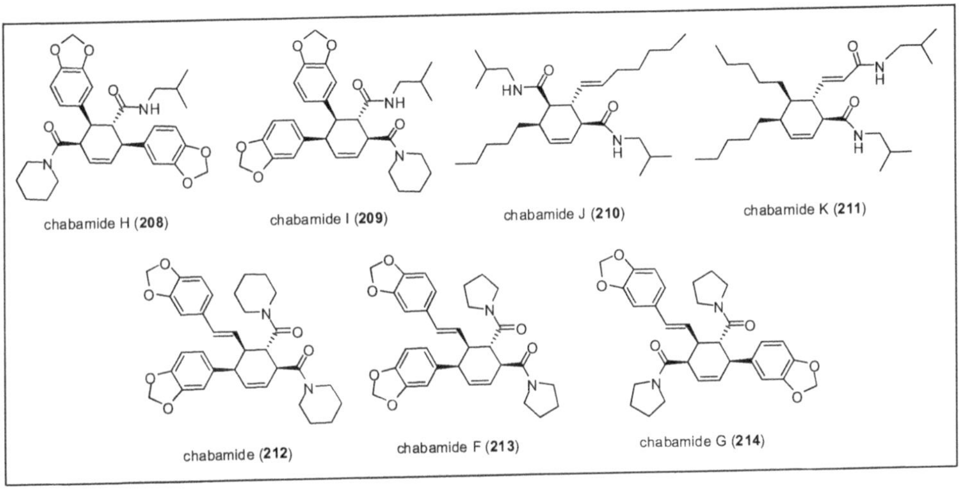

chabamide H (**208**)   chabamide I (**209**)   chabamide J (**210**)   chabamide K (**211**)

chabamide (**212**)   chabamide F (**213**)   chabamide G (**214**)

Fig. 5. Dimeric [4+2] alkamides from *Piper chaba.*

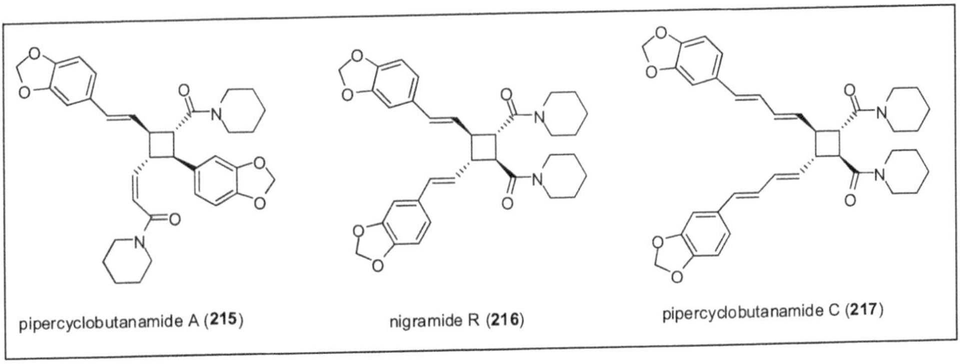

pipercyclobutanamide A (**215**)   nigramide R (**216**)   pipercyclobutanamide C (**217**)

Fig. 6. Dimeric [2+2] alkamides from *Piper nigrum.*

The *Piper* species have been used in traditional medicine for thousands of years in China, India and Mexico, among other countries, for the treatment of several diseases and ailments. For example, *P. longum* is used for treatment of gonorrhea, menstrual and chronic intestinal pain, tuberculosis, sleeping problems, respiratory infections such as coughs, bronchitis and asthma, malarial fever, diarrhea, jaundice and arthritis. The beneficial effects of this species include analgesic and diuretic activities, relaxation of muscle tension, and the alleviation of anxiety.

Species	Alk	Name	R₁	R₂	Reference
Ottonia corcovadensis	218	piperlonguminine	5-(MDP)-2E,4E-pentadienyl	N-isobutyl	(Costa & Mors, 1981).
	219	isopiperlonguminine	5-(MDP)-2Z,4Z-pentadienyl	N-isobutyl	
	220	corcovadine	5-(MDP)-2E,4E-pentadienyl	N-3-acetoxy-isobutyl	
	221	isocorcovadine	5-(MDP)-2Z,4Z-pentadienyl	N-3-acetoxy-isobutyl	
	222	piperovatine	6-(p-MP)-2Z,4Z-hexadienyl	N-isobutyl	
Ottonia propinqua	223	N-isobutyl-6-(p-methoxyphenyl)-2E,4E-hexadieneamide	6-(p-MP)-2E,4E-hexadienyl	N-isobutyl	(Antunes et al., 2001)
Piper chaba	224	pellitorine	2E,4E-decadienyl	N-isobutyl	(Patra & Ghosh, 1974) (Rao et al., 2011)
	218	piperlonguminine	5-(MDP)-2E,4E-pentadienyl	N-isobutyl	
	225	4,5-dihydropiperlonumine	5-(MDP)-2E-pentenyl	N-isobutyl	
	226	guineensine	13-(MDP)-2E,4E,14E-tridecatrienyl	N-isobutyl	
	227	brachystamide B	15-(MDP)-2E,4E,14E-pentadecatrienyl	N-isobutyl	
	228	sylvatine	5-(MDP)-2E,4E-pentadienyl	N-10-methyl-6E-undecenyl	
	229	trichostachine	5-(MDP)-2E,4E-pentadienyl	pyrrolidinyl	
	230	piperine	5-(MDP)-2E,4E-pentadienyl	5,6-dihydro-2(1H)pyridinone	
	231	piplartine	3-(TMP)-2E-propenyl	5,6-dihydro-2(1H)pyridinone	
Piper hispidum	232	(3Z,5Z)-N-isobutyl-8-(3',4'-methylenedioxy-phenyl)-heptadienamide	7-(MDP)-2Z,4Z-heptadienyl	N-isobutyl	(Navickiene et al., 2000)
	233	N-[3-(6'-methoxy-3',4'-methylenedioxyphenyl)-2Z-propenoyl]pyrrolidine	3-(MDP)-2Z-propenyl	pyrrolidinyl	
	234	piperamine	5-(MDP)-2E-pentenyl	pyrrolidinyl	
Piper longum			**224, 228**		
	235	sarmentine	2E,4E-decadienyl	pyrrolidinyl	(Das et al., 1996)
	236	piperrolein B	9-(MDP)-8E-nonenyl	piperidinyl	(Lee et al., 2006)
	237	retrofractamide C	9-(MDP)-2E,8E-nonadienyl	N-isobutyl	(H. Huang et al, 2010)
	238	pipernonaline	9-(MDP)-2E,8E-nonadienyl	piperidinyl	
	239	(2E,4Z,8E)-N-[9-(3,4-methylenedioxyphenyl)-2,4,8-nonatrienoyl]piperidine	9-(MDP)-2E,4Z,8E-nonatrienyl	piperidinyl	(P.L. Huang et al.,2010)

Species	Alk	Name	R$_1$	R$_2$	Reference
	240	dehydropipernonaline	9-(MDP)-2E,4E,8E-nonatrienyl	piperidinyl	(Cotinguiba et al., 2009)
	241	guineensine	13-(MDP)-2E,4E,12E-tridecatrienyl	N-isobutyl	(Navickiene et al., 2000)
	242	(+)-sesamine	11-(MDP)-2E,10E-undecadienyl	N-isobutyl	
	243	piperchabamide D	9-(MDP)-2E,8E-nonadienyl	piperidinyl	
Piper scatorum	223	N-isobutyl-6-(p-methoxyphenyl)-2E,4E-hexadieneamide	6-(p-MP)-2E,4E-hexadienyl	N-isobutyl	
			224, 228		
	244	(Z)-piplartine	3-(TMP)-2Z-propenyl	5,6-dihydro-2(1H)pyridinone	
Piper tuberculatum	231	(E)-piplartine	3-(TMP)-2E-propenyl	5,6-dihydro-2(1H)pyridinone	
	245	8,9-dihydropiplartine	3-(TMPI)-propanyl	5,6-dihydro-2(1H)pyridinone	
	246	10,11-dihydropiperine	5-(MDP)-2E,4E-pentadienyl	piperidinyl	
	247	5,6-dihydropiperlonguminine	5-(MDP)-2E-pentenyl	N-isobutyl	
	248	fagaramide	3-(MDP)-2E-propenyl	N-isobutyl	
			224, 228, 234, 236, 238		
	249	2E-octadec-2-enoic acid piperidide	2E-octadecenyl	piperidinyl	
	250	N-cinnamoylpiperidine	2E-phenethenyl	piperidinyl	
	251	feruperine	5-(HMP)-2E,4E-pentadieyl	pyrrolidinyl	
	252	piperylin	5-(MDP)-2E,4E-pentadienyl	piperidinyl	
	253	piperrolein A	7-(MDP)-6E-heptenyl	pyrrolidinyl	
Piper nigrum	254	piperamide-C7:1(6E)	7-(MDP)- 6E-heptenyl	piperidinyl	(Subehan et al., 2006)
	255	piperamide-A6:2 (2E,6E)	7-(MDP)-2E,6E-heptadienyl	pyrrolidinyl	
	256	piperamide-C9:1(8E)	9-(MDP)-8E-nonenyl	piperidinyl	
	257	retrofractamide C	9-(MDP)-2E,8E-nonadienyl	N-isobutyl	
	258	dehydropipernonaline	9-(MDP)-2E,4Z,8E-nonatrienyl	piperidinyl	
	250	piperamide-C9:3	9-(MDP)-2E,4E,8E-nonatrienyl	piperidinyl	
	260	(2E,4E,8E)piperide	9-(MDP)-2E,4E,8E-nonatrienyl	pyrrolidinyl	
Peperomia duclouxii	261	pipercallosine	9-(MDP)-2E,4E-nonadienyl	N-isobutyl	(Li et al., 2007)
	262	pipercallosidine	7-(MDP)-2E-heptenyl	N-isobutyl	

Table 6. Alkamides from the Piperaceae family. MDP=3',4'-methylenedioxyphenyl; p-MP=p-methoxyphenyl; TMP= 3',4',5'-trimethoxyphenyl; HMP=4´-hydroxy-3´-methoxyphenyl.

In contrast, *P. hispidum* and *P. tuberculatum* exhibit antifungal activity and produce amides with the *cis* geometry in their side chains, a structural feature quite rare in nature (table 6, Navickiene et al., 2000).

Pipernonaline (**238**) is an alkamide possessing mosquito larvicidal activity that has been isolated from *P. longum* (Huang et al., 2010), whereas some piperamides, such as (Z)-piplartine (**244**), (E)-piplartine (**231**), 8,9-dihydropiplartine (**245**) and pellitorine (**228**), isolated from P. *tuberculatum* seeds have been shown to inhibit the proliferation of *Trypanosoma cruzi* parasites. These alkamides are considered to be templates for the design of novel and potent hit compounds for the treatment of Chagas' disease (Cotinguiba et al., 2009).

Piperine (*E,E* isomer of 1-piperolypiperidine, **224**) is the major component in the fruits of several species of *Piper*, particularly *P. longum* and *P. nigrum*. This compound showed diverse biological activities such as antioxidant, anti-inflammatory, analgesic, antiplatelet aggregation, antihyperlipidemic, antihypertensive, cytoprotective, antitumor, antimicrobial, hepatoprotective and antidepressant activities. The structure of piperine resembles that of Capsaicin (158, table 3), the pungent component in the majority of the chilli peppers species. Similar to capsaicin, piperine also serves as a natural agonist of the vanilloid receptor (TRPV1 channel), which is involved in the neurotransmission of thermal and nociceptive stimuli.

Piplartine   (5,6-dihydro-1-[(2E)-1-oxo3-(3',4',5'-trimethoxyphenyl)-2-propen-1-yl]-2(1H)-pyridinone, **244**, table 6) is another important alkamide isolated from the *Piper* species. This compound exhibits antifungal properties and has demonstrated antiplatelet aggregation, anxiolytic, antidepressant and antitumor activities in murine models. This naturally occurring alkamide is also a cytotoxic agent against cultured tumor cells, exhibiting promising anticancer properties. However, piplartine also shows mutagenic activity in yeast and cultured mammalian cells, inducing *in vitro* and *in vivo* chromosomal damage, potentially due to DNA breaks (Bezerra et al., 2009). The alkamides isolated from plants that belong to the Piper family are shown in table 6.

4. Other family plants - Alkamides with both fragments including aromatic residues

The cinnamoylbenzylamide tribulusimide (**263**, fig. 7) and several cinnamoylphenethylamides (table 7) and benzylphenethylamides (table 8) are the condensation products of cinnamic acid and benzylamine derivatives, cinnamic acid and phenethylamine and benzylic acid and phenethylamine, respectively. These alkamides have been isolated from a broad variety of plants that belong to at least 28 families. A selection of these alkamides are shown in table 9.

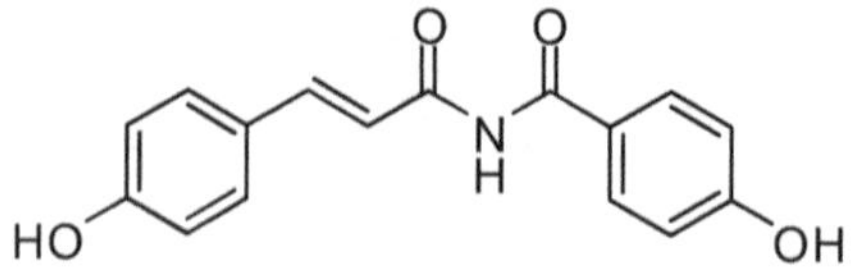

tribulusimide (**263**)

Fig. 7. Cinnamoylbenzylamide.

Alkamide	Name	R_1	R_2	R_3	R_4	R_5	R_6
264	p-coumaroyltyramine	H	OH	H	H	H	OH
265	caffeoyltyramine	OH	OH	H	H	H	OH
266	feruloyltyramine	OCH$_3$	OH	H	H	H	OH
267	dihydro-feruloyltyramine	OCH$_3$	OH	H	H	H	OH
268	sinapoyltyramine	OCH$_3$	OH	OCH$_3$	H	H	OH
269	feruloylmethoxytyramine	OCH$_3$	OH	H	H	OCH$_3$	OH
270	terrestriamide	OCH$_3$	OH	H	=O	H	OH
271	feruloyldopamine	OCH$_3$	OH	H	H	OH	OH
272	coumaroyldopamine	H	OH	H	H	OH	OH
273	feruloyl-4-O-methyldopamine	OCH$_3$	OH	H	H	OH	OCH$_3$
274	feruloyl-3-O-methyldopamine	OCH$_3$	OH	H	H	OCH$_3$	OH
275	p-coumaroyl-3-O-methyldopamine	H	OH	H	H	OCH$_3$	OH
276	2-(4'-hydroxyphenyl) ethylcaffeic amide	OH	OH	H	H	H	OH
277	N-cis-feruloyloctopamine	OCH$_3$	OH	H	OH	H	OH
278	coumaroyloctopamine	H	OH	H	OH	H	OH
279	β-(p-hydroxy-phenylethyl) p-hydroxycinnamamide	H	OH	H	H	H	OH
280	3-methoxyaegeline	H	H	H	OH	OCH$_3$	OCH$_3$
281	3-methoxy-7-acetylaegeline	H	H	H	OAc	OCH$_3$	OCH$_3$
282	3-methoxy-7-cinnamoylaegeline	H	H	H	Ocinnamoyl	OCH$_3$	OCH$_3$

Table 7. Cinnamoylphenethylamides isolated from diverse plants.

Alk	Name	Δ	R_1	R_2
283	N-[2-(3,4-dihydroxyphenyl)ethyl]-3,4-dihydroxybenzamide	---	OH	OH
284	alatamide [N-(E)-(p-methoxystyryl)-benzamide]	2E	OCH$_3$	H
285	dihydroalatamide [N-benzoyltyramine methyl ether]	---	OCH$_3$	H

Table 8. Benzylphenethylamides isolated from diverse plants.

Despite the broad distribution of alkamides with both fragments, including aromatic residues among a wide variety of plant families, the presence of feruloyltyramine (266) is exceptionally important because it is a common compound found in the majority of alkamide-producing plants. The Z- and E-stereoisomers of feruloyltyramine have been isolated and are two of the most frequently characterized alkamides. The second most important alkamide is p-coumaroyltyramine (264), which is isolated also in both stereoisomeric forms, the E-stereoisomer being the most common (table 9).

Family	Species		Alkamide	Reference
Alliaceae	*Allium fistulosum*		**264**	(Nishioka et al., 1997)
Amaranthaceae	*Amaranthus*	*hypochondriacus*	**264, 265, 266, 268, 271, 273**	(Pedersen et al., 2010)
		mantegazzianus	**264, 265, 266, 268, 271, 273**	
	Achyranthes ferruginea		***trans*-273**	(Alam et al, 2003)
Anacardiaceae	*Mangifera indica*		**276**	(Ghosal & Chakrabarti, 1988)
Annonaceae	*Annona cherimola*		**264, *cis*-265, *cis*-266, 267, *cis*-269, *trans*-269**	(Chen et al., 1998)
Aristolochiaceae	*Aristolochia*	*gehrtii*	***cis*-264, *trans*-264, *cis*-266, *trans*-266, *cis*-275, *trans*-275**	(Navickiene & Lopes, 2001)
		gigantea	***trans*-264, *trans*-266, *cis*-275, 276, *cis*-277**	(Holzbach & Lopes, 2010)
Cannabidaceae	*Cannabis sativa*		**264, *trans*-265, *trans*-266**	(Sakakibara et al, 1991)
Chenopodiaceae	*Chenopodium album*		***trans*-273, *cis*-275**	(Horio et al., 1993)
Concolvulaceae	*Ipomoea aquatica*		***cis*-266, *trans*-266**	(Tseng et al., 1992)
Euphobiaceae	*Antidesma membranaceum*		***trans*-266, *cis*-277, *trans*-277**	(Buske et al., 1997)
Flacourtiaceae	*Casearia membranacea*		***cis*-266, *trans*-266**	(Chang et al., 2003)
Fumariaceae	*Dactylicapnos torulosa*		***trans*-266**	(Rucker et al., 1994)
Hernandiaceae	*Sparattanthelium tupiniquinorum*		***trans*-264, *trans*-266**	(Pereira et al., 2007)
Lauraceae	*Actinodaphne longifolia*		***trans*-266, *trans*-273**	(Tanaka et al., 1989)
Leguminosae	*Mucuna birdwoodiana*		***trans*-266**	(Goda et al., 1987)
Magnoliaceae	*Michelia alba*		***cis*-266, *trans*-266**	(Chen et al., 2008)
Malvaceae	*Hibiscus taiwanensis*		***cis*-266, *trans*-266**	(Wu et al., 2005)
Menispermaceae	*Sinomenium acutum*		**266**	(Otsuka et al., 1993)
Nyctagenaceae	*Mirabilis jalapa*		***trans*-273**	(Michalet et al., 2007)
Papaveraceae	*Hypecoum*	*imberbe*	***trans*-266**	(Hussain et al., 1982)
		parviflorum	***trans*-266**	
Piperaceae	*Peperomia duclouxii*		**268, *trans*-274, *trans*-271, 283**	(Li et al., 2007)
Plumbaginaceae	*Ceratostigma willmottianum*		***trans*-265, *trans*-266**	(Yue et al., 1997)
Polygonaceae	*Eskemukerjea megacarpum*		***trans*-266**	(Miyaichi et al., 2006)
Portulacaceae	*Portulaca oleracea*		***trans*-266**	(Mizutani et al., 1998)
Rutaceae	*Evodia belahe*		**279**	(Pedersen et al. , 2010)
	Pleiospermium alatum		**284, 285**	(Chatterjee et al., 1975)
	Zanthoxylum syncarpum		**280, 281, 282**	(Ross et al., 2005)
Solanaceae	*Solanum*	*khasianum*	***cis*-264, *trans*-264, *cis*-266, *trans*-266, *cis*-277, *trans*-277, *cis*-278, *trans*-278**	(Muhlenbeck et al., 1996)
		lycopersicum	**264, 266, 272, 273**	(Zacares et al., 2007)
		citrullifolium	***trans*-266**	(Turnock et al., 2001)
	Cestrum lanatum		***trans*-266**	
Zygophyllaceae	*Tribulus terrestris*		**24, *trans*-265, 271, 263**	(Lv et al., 2008)

Table 9. Distribution of alkamides including both acid and amide residues.

These alkamides have been associated with diverse biological activities, such as the potentiation of antibiotics, inhibition of prostaglandin biosynthesis, antioxidant activity and more. Furthermore, cinnamoylphenethylamines have been suggested to have an impact on human health if present in the diet (Pedersen et al., 2010).

Some dimeric alkamides have been isolated from *Cannabis sativa* (Cannabinaceae, Sakakibara et al., 1991) (fig. 8).

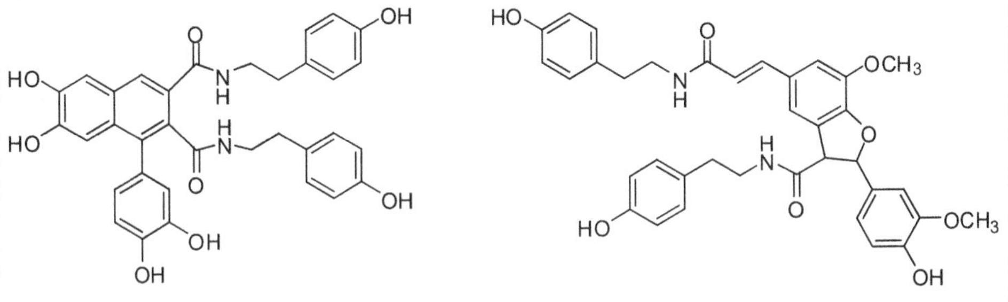

cannabisin A (**288**)   Grossamine (**289**)

Fig. 8. Dimeric alkamides from *Cannabis sativa*.

5. Conclusion

Alkamides are natural products distributed among several medicinal plants that are a part of at least 33 families. These plants are used for a variety of medicinal purposes in many places throughout the world. Chemical and pharmacological research of these plants have established that alkamides contribute to the notable bioactivity of these plants. Asteraceae, Solanaceae, Rutaceae and Piperaceae are plant families that specialize in the biosynthesis of these natural products. Importantly, alkamides are chemical markers for plants in each family and genus.

Alkamides with both acid and amine aliphatic residues are characteristic compounds produced by the Asteraceae family, especially from the *Achillea*, *Acmella*, *Spilanthes*, *Echinaceae* and *Heliopsis* genera. Alkamides with one aromatic residue can be classified in the following two groups: (1) alkamides with an aromatic residue at the amine core and (2) alkamides with an aromatic residue at the acid. The first group has been isolated from the Solanaceae family, specifically from the *Capsicum* genus for which those alkamides are named "capsaicinoids". Other alkamides that belong to this group have been isolated from the *Lepidium* (Brassicaceae) and *Glycosmis* (Rutaceae) genera. *Glycosmis* alkamides are rare and have characteristic sulfur-containing structures. The second group corresponds to piperine and its analogs. These compounds are characteristic of the *Piper* genus (Piperaceae). Furthermore, the alkamides with both acid and amine aromatic residues are widely distributed among at least 28 plant families. Feruloyltyramine and *p*-coumaroyltyramine are the most commonly isolated alkamides that belong to this group of compounds.

Pure alkamides and plants that produce alkamides have a pungent and/or irritating taste as well as analgesic and anesthetic effects. Many alkamides are used to treat dental, muscular and arthritic pain. Some alkamides are also consumed to enhance immune response and to relieve colds, respiratory infections and influenza. Anti-inflammatory activity is associated with all of these natural products. Despite the relatively simple structures of alkamides, these compounds have attracted several research groups to study their diversity, distribution and chemical and pharmacological behaviours. Additionally, alkamides have been observed to exhibit many other bioactivities, making these compounds a relatively new and promising family of natural products.

6. Acknowledgments

To CONACyT (Grant number 79584-Q). I am grateful to Enrique Salazar Leyva for technical assistance. I apologize to all colleagues whose studies were not cited due to space limitations.

7. References

Acosta-Madrid, I.I.; Castañeda-Hernández, G.; Cilia-López, V.G.; Cariño-Cortés, R.; Pérez-Hernández, N. Fernández-Martínez, E. & Ortiz, M.I. (2009). Interaction between *Heliopsis longipes* extract and diclofenac on the thermal hyperalgesia test. *Phytomedicine*, Vol.16, No.4, (April 2009), pp. 336–341, doi:10.1016/j.phymed.2008.12.014

Alam, A.H.M.K.; Sadik, G.; Harun, O.R.; Hasan, C.M. & Rashid, M.A. (2003). *N-trans*-feruloyl-4-methyldopamine from *Achyranthes ferruginea*. *Biochemical Systematics and Ecology*, Vol.31, No.11, (November 2003), pp. 1345–1346, doi:10.1016/S0305-1978(03)00115-7

Antunes, P.A.; Chierice, G.O.; Constantino, C.J.L. & Aroca, R.F. (2001). Spectroscopic characterization of N-isobutyl-6-p-methoxyphenyl) 2E,4E-hexadieneamide extracted from *Ottonia propinqua*. *Vibrational Spectroscopy*, Vol.27, No.2, (December 1989), pp. 175–181, doi:10.1016/S0924-2031(01)00132-1

Bauer, R. & Remiger, P. (1989a). TLC and HPLC analysis of alkamides in *Echinaceae* drugs. *Planta Medica*, Vol.55, No.4, (January 1989), pp. 367–371, doi:10.1055/s-2006-962030

Bauer, R.; Remiger, P. & Wagner, H. (1989b). Alkamides from the roots of *Echinaceae angustifolia*. *Phytochemistry*, Vol.28, No.2, (September 1989), pp. 505–508, doi:10.1016/0031-9422(89)80042-1

Bauer, R. & Foster, S. (1991). Analysis of alkamides and caffeic acid derivatives from *Echinaceae simulata* and *Echinaceae paradoxa* roots. *Planta Medica*, Vol.57, No.5, (October 1991), pp. 447–449, doi:10.1055/s-2006-960147

Bauer, R.; Reming, P. & Alstat, E. (1990). Alkamides and caffeic acid derivatives from the roots of *Echinaceae tennesseensis*. *Planta Medica*, Vol.67, No.6, (December 1990), pp. 533–534

Bezerra, D.P.;Vasconcellos, M.C.; Machado, M.S.; Villela, I.V. ; Rosa, R.M.; Moura, D.J.; Pessoa, C.; Moraes, M.O.; Silveira, E.R.; Lima M.A.S.; Aquino, N.C.; Henriques, J.A.P.; Saffi, J. & Costa-Lotufo, L.V. (2009). Piplartine induces genotoxicity in eukaryotic but not in prokaryotic model systems. *Mutation Research*, Vol.677, No.1-2, (June-July 2009), pp. 8–13, doi: 10.1016/j.mrgentox.2009.04.007

Binns, S.E.; Hudson, J. ; Merali, S. & Arnason, J.T. (2002). Antiviral activity of characterized extracts from *Echinaceae* spp. (Heliantheae : Asteraceae) against *Herpes simplex* virus (HSV-1). *Planta Medica*, Vol 68, No.9, (September 2002), pp. 780–783, doi:10.1055/s-2002-34397

Bohlmann, F.; Ziesche, J.; Robinson, H. & King, M.R. (1980). Neue amide aus *Spilanthes alba*. *Phytochemistry*, Vol.19, No.7, (July 1980), pp. 1535–1537, doi: 10.1016/0031-9422(80)80212-3

Bohlmann, F.; Hartono, L. & Jakupovic, J. (1985). Highly unsaturated amides from *Salmea scandens*. *Phytochemistry*, Vol.24, No.3, (March 1985), pp. 595–596, doi: 10.1016/S0031-9422(00)80774-8

Booonen, J.; Baert, L.; Burvenich, C.; Blondeelc, P.; De Saegerd, S. & De Spiegeleera B. (2010). LC–MS profiling of *N*-alkylamides in *Spilanthes acmella* extract and the transmucosal behaviour of its main bioactive spilanthol. *Journal of Pharmaceutical and Biomedical Analysis*, Vol.53, No.3, (November 2010), pp. 243–249, doi:10.1016/j.jpba.2010.02.010

Buske, A.; Schmidt, J.; Porzel, A. & Adam, G. (1997). Benzopyranones and ferulic acid derivatives from *Antidesma membranaceum*. *Phytochemistry*, Vol.46, No.8, (December 1997), pp. 1385–1388, doi:10.1016/S0031-9422(97)00488-3

Calle, J.; Rivera, A. ; Reguero, M.T. ; del Rio, R.E. & Joseph-Nathan, P. (1988). Estudio del espilantol usando técnicas de resonancia magnética nuclear en dos dimensiones. *Revista Latinoamericana de Quimica*, Vol.19, pp. 94–97

Campos-Cuevas, J.C; Pelagio-Flores, R.; Raya-Gonzalez, J.; Mendez-Bravo, A.; Ortiz-Castro, R. & Lopez-Bucio, J. (2008). Tissue culture of *Arabidopsis thaliana* explants reveals a stimulatory effect of alkamides on adventitious root formation and nitric oxide accumulation. *Plant Science*, Vol.174, No.2, (February 2008), pp. 165–173, doi:10.1016/j.plantsci.2007.11.003

Cariño-Cortés, R.; Gayosso-De-Lucio, J.A.; Ortiz, M.I.; Sánchez-Gutiérrez, M.; García-Reyna, P.B.; Cilia-López, V.G.; Pérez-Hernández, N.; Moreno, E. & Ponce-Monter H. (2010). Antinociceptive, genotoxic and histopathological study of *Heliopsis longipes* S.F. Blake in mice. *Journal of Ethnopharmacology*, Vol.130, No.2, (July 2010), pp. 216–221, doi:10.1016/j.jep.2010.04.037

Casado, M.; Ortega, M.G. ; Peralta, M.; Agnese, A.M. & Cabrera, J.L. (2009). Two new alkamides from roots of *Acmella decumbens*. *Natural Product Research*, Vol.23, No.14, (September 2009), pp. 1298–1303, doi:10.1080/14786410802518201

Cech, N.B.; Tutor, K.; Doty, B.A.; Spelman, K.; Sasagawa, M.; Raner, G.M. & Wenner, C.A. (2006). Liver enzyme-mediated oxidation of *Echinacea purpurea* alkylamides: Production of novel metabolites and changes in immunomodulatory activity. *Planta Medica*, Vol.72, No.15, (December 2006), pp. 1372–1377, doi:10.1055/s-2006-951718

Chang, K.C.; Duh, C.Y.; Chen, I.S. & Tsai, I.L. (2003). A cytotoxic butenolide, two new dolabellane diterpenoids, a chroman and a benzoquinol derivative Formosan *Casearia membranacea*. *Planta Medica*, Vol.69, No.7, (July 2003), pp. 667–672, doi:10.1055/s-2003-41120

Chatterjee, A.; Chakrabarty, M. & Kundu, A.B. (1975). Constituenys of *Pleiospermium alatum*: alatamide and *N*-benzoyltyramine methyl ether. *Australian Journal Chemistry*, Vol.28, No.2, (March 1975), pp. 457–460, doi:10.1071/CH9750457

Chen, C.Y.; Chang, F.R.; Yen, H.F. & Wu, Y.C. (1998). Amides from stems of *Annona cherimola*. *Phytochemistry*, Vol.49, No.5, (November 1998), pp. 1443–1447, doi:10.1016/S0031-9422(98)00123-X

Chen, I.-S.; Chen, T.-L.;Lin, W.-Y.; Tsai, I.-L. & Chen, Y.-Ch.(1999). Amides from stems of Isobutylamides from the fruit of *Zanthoxylum integrifoliolum*. *Phytochemistry*, Vol.52, No.2, (September 1999), pp. 357–360, doi: 10.1016/S0031-9422(99)00175-2

Chen, C.Y.; Huang, L.Y.; Chen, L.J.; Lo, W.L.; Kuo, S.Y.; Wang, Y.D.; Kuo, S.H. & Hsieh, T.J. (2008). Chemical constituents from the leaves of *Michelia alba*. *Chemistry of Natural Compounds*, Vol.44, No.1, (January 2008), pp. 137–139, doi: 10.1007/s10600-008-0043-7

Chen, Y.; Fu, T.; Tao, T.; Yang, J.; Chang, Y.; Wang, M.; Kim, L.; Qu, L.; Cassdy, J.; Scalzo, R. & Wang, X. (2005). Macrophage Activating Effects of New Alkamides from the Roots of *Echinacea* Species. *Journal of Natural Products*, Vol.68, No.5, (April 2005), pp. 773–776, doi:10.1021/np040245f

Claros, B.M.G.; da Silva, A.J.R.; Vasconcellos, M.L.A.A.; de Brito, A.P.P. & Leitao, G.G. (2000). Chemical constituents of two *Mollinedia* species. *Phytochemistry*, Vol.55, No.7, (December 2000), pp. 859–862, doi:10.1016/S0031-9422(00)00294-6

Continguiba, F.; Regasini, L.O.; Bolzani, V.S.; Debonsi, H.M.; Passerina G.D.; Barreto, R.M. ; Kato, M.J. & Furlan, M. (2009). Piperamides and their derivatives as potential anti-trypanosomal agents. *Medicinal Chemistry Research*, Vol.18, No.9, (December 2009), pp. 703–711, doi:10.1007/s00044-008-9161-9

Costa, S.S. & Mors, W.B. (1981). Amides from *Ottonia corcovadensis*. *Phytochemistry*, Vol.20, No.6, (June 1981), pp. 1305–1305, doi:10.1016/0031-9422(81)80027-1

Das, B. ; Kashinatham, A. & Srinivas, N.S. (1996). Alkamides and other constituents of *Piper longum*. *Planta Medica*, Vol.62, No.6, (December 1996), pp. 582–582

Déciga-Campos, M.; Rios, M.Y. & Aguilar-Guadarrama, B. (2010). Antinociceptive effect of *Heliopsis longipes* extract and affinin in mice. *Planta Medica*, Vol.76, No.7, (May 2010), pp. 665–670, doi:10.1055/s-0029-1240658

Dominguez, X.A. ; Sánchez, H. ; Slim, J.S. ; Jakupovic, J. ; Lehmann, L. & Bohlmann, F. (1987). Highly unsaturated amides from *Sanvitalia oxymoides*. *Revista Latinoamericana de Quimica*, Vol.18, pp. 114–115

Goda, Y.; Shibuya, M. & Sankawa, U. (1987). Inhibitors of prostaglandin biosynthesis from *Mucuna birdwoodiana*. *Chemical & Pharmaceutical Bulletin*, Vol.35, No.7, (July 1987), pp. 2675–2677

Greger, H.; Hofer, O. & Werner, A. (1985). New amides from *Sphilanthes oleracea*. *Monatshefte fur Chemie*, Vol.116, No.2, (February 1985), pp. 273–277, doi:10.1007/BF00798463

Greger, H.; Hofer, O. & Werner, A. (1987a). Biosynthetically simple C_{18}-alkamides from *Achillea* species. *Phytochemistry*, Vol.26, No.8, (December 1986), pp. 2235–2242, doi:10.1016/S0031-9422(00)84690-7

Greger, H.; Zdero, C. & Bolhmann, F. (1987b). Pyrrole amides from *Achillea ageratifolia*. *Phytochemistry*, Vol.26, No.8, (December 1986), pp. 2289–2291, doi:10.1016/S0031-9422(00)84703-2

Greger, H. (1987c). Highly unsaturated isopentyl amides from *Achillea wilhelmsii*. *Journal of Natural Products*, Vol.50, No.6, (November 1987), pp. 1100–1107, doi:10.1021/np50054a015

Greger, H. & Hofer, O. (1989). Polyenic acid piperideides ando other alkamides from *Achillea millefolium*. *Phytochemistry*, Vol.28, No.9, (September 1989), pp. 2363–2368, doi:10.1016/S0031-9422(00)97985-8

Greger, H. & Hofer, O. (1990). Alkamides and polyacetylenes: two different biogenetic trends in the European *Achillea millefolium* group. *Planta Medica*, Vol.56, No.6, (December 1990), pp. 531–532, doi:10.1055/s-2006-961094

Greger, H. & Werner, A. (1990). Comparative HPLC analyses of alkamides within the *Achillea millefolium* group. *Planta Medica*, Vol.56, No.5, (October 1990), pp. 482–486, doi:10.1055/s-2006-961017

Greger, H.; Hadacek, F.; Hofer, O.; Wurz, G.; & Zechner, G. (1993a). Different types of sulphur-containing amides from *Glycosmis* cf. *chlorosperma*. *Phytochemistry*, Vol.32, No.4, (March 1993), pp. 933–936, doi:10.1016/0031-9422(93)85232-G

Greger, H.; Zechner, G.; Hofer, O.; Hadacek, F.; & Wurz, G. (1993b). Sulphur-containing amides from *Glycosmis* species with different antifungal activity. *Phytochemistry*, Vol.34, No.1, (August 1993), pp. 175–179, doi:10.1016/S0031-9422(00)90802-1

Greger, H.; Hofer, O.; Zechner, G.; Hadacek, F. & Wurz, G. (1994). Sulphones derived from methylthiopropenoic acid amides from *Glycosmis angustifolia*. *Phytochemistry*, Vol.37, No.5, (November 1994), pp. 1305–1310, doi:10.1016/S0031-9422(00)90403-5

Greger, H. & Hofer, O. (1996). Bioactive amides from *Glycosmis* species. *Journal of Natural Products*, Vol.59, No.12, (December 1996), pp. 1163–1168, doi:10.1021/np9604238

Ghosal, S.; Chakrabarti, D.K. (1988). Differences in phenolic and steroidal constituents between healthy and infected florets of *Mangifera indica*. *Phytochemistry*, Vol.27, No.5, (August 1987), pp. 1339–1343, doi:10.1016/0031-9422(88)80189-4

Herz, W. & Kulanthaivel, P. (1985). An amide from *Salmea scandens*. *Phytochemistry*, Vol.24, No.1, (January 1985), pp. 173–174, doi:10.1016/S0031-9422(00)80830-4

Holzbach J.C. & Lopes L.M.X. (2010). Aristolactams and Alkamides of *Aristolochia gigantea*. *Molecules*, Vol.15, No.12, (December 2010), pp. 9462-9472; doi:10.3390/molecules15129462

Horio, T.; Yoshida, K.; Kikuchi, H.; Kawabata, J. & Mizutani, J. (1993). A phenolic amide from roots of *Chenopodium album*. *Phytochemistry*, Vol.33, No.4, (July 1993), pp. 807–808, doi:10.1016/0031-9422(93)85278-Y

Huang, H.; Morgan, C.M.; Asolkar, R.N.; Kiovunen, M.E. & Marrone, P.G. (2010). Phytotoxicity of Sarmentine Isolated from Long Pepper (*Piper longum*) Fruit. *Journal of Agricultural and Food Chemistry*, Vol.58, No.18, (August 2010), pp. 9994–10000, doi:10.1021/jf102087c

Hussain, S.F.; Gozler, B.; Shamma, M.; Gozler, T. (1982). Feruloyltyramine from *Hypecoum*. *Phytochemistry*, Vol.21, No.12, (December 1982), pp. 2979–2980, doi:10.1016/0031-9422(80)85081-3

Islam, T.; Hashidoko, Y.; Ito, T.; Tahara, S. (2004). Interruption of the homing events of phytopathogenic Aphanomyces cochlioides zoospores by secondary metabolites from nonhost *Amaranthus gangeticus*. *Journal of Pesticide Science*, Vol.29, No.1, (January 2004), pp. 6–14, doi:10.1584/jpestics.29.6

Johns, T. ; Graham, K. & Towers, G.H.N. (1982). Molluscicidal activity of affinin and other isobutylamides from the Asteraceae. *Phytochemistry*, Vol.21, No.11, (November 1982), pp. 2737–2738, doi:10.1016/0031-9422(82)83110-5

Kim, D.K.; Lim, J.P.; Kim, J.W.; Park, H.W. & Eun, J.S. (2005). Antitumor and antiinflammatory constituents from *Celtis sinensis. Archives of Pharmacal Research*, Vol.28, No.1, (January 2005), pp. 39–43, doi:10.1007/BF02975133

Kobata, k.; Saito, K.; Tate, H.; Nashimoto, A.; Okuda, H.; Takemura, I.; Miyakawa, K.; Takahashi, M.; Iwai, K. & Watanabe, T. (2010). Long-Chain N-Vanillyl-acylamides from. *Journal of Agricultural and Food Chemistry*, Vol.58, No.6, (March 2010), pp. 3627–3631, doi:10.1021/jf904280z

Kozukue, N.; Han, J.-S.; Kozukue, E.; Lee, S.-J.; Kim, J.-A.; Lee, K.-R.; Levin, C.E. & Friedman, M. (2005). Analysis of Eight Capsaicinoids in Peppers and Pepper-Containing Foods by High-Performance Liquid Chromatography and Liquid Chromatography–Mass Spectrometry. *Journal of Agricultural and Food Chemistry*, Vol.53, No.23, (October 2005), pp. 9172–9181, doi:10.1021/jf050469j

Lazarevic, J.; Radulovic, N.; Zlatkovic. B. & Palic, R. (2010). Composition of *Achillea distans* Willd. subsp. *distans* root essential oil. *Natural Product Research*, Vol.24, No.8, (May 2010), pp. 718–731, doi:10.1080/14786410802617292

Lalone, C.A.; Huang, N.; Rizshsky, L.; Yum, M.-Y.; Singh, N.; Hauck, C.; Nicolau, B.J.; Wurtele, E.S.; Kohut, M.L.; Murphy, P.A. & Birt, D.F (2010). Enrichment of *Echinacea angustifolia* with Bauer alkylamide 11 and Bauer ketone 23 increased anti-inflammatory potential through interference with COX-2 enzyme activity. *Journal of Agricultural and Food Chemistry*, Vol.58, No.15, (December 2010), pp. 8573–8584, doi:10.1021/jf1014268

Lee, S.W.; Rho, M.-Ch.; Nam. J.Y.; Lim, E.H.; Kwon, O.E.; Kim, Y.H.; Lee, H.S. & Kim, Y.K. (2004). Guineensine, an acyl-CoA: cholesterol acyltransferase inhibitor, from the fruits of *Piper longum. Planta Medica*, Vol.70, No.7, (July 2004), pp. 678–679, doi:10.1055/s-2004-827193

Lee, S.W.; Kim, Y.K.; Kim, K.; Lee, H.S.; Choi, J.H.; Lee, W.S.; Jun, Ch.-D.; Park, J.H.; Lee, J.M.; & Rho, M.-Ch. (2008). Alkamides from the fruits of *Piper longum* and *Piper nigrum* displaying potent cell adhesion inhibition. *Bioorganic & Medicinal Chemistry Letters*, Vol.18, No.16, (August 2008), pp. 4544–4546, doi:10.1016/j.bmcl.2008.07.045

Lee, S.W.; Rho, M.-Ch.; Park, H.R.; Choy, J.-H.; Kang, J.Y.; Lee, J.W. & Kim, Y.K. (2006). Inhibition of Diacylglycerol Acyltransferase by Alkamides Isolated from the Fruits of *Piper longum* and *Piper nigrum. Journal of Agricultural and Food Chemistry*, Vol.54, No.26, (December) 2006, pp. 9759–9763, doi:10.1021/jf061402e

Li, N.; Wu, J.L.; Hasegawa, T.; Sakai, J.; Bai, L.M.; Wang, L.Y.; Kakuta, S.; Furuya, Y.; Ogura, H.; Kataoka, T.; Tomida, A.; Tsuruo, T. & Ando, M. (2007) Bioactive polyketides from *Peperomia duclouxii. Journal of Natural Products*, Vol.70, No.6, (June 2007), pp. 998–1001, doi:10.1021/np070089n

Lv, A.L.; Zhang, N.; Sun, M.G.; Huang, Y.F.; Sun, Y.; Ma, H.Y.; Hua, H.M. & Pei, Y.H. (2008). One new cinnamic imide derivative from the fruits of *Tribulus terrestris. Natural Products Research*, Vol.22, No.11, (July 2008), pp. 1007–1010, doi:10.1080/14786410701654867

López-Martínez, S.; Aguilar-Guadarrama, A.B. & Rios, M.Y. (2011). Minor alkamides from *Heliopsis longipes* S.F. Blake (Asteraceae) fresh roots. *Phytochemistry Letters*, Vol.4, No.3, (September 2011), pp. 275–279, doi:10.1016/j.phytol.2011.04.014

Martin, R. & Becker, H. (1984). Sphilanthol related amides from *Acmella ciliata*. *Phytochemistry*, Vol.23, No.8, (August 1984), pp. 1781–1783, doi:10.1016/S0031-9422(00)83490-1

Martin, R. & Becker, H. (1985). Amides and other constituents from *Acmella ciliata*. *Phytochemistry*, Vol.24, No.10, (October 1985), pp. 2295–3000, doi:10.1016/S0031-9422(00)83030-7

McFerren, M.A.; Cordova, D.; Rodriguez, E; & Rauh, J.J. (2002). In vitro neuropharmacological evaluation of piperovatine, an isobutylamide from *Piper piscatorum* (Piperaceae). *Journal of Ethnopharmacology*, Vol.83, No.3, (December 2002), pp. 201–207, doi:10.1016/S0378-8741(02)00224-6

Meghvansi, M.K.; Siddiqui, S.; Khan, Md. H.; Gupta, V.K.; Vairale, M.G.; Gogoi, H.K.; & Singh, L. (2010). Naga chilli: A potential source of capsaicinoids with broadspectrum ethnopharmacological applications. *Journal of Ethnopharmacology*, Vol.132, No.1, (October 2010), pp. 1–14, doi:10.1016/j.jep.2010.08.034

Michalet, S.; Cartier, G.; David, B.; Mariotte, A.M.; Dijoux-Franca, M.G.; Kaatz, G.W.; Stavri, M. & Gibbons, S. (2007). N-Caffeoylphenalkylamide derivatives as bacterial efflux pump inhibitors. *Bioorganic & Medicinal Chemistry Letters*, Vol.17, No.6, (March 2007), pp.1755–1758, doi:10.1016/j.bmcl.2006.12.059

Miyaichi, Y.; Nunomura, N.; Kawata, Y.; Kizu, H.; Tomimori, T.; Watanabe, T.; Takano, A. & Malla, K.J. (2006). Studies on Nepalese crude drugs. XXVIII. Chemical constituents of Bhote Khair, the underground parts of *Eskemukerjea megacarpum* HARA. *Chemical & Pharmaceutical Bulletin*, Vol.54, No.1, (January 2006), pp. 136–138, doi:10.1248/cpb.54.136

Mizutani, M.; Hashidoko, Y.; Tahara, S. (1998). Factors responsible for inhibiting the motility of zoospores of the phytopathogenic fungus Aphanomyces cochlioides isolated from the non-host plant *Portulaca oleracea*. *FEBS Letters*, Vol.438, No.3, (November 1998), pp. 236–240, doi:10.1016/S0014-5393(98)01308-8

Molina, J.; Salgado, R.; Ramírez, E. & del Río, R.E. (1996). Purely olefinic alkamides in *Heliopsis longipes* and *Acmella* (Spilanthes) *oppositifolia*. *Biochemical Systematics and Ecology*, Vol. 24, No.1, (January 1996), pp. 43–47, doi:10.1016/0305-1978(95)00099-2

Muhammad, I.; Zao, J.; Dumbar, D.C. & Khan, I.A. (2002). Constituents of *Lepidium meyenii* 'maca'. *Phytochemistry*, Vol.59, No.1, (January 2002), pp. 105–110, doi:10.1016/S0031-9422(01)00395-8

Muller-Jakic, B.; Breu, W.; Probstle, A.; Redl, K.; Greger, H. & Bauer, R. (1994). In vitro inhibition of cyclooxygenase and 5-lipoxygenase by alkamides from *Echinaceae* and *Achillea* species. *Planta Medica*, Vol.60, No.1, (February 1994), pp. 37–40, doi:10.1055/s-2006-959404

Muhlenbeck, U.; Kortenbusch, A. & Barz, W. (1996). Formation of hydroxycinnamoylamides and α-hydroxyacetovanillone in cell cultures of *Solanum khasianum*. *Phytochemistry*, Vol.42, No.6, (August 1996), pp. 1573–1579, doi:10.1016/0031-9422(96)00173-2

Navickiene, H.M.D.; Alecio, A.C.; Kato, M.J.; Bolzani, V.S.; Young, M.C.M.; Cavalheiro, A.J. & Furlan, M. (2000). Antifungal amides from *Piper hispidum* and *Piper tuberculatum*. *Phytochemistry*, Vol.55, No.6, (November 2000), pp. 621–626, doi:10.1016/S0031-9422(00)00226-0

Navickiene, H.M.D. & Lopes, L.M.X. (2001). Alkamides and phenethyl derivatives from *Aristolochia gehrtii*. *Journal of the Brazilian Chemical Society*, Vol. 12, No.4, (August 2001), pp. 467–472, doi:10.1590/S0103-50532001000400004

Nishioka, T.; Watanabe, J.; Kawabata, J. & Niki, R. (1997). Isolation and activity of *N*-p-coumaroyltyramine, an α-glucosidase inhibitor in Welsh onion (*Allium fistulosum*). *Bioscience, Biotechnology, and Biochemistry*, Vol.61, No.7, (July 1997), pp. 1138–1141, doi:10.1271/bbb.61.1138

Otsuka, H.; Ito, A.; Fujioka, N.; Kawamata, K.I.; Kasai, R.; Yamasaki, K. & Satoh, T. (1993). Butenolides from *Sinomenium acutum*. *Phytochemistry*, Vol.33, No.2, (May 1993), pp. 389–392, doi:10.1016/0031-9422(93)85525-V

Pandey, V.; Chopra, M. & Agrawal, V. (2011). In vitro isolation and characterization of biolarvicidal compounds from micropropagated plants of *Spilanthes acmella*. *Parasitol Research*, Vol.108, No.2, (February 2011), pp. 297–304, doi:10.1007/s00436-010-2056-y

Patnaik, T.; Dey, R.K. & Gouda, P. (2008). Antimicrobial activity of friedelan-3-β-ol and *trans-N*-caffeoyltyramine isolated from the root of *Vitis trifolia*. *Asian Journal Chemistry*, Vol.20, No.1, pp. 417–421

Patra, A. & Ghosh, A. (1974). Amides of *Piper chaba*. *Phytochemistry*, Vol.13, No.12, (December 1974), pp. 2889–2890, doi:10.1016/0031-9422(74)80272-4

Perry, N.B.; van Klink, J.W.; Burgess E.J. & Parmenter, G.A. (2000). Alkamide levels in *Echinaceae purpurea*: effects of processing, drying and storage. *Planta Medica*, Vol.66, No.1, (February 2000), pp. 54-56, doi:10.1055/s-2000-11111

Pedersen, H.A.; Steffenses S.K.; Christopherses C.; Mortensen, A.G.; Jorgensen L.N.; Niveyro, S.; de Troiani R.M.; Rodriguez-Enriquez, R.J.; Barba-de la Rosa, A.P. & Fomsgaard, I.S. (2010). Synthesis and Quantitation of Six Phenolic Amides in *Amaranthus* spp. *Journal of the Agricultural and Food Chemistry*, Vol.58, No.10, (May 2010), pp. 6306-6311, doi:10.1021/jf100002v

Pereira, C.A.B.; Oliveira, F.M.; Conserva, L.M.; Lemos, R.P.L. & Andrade, E.H.A. (2007). Cinnamoyltyramine derivatives and other constituents from *Sparattanthelium tupiniquinorum* (Hernandiaceae). *Biochemical Systematics and Ecology*, Vol.35, No.9, (September 2007), pp. 637–639, doi:10.1016/j.bse.2007.03.014

Perry, N.B.; van Klink, J.W.; Burgess E.J. & Parmenter, G.A. (1997). Alkamide levels in *Echinaceae purpurea*: a rapid analytical method revealing differences among roots, rhizomes, steams, leaves and flowers. *Planta Medica*, Vol.63, No.1, (February 1997), pp. 58-62, doi:10.1055/s-2006-957605

Rao, V.R.S.; Suresh, G.; Banu, K.S.; Raju, S.S.; Vishnu vardhan, M.V.P.S.; Ramakrishna, S. & Rao, M. (2011). Novel dimeric amide alkaloids from Piper chaba Hunter: isolation, cytotoxic activity, and their biomimetic synthesis. *Tetrahedron*, Vol.67, No.10, (March 2011), pp. 1885-1892, doi:10.1016/j.tet.2011.01.015

Ramsewak, R.S.; Erickson, A.J. & Nair, M.G. (1999). Bioactive *N*-isobutylamides from the flower buds of *Spilanthes acmella*. *Phytochemistry*, Vol.51, No.6, (July 1999), pp. 729–732, doi:10.1016/S0031-9422(99)00101-6

Rios-Chavez, P.; Ramirez-Chavez, E.; Armenta-Salinas, C. & Molina-Tores, J. (2003). Acmella radicans var. radicans: in vitro culture establishment and alkamide content. *In Vitro Cellular & Developmental Biology – Plant*. Vol.39, No.1, (January–February 2003), pp. 37–41, doi:10.1079/IVP2002354

Rios, M.Y.; Aguilar-Guadarrama, A.B. & Gutiérrez, M.C. (2007). Analgesic activity of affinin, an alkamide from *Heliopsis longipes* (Compositae). *Journal of Ethnopharmacology,* Vol.110, No.2, (March 2007), pp. 364-367, doi:10.1016/j.jep.2006.09.041

Rosario, S.L.; da Silva, A.J. & Parente, J.P. (1996). Alkamides from *Cissampelos glaberrima. Planta Medica,* Vol.62, No.4, (August 1996), pp. 376-377, doi:10.1055/s-2006-957913

Ross, S.A.; Al-Azeib, M.A.; Krishnaveni, K.S.; Fronczek, F.R. & Burandt, Ch.L. (2005). Alkamides from the Leaves of *Zanthoxylum syncarpum. Journal of Natural Products,* Vol.68, No.8, (August 2005), pp. 1297-1299, doi:10.1021/np0580558

Rucker, G.; Breitmaier, E.; Zhang, G.L. & Mayer, R. (1994). Alkaloids from *Dactylicapnos torulosa. Phytochemistry,* Vol.36, No.2, (May 1994), pp. 519–523, doi:10.1016/S0031-9422(00)97106-1

Saadali, B.; Boriky, D.; Blaghen, M.; Vanhaelen, M. & Talbi, M. (2001). Alkamides from *Artemisia dracunculus. Phytochemistry,* Vol.58, No.7, (December 2001), pp. 1083–1086, doi:10.1016/S0031-9422(01)00347-8

Sailaja, R. & Setty, O.H. (2006). Protective effect of *Phyllanthus fraternus* against allyl alcohol-induced oxidative stress in liver mitochondria. *Journal of Ethnopharmacology,* Vol.105, No.1-2, (April 2006), pp. 201–209, doi:10.1016/j.jep.2005.10.019

Sakakibara, I.; Katsuhara, T.; Ikeya, Y.; Hayashi, K. & Mitsuhashi, H. (1991). Cannabisin-A, an arylnaphthalene lignanamide from fruits of *Cannabis sativa. Phytochemistry,* Vol.30, No.9, (September 1991), pp. 3013–3016, doi:10.1016/S0031-9422(00)98242-6

Schulthess, B.H; Giger, E. & Baumann T.W. (1991). Echinaceae: anatomy, phytochemical patern, and germination of the achene. *Planta Medica,* Vol.57, No.4, (August 1991), pp. 384–388, doi:10.1055/s-2006-960123

Senchina, D.S.; Wu, L.; Flinn, G.N.; Konopa, D.L.; McCoy, J.-A.; Widrelechner, M.P.; Wurtele, E.S. & Kohut, M.L. (2006). Year-and-a-half old, dried Echinaceae roots retain cytokine-modulating capabilities in an in vitro human older adult model of influenza vaccination. *Planta Medica,* Vol.72, No.15, (December 2006), pp. 1207–1215, doi:10.1055/s-2006-957078

Sittie, A.A.; Lemmich, E.; Olsen, C.E.; Hviid, L. & Chistensen, S.B. (1998). Alkamides from *Phyllanthus fraternus. Planta Medica,* Vol.64, No.2, (March 1998), pp. 192–193, doi:10.1055/s-2006-957405

Subehan; Usia, T.; Kadota, S. & Tezika, Y. (2006). Mechanism-based inhibition of human liver microsomal cytochrome P450 2D6 (CYP2D6) by alkamides of *Piper nigrum. Planta Medica,* Vol. 72, No.6, (April 2006), pp. 527–532, doi:10.1055/s-2006-931558

Tanaka, H.; Nakamura, T.; Ichino, K. & Ito, K. (1989). A phenolic amide from *Actinodaphne longifolia. Phytochemistry,* Vol.28, No.9, (September 1989), pp. 2516–2517, doi:10.1016/S0031-9422(00)98022-1

Tofern, B.; Manna, P.; Kalogaa, M.; Jenett-Siemsa, K.; Witte, L. & Eicha, E. (1999). Aliphatic pyrrolidine amides from two tropical convolvulaceous species. *Phytochemistry,* Vol.52, No.8, (December 1999), pp. 1437–1441, doi:10.1016/S00319422(99)00245-9

Tseng, C.F.; Iwakami, S.; Mikajiri, A.; Shibuya, M.; Hanaoka, F.; Ebizuka, Y.; Padmawinata, K. & Sankawa, U. (1992). Inhibition of *in vitro* prostaglandin and leukotriene biosyntheses by cinnamoyl-β-phenethylamine and *N*-acyldopamine derivatives. *Chemical & Pharmaceutical Bulletin,* Vol.40, No.2, (February 1992), pp. 396–400

Turnock, J.; Cowan, S.; Watson, A.; Bartholomew, B.; Bright, C.; Latif, Z.; Sarker, S.D.; Nash, R.J. (2001). *N-trans*-feruloyltyramine from two species of the *Solanaceae. Biochemical*

Systematics and Ecology, Vol.29, No.2, (February 2001), pp. 209–211, doi:10.1016/S0305-1978(00)00030-2

Woelkar, K.; Xu, W.; Pei, Y.; Makriyannis, A.; Picone, R.P. & Bauer, R. (2005). The endocannabinoid system as a target for alkamides from *Echinaceae angustifolia* roots. *Planta Medica*, Vol.71, No.8, (August 2005), pp. 701-705, doi:10.1055/s-2005-871290

Wu, P.L.; Wu, T.S.; He, C.X.; Su, C.H. & Lee, K.H. (2005). Constituents from the stems of *Hibiscus taiwanensis*. *Chemical & Pharmaceutical Bulletin*, Vol.53, No.1, (January 2005), pp. 56–59, doi:10.1248/cpb.53.56

Wu, L.C.; Fan, N.C.; Lin, M.H.; Chu, I.R.; Huang, S.J.; Hu, C.Y. & Han, S.Y. (2008). Anti-inflammatory effect of spilanthol from *Spilanthes acmella* on murine macrophage by down-regulating LPS-induced inflammatory mediators. *Journal of the Agricultural and Food Chemistry*, Vol.56, No.7, (March 2008), pp. 2341–2349, doi:10.1021/jf073057e

Wu, T.-S..; Chang, F.-C. & Wu, P.-L. (1995). Flavonoids, amidosulfoxides and an alkaloid from the leaves of *Glycosmis citrifolia*. *Phytochemistry*, Vol.39, No.6, (August 1995), pp. 1453-1457, doi:10.1016/0031-9422(95)00171-3

Yue, J.M.; Xu, J.; Zhao, Y.; Sun, H.D. & Lin, Z.W. (1997). Chemical components from *Ceratostigma willmottianum*. *Journal of Natural Products*, Vol.60, No.10, (October 1997), pp. 1031–1033, doi:10.1021/np97004

Zacares, L.; Lopez-Gresa, M.P.; Fayos, J.; Primo, J.; Belles, J.M. & Conejero, V. (2007). Induction of *p*-coumaroyldopamine and feruloyldopamine, two novel metabolites, in tomato by the bacterial pathogen *Pseudomonas syringae*. *Mol. Plant-Microbe Interact.*, Vol.20, No.11, (November 2007), pp. 1439–1448, doi:10.1094/MPMI-20-11-1439

Zhao, J.; Muhammad, I.; Dunbar, D.Ch.; Mustafa, J. & Khan, I.A. (2005). New Alkamides from Maca (*Lepidium meyenii*). *Journal of the Agricultural and Food Chemistry*, Vol.53, No.3, (January 2005), pp. 690−693, doi:10.1021/jf048529t

7

Medicinal and Edible Plants as Cancer Preventive Agents

Ken Yasukawa
School of Pharmacy, Nihon University
Japan

1. Introduction

Cancer chemoprevention is currently one of the most urgent projects in public health. According to epidemiological surveys, the majority of human cancers are related to two factors; diet and smoking (Banning, 2005; Hirayama, 1984). However, in the general population, dairy consumption of certain foods has also been shown to have anticancer effects. This highlights the importance of environmental factors such as diet in cancer chemoprevention (Banning, 2005). It is also evident that an understanding of the mechanisms of carcinogenesis is essential for cancer chemoprevention. Most cancer prevention research is based on the concept of multistage carcinogenesis (Fig. 1.): initiation→promotion→progression (Piot & Dragan, 1991; Morse & Stoner, 1993). In contrast to both the initiation and progression stages, animal studies indicate that the promotion stage occurs over a long time period and may be reversible, at least early on. Therefore, the inhibition of tumor promotion is expected to be an efficient approach to cancer control (Sporn, 1976; Murakami, et al., 1996). Cancer chemoprevention is defined as the use of specific natural and synthetic chemical agents to reverse or suppress carcinogenesis and prevent the development of invasive cancers. There has been a growing awareness in recent years that dietary non-nutrient compounds can have important effects as chemopreventive agents, and considerable work on the cancer chemopreventive effects of such compounds in animal models has been undertaken. In the course of our research on potential antitumor-promoters (cancer chemopreventive agents) from edible plants and fungi, and from crude drugs, we have found that various triterpene alcohols and sterols and their oxygenated derivatives showed inhibitory effects on mouse ear inflammation induced by 12-*O*-tetradecanoylphorbol-13-acetate (TPA). We have recently reviewed the chemopreventive activities of naturally occurring terpenoids (Akihisa & Yasukawa, 2001; Akihisa, et al., 2003; Yasukawa, 2010). Primary prevention of cancer aims to avoid the development of cancer. Thus, it is important to inhibit the initiation and/or promotion of carcinogenesis. However, the adult population bears tumor cells that cannot revert to normal cells, and thus effective strategies to prevent cancer include avoiding continuous contact between these cells and promoters and/or aggressively inhibiting the tumor promoter effects. Therefore, to prevent cancer, it is essential to find effective compounds (anti-tumor promoters) that delay, inhibit or block tumor promotion, which is a reversible and long-term process. Active research is now being conducted using animal carcinogenesis models on cancer preventing substances contained in plants and vegetables. In this chapter I review the chemopreventive activity of natural sources, foods, supplements, crude drugs and Kampo medicines (traditional Japanese herbal prescriptions).

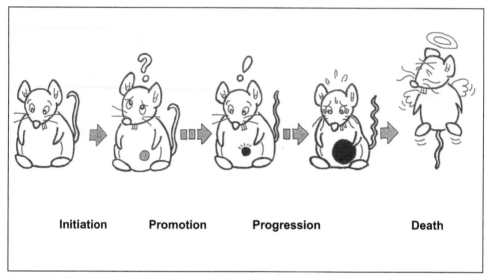

Initiation   **Promotion**   **Progression**   **Death**

Fig. 1. The theory of two-stage carcinogenesis.

2. Primary screening of antitumor promoters

In general, carcinogenesis has three stages: initiation, promotion and progression (Fig.1). Various bioassay systems are available in the literature for the screening of potentially chemopreventive compounds. Several convenient primary screening tests have been developed to evaluate compounds for their ability to inhibit tumor promotion. These tests are based on the activity of the tumor promoter TPA which has a wide range of activities. For example, at the biochemical level, TPA induces ornithine decarboxylase (ODC) in skin, activates protein kinase C (PKC), stimulates arachidonic acid release and prostaglandin synthesis, and generates superoxide anion radicals. At the cellular and tissue levels, TPA induces inflammation, blocks intercellular signal transduction, stimulates HL-60 cell aggregation and differentiation, and activates Epstein-Barr virus (EBV) (Ohigashi, et al., 1986). Screening tests for tumor promotion inhibition are based on these multiple activities, and based on inhibition of TPA-induced activity, a compound is presumed to be an anti-tumor promoter.

In addition, other tests using cells and enzymes are based on biochemical reactions. These include apoptosis induction, cell proliferation inhibition, cyclooxygenase-2 (COX-2) inhibition, cell differentiation enhancement, farnesyl protein transferase inhibition, phase II detoxification enzyme induction, lipoxygenase inhibition, ODC induction inhibition and superoxide production inhibition. The commonly used primary screening tests are described below.

2.1 Inhibition of TPA-induced inflammation

When TPA is applied to the auricle of mice, erythema and inflammation peak in 6 to 8 h, however erythema can still be observed after 24 h. Based on this phenomenon, testing is performed by applying the test substance before and after TPA application, then measuring auricular edema 6 h after TPA application to evaluate inhibitory activity (Yasukawa, et al., 1989).

2.2 Epstein-Barr virus activation inhibition test

In this test, using EBV non-producing Raji cells (human B lymphocytes) derived from Burkitt's lymphoma containing the EBV genome, TPA and the test substance are added in the presence of *n*-butanoic acid. After culturing for 48 h, indirect immunofluorescence is used to detect early antigen (EA) on the cell surface as an index of EBV activation inhibition by the test substance (Ohigashi, et al., 1986).

3. Anti-carcinogenic tests in animals

Compounds that show effectiveness in primary screening studies, particularly those with potent activity that are available in sufficient quantities, are then evaluated for inhibitory effects in animal model studies. In mice, application of the initiator 7,12-dimethylbenz[*a*]anthracene (DMBA) at trace amounts does not cause skin cancer, however subsequent application of the tumor promoter TPA eventually results in skin cancer (Skin-1; Table 1). Further studies with animal models have been performed for carcinogenesis of skin (Skin-2~Skin-7), bladder (Bladder), colon (Colon-1~Colon-3), liver (Liver-1~Liver-3), lung (Lung-1 and Lung-2), mammary (Mammary-1~Mammary-3), pancreas (Pancreas), tongue (Tongue), uterus (Uterus) and multi-organs (Multi), using natural sources (Table 1).

4. Supplemental and edible plants

While numerous anticarcinogens exist in the diet, an important question is how to use such substances in an effective, directed manner to reduce the cancer risk in humans. The concept of designer foods is one approach for accomplishing this goal, whereby foods would be engineered to contain effective levels of anticarcinogens. This approach is limited by the level of scientific knowledge on which to base such food design. Below, I describe a number of supplemental and edible plants that inhibited cancerogenesis in animal experiment.

4.1 Edible plants

Humans have used leaves as food since time immemorial. Different types of leaves, depending on location and season, have been part of the human diet since prehistoric times. There is historical documentation of certain edible leaves in ancient Greece and Rome and in the Middle ages. Plants of the families *Compositae, Cruciferae, Cucurbitaceae, Leguminosae, Liliaceae, Rutaceae* and *Zingiberaceae* have many kinds to use as vegetables. The following is an outline of the sources of these plants as well as edible fungi and mushrooms.

Code	Bioassay system	Reference
Bladder	Inhibition of N-butyl-N-(4-hydroxybutyl)-nitrosamine (BHBN)/sodium saccharin (SS) induced urinary tumors	Sugiyama, et al., 1994
Colon-1	Inhibition of azoxymethane (AOM) induced colon tumors	Vanamala, et al., 2006
Colon-2	Inhibition of 1,2-dimethylhydrazin (DMH) induced colon tumors	Fukushima, et a., 2001
Colon-3	Inhibition of N-methyl-N-nitrosourea (MNU) induced colon tumor	Narisawa, et al., 1991
Liver-1	Inhibition of diethylnitrosamine (DEN) induced hepatic tumors	Ognanesian, et al., 1997
Liver-2	Inhibition of Aflatoxin B$_1$ induced liver tumors	Manson,et al., 1998
Liver-3	Inhibition of DEN/phenobarbital induced liver tumors	Kapadia, et al., 2003
Lung-1	Inhibition of 4-(methylnitrosamino)-1-(3-pyridyl)-1-butanone (PhIP) induced lung tumors	Kohno, et al., 2001
Lung-2	Inhibition of 4-NQO/glycerol induced lung tumors	Konoshima, et al., 1994
Mammary-1	Inhibition of 2-amino-1-methyl-6-phenylimidazol[4,5-b]-pyridine induced mammary tumors	Ohta, et al., 2000
Mammary-2	Inhibition of 7,12-dimethylbenz[a]anthracene (DMBA) induced mammary tumors	Tanaka, et al., 1997a
Mammary-3	Inhibition of N-methyl-N-nitrosourea (MNU) induced mammary tumors	Bresnick, et al., 1990
Multi	Induction DEN, dihydroxy-di-N-propylnitrosamine (DHPN), MNU induced multi organ tumors	Kim, et al., 1997
Pancreas	Inhibition of N-nitrosobis-(2-oxopropyl)amine (BOP) induced pancreatic tumors	Birt, et al., 1987
Skin-1	Inhibition of DMBA/ 12-O-tetradecanoylphorbol-13-acetate (TPA) induced skin tumors	Slaga, et al., 1980
Skin-2	Inhibition of benzo[a]pyrene/croton oil induced skin tumors	Sadhana, et al., 1988
Skin-3	Inhibition of DMBA/ teleocidin induced skin tumors	Yoshizawa, et al., 1984
Skin-4	Inhibition of DMBA/ TPA+mezerein induced skin tumors	Perchellet, et al., 1990
Skin-5	Inhibition of DMBA/ ultra violet B (UVB) induced skin tumors	Kapadia, et al., 2003
Skin-6	Inhibition of DMBA/fumonisin B1 induced skin tumors	Takasaki, et al.,1999a
Skin-7	Inhibition of (+)-(E)-4-methyl 2[(E)-hydroxyimino]-5-nitro-6-methoxy-3-hexenamido (NOR-1)/TPA induced skin tumors	Konoshima, et al., 1999
Tongue	Inhibition of 4-NQO induced tongue tumors	Tanaka, et al., 1992
Uterus	Inhibition of MNU/estradiol-17β induced endometrial tumor	Niwa, et al., 2001

Table 1. Bioassay systems related to cancer chemopreventive activities described in this chapter.

4.1.1 *Compositae* plants and their components

Seventy-five methanol extracts obtained from 53 species in 11 tribes of *Compositae* plants were assayed, and *Carthmus tinctorius* (safflower), *Chrysanthemum morifolium* var. *sinensis* forma *esculentum* (edible chrysanthemum) and *Taraxacum officinale* (dandelion) markedly inhibited TPA-induced inflammation in mice (Yasukawa, et al., 1998a).

The artichoke (*Cynara cardunculus* L.) is a perennial thistle originating in Southern Europe around the Mediterranean. The total antioxidant capacity of artichoke flower heads is one of the highest reported for vegetables. Artichokes can also be made into a herbal tea. Topical application of the methanol extract of artichoke flowers suppressed tumor promotion by DMBA/TPA in mouse skin (Yasukawa, et al., 2010). Four triterpenes, α- and β-amyrin, taraxasterol and ψ-taraxasterol, and their acetates were isolated from the active fraction of this extract.

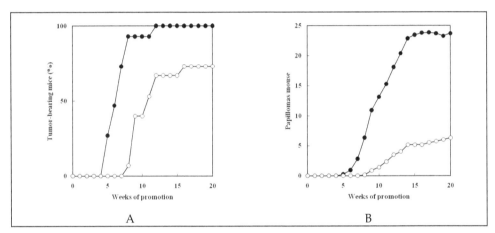

Fig. 2. Inhibitory effects of an artichoke methanol extract on skin papilloma promotion by DMBA/TPA in mice. One week after initiation with a single topical application of DMBA (50 μg), 1 μg of TPA was applied twice weekly. Topical application of the methanol extract (1 mg) and vehicle was performed 30 min before each TPA treatment. Data are expressed as the percentage of mice bearing papillomas (A), and as the average number of papillomas per mouse (B). ●, +TPA with vehicle alone; ○, +TPA with an artichoke methanol extract. (Yasukawa, et al., 2010).

Fig. 2A illustrates the time course of skin tumor formation in the groups treated with DMBA/TPA, with and without the methanol extract of artichoke flowers. The first tumor appeared at week 6 in the group treated with DMBA/TPA and all 15 mice had tumors at week 12. In the group treated with DMBA/TPA and a methanol extract of artichoke flowers, the first tumor appeared at week 8. The percentage of tumor-bearing mice treated with DMBA/TPA and a methanol extract of artichoke flowers was 73% at week 20. The group treated with DMBA/TPA produced 23.7 tumors per mouse at week 20, while the group treated with DMBA/TPA and a methanol extract of artichoke flowers had 6.3 tumors per mouse (Fig. 2B). Treatment with the methanol extract resulted in a 73% reduction in the average number of tumors per mouse at week 20 (Yasukawa, et al., 2010).

Edible chrysanthemum is a bitter aromatic herb that has been experimentally shown to lower fever, soothe inflammation, dilate the coronary arteries (increasing blood flow to the heart), and inhibit the growth of pathogens. It is used in folk medicine for hypertension, coronary artery disease, angina, feverish colds, and liver-related disorders. Triterpenoids were isolated from edible chrysanthemum flowers, and heliantriol C was found to be the major compound (Yasukawa, et al., 1996d). The activity of heliantriol C was ten times greater than other pentacyclic triterpenes against TPA-induced tumor promotion in mouse skin (Yasukawa, et al., 1998b).

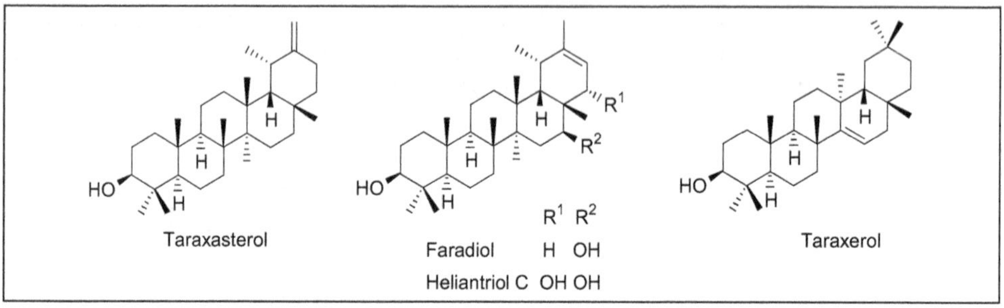

Taraxasterol

Faradiol   H   OH
Heliantriol C OH OH
R¹ R²

Taraxerol

Fig. 3. The chemical structures of triterpenoids from *Compositae* plants.

4.1.2 *Labiatae* plants and their components

Perilla is a very popular herb in Japan; it is mainly used as a garnish in the same way that parsley is used in Europe. The nettle-like leaves are bright green, reddish or purple. *Perilla frutescens* Britton var. *crispa* Decaisne is a bushy annual, native to southeast Asia, and has long been grown in China for the oil extracted from the its seeds. Perilla oil has been shown to inhibit colon carcinogenesis by MNU in rat (Narisawa, et al., 1991; 1994).

Rosmarinus officinalis L., commonly called rosemary, is a woody perennial herb with fragrant evergreen needle-like leaves that are often used in cooking. It has been found to act both as a stimulant and as a mild analgesic, and has been in folk use to treat headaches and epilepsy. Rosemary methanol extract suppressed tumor promotion by DMBA/TPA in mouse skin (Huang, et al., 1994). The active components, ursolic acid and carnosol, were isolated from the methanol extract, and were shown to inhibit DMBA/TPA-promoted two-stage carcinogenesis in mouse skin (Huang, et al., 1994).

Carnosol   Ursolic acid

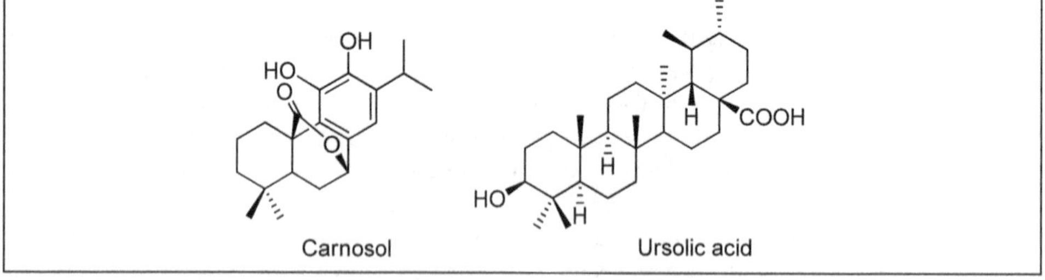

Fig. 4. The chemical structures of terpenoids from rosemary.

4.1.3 Grape and its components

Comparing diets among Western countries, researchers have discovered that although the French tend to eat higher levels of animal fat, their incidence of heart disease remains surprisingly low. This phenomenon has been termed the French Paradox, and is thought to occur from the protective benefits of regularly consuming red wine. Apart from the potential benefits of alcohol itself, including reduced platelet aggregation and vasodilation, polyphenols (e.g., resveratrol), found mainly in the grape skin, provide other suspected health benefits. The ethanol extract of grapes (*Vitis vinifera* L., *Vitaceae*) inhibited tumor promotion by DMBA/TPA in mouse skin (Alam, et al., 2002). In a model of liver carcinogenesis, tumor initiation was performed by a single intraperitoneal injection of DENA, followed by promotion with phenobarbital in the drinking water. Resveratrol dose-dependently reduced the incidence, total number and multiplicity of visible hepatocyte nodules (Bishayee & Dhir, 2009).

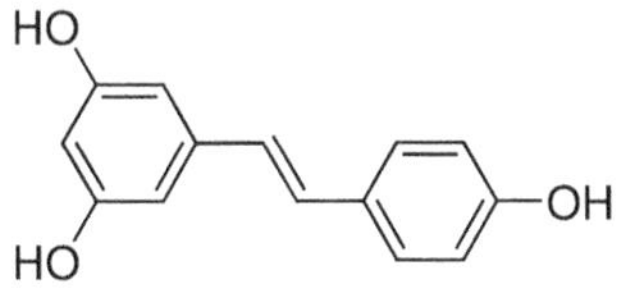

Resveratrol

Fig. 5. The chemical structure of resveratrol from grape.

On the other hand, grape seeds are a rich source of monomeric, dimeric and oligomeric proanthocyanidins. Commercial preparations of grape seed extracts are currently marketed as supplements due to their perceived potential health benefits, particularly as antioxidants. The polyphenolic fraction of grape seeds suppressed tumor promotion by DMBA/TPA in mouse skin (Bomser, et al., 1999; Zhao, et al., 1999). The mechanism of its activity is due, in part, to the inhibition of TPA-induced epidermal ODC and myeloperoxidase activities (Bomser, et al., 1999).

4.1.4 *Citrus* plants and their components

Citrus unshiu Marc. (*Rutaceae*) is a seedless, easy-peeling citrus mutant of Japanese origin. In Japan, it is known as mikan or formally unshu mikan. Its fruit is sweet, about the size of the mandarin orange *Citrus reticulate* Blanco. The peel has been used as a crude drug for gastric secretion promotion, anti-allergic action, inhibition of airway contraction, and sedative effect. Oral administration of unshu mikan juice inhibited colon carcinogenesis by azoxymethane (AOM) (Tanaka, et al., 2000), and lung carcinogenesis by 4-(methylnitrosamino)-1-(3-pyridyl)-1-butanone (NNK) in mice (Kohno, et al., 2001). Unshu mikan contains high amounts of β–cryptoxanthin and hesperidin. β–Cryptoxanthin was shown to inhibit colon carcinogenesis induced by MNU (Narisawa, et al., 1999), while hesperidin inhibited AOM-induced colon carcinogenesis in rat (Tanaka, et al., 1997b).

The grapefruit (*Citrus* × *paradisi* Macfad.), is a subtropical citrus tree known for its bitter fruit, an 18th-century hybrid first bred in Barbados. It is a good source of vitamin C, contains the fiber pectin, and the pink and red hues contain the antioxidant lycopene. Grapefruit pulp suppressed AOM-induced colon carcinogenesis in rat (Vanamala, et al., 2006). The active components limonin and naringin protected against AOM-induced aberrant crypt foci by suppressing proliferation and elevating apoptosis through anti-inflammatory activities.

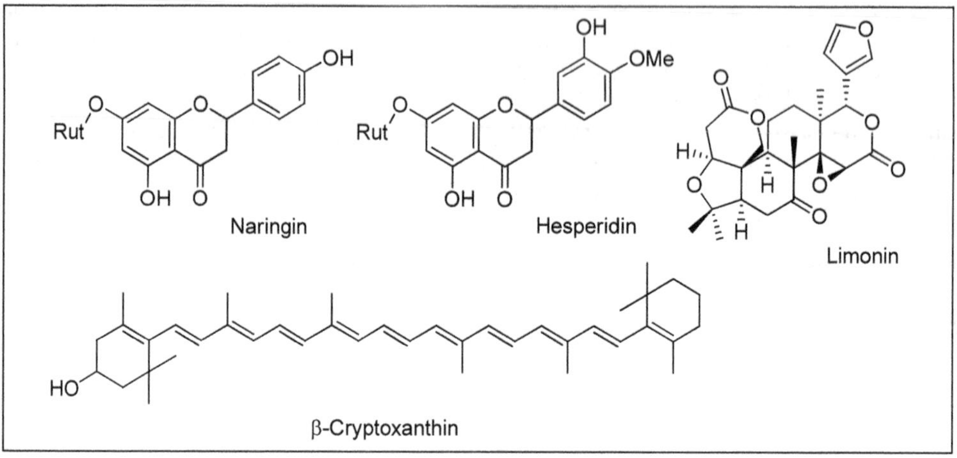

Fig. 6. The chemical structures of flavanons and terpenoids from *Citrus* spp.

4.1.5 Soy milk

Soy milk, sometimes referred to as soy drink/beverage, is a beverage made from soybean (*Glycine max* L., *Leguminosae*). Soy milk contains about the same proportion of protein as cow's milk. The coagulated protein from soy milk can be made into "tofu", just as milk can be made into cheese. Soy milk inhibited 4-(methylnitrosamino)-1-(3-pyridyl)-1-butanone-induced mammary carcinogenesis in rats (Ohta, et al., 2000). Soy beans contain high amounts of isoflavonoids and saponins; isoflavonoids have been shown to have phytoestrogenic activity (Moliteni, et al., 1995).

4.1.6 Cabbage and its components

The leafy green vegetable cabbage is a popular cultivar of the species *Brassica oleracea* L. (*Cruciferae*). It is a herbaceous, biennial, dicotyledonous flowering plant distinguished by a short stem upon which is crowned a mass of leaves, usually green but in some varieties red or purplish, and which forms a characteristic compact, globular cluster while immature. Cabbage is an excellent source of vitamin C and also contains significant amounts of glutamine, an amino acid that has anti-inflammatory properties. Along with broccoli and other brassica vegetables have been shown to include indole-3-carbinol (I3C). In European folk medicine, cabbage leaves are used to treat acute inflammation, and fresh cabbage juice has been shown to promote rapid healing of peptic ulcers. Oral administration of cabbage inhibited N-nitrosobis-(2-oxopropyl)amine (BOP)-induced pancreatic carcinogenesis in hamsters; however cabbage was not observed to inhibit tumor promotion by DMBA/TPA in mouse skin (Birt, et al., 1987). Oral intake of cabbage suppressed mammary carcinogenesis by N-methyl-N-nitrosourea (MNU) in rat (Bresnick, et al., 1990). In addition, I3C inhibited tumor promotion by DMBA/TPA in mouse skin (Srivastava & Shukla, 1998). DMBA-induced mammary carcinogenesis in rat (Grubbs, et al., 1995), tongue carcinogenesis in rat (Tanaka, et al., 1992), aflatoxin B_1-induced liver carcinogenesis in rat (Manson, et al., 1998), and DEN-induced liver carcinogenesis in mice (Oganesian, et al., 1997). However, I3C enhanced liver and thyroid gland neoplastic development when given during the promotion stage in a rat medium-term multi-organ carcinogenesis model (Kim, et al., 1997).

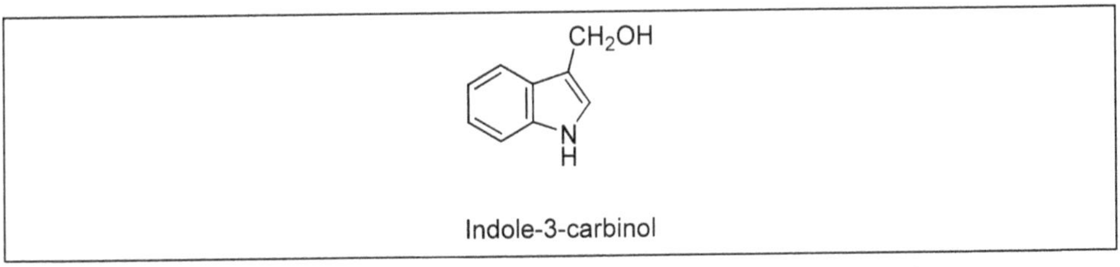

Indole-3-carbinol

Fig. 7. The chemical structure of indole-3-carbinol from cruciferous vegetables.

4.1.7 Green tea and its components

Green tea (the leaves of *Camellia sinensis* L., *Theaceae*) is derived from a perennial herbaceous plant native to southeastern Asia. Fujiki, et al. first reported that (-)-epigallocatechin gallate (EGCG), a component of green tea, inhibited tumor promotion by DMBA/teleocidin in mouse skin (Yoshizawa, et al., 1987). The polyphenolic fraction of green tea inhibited TPA-induced tumor promotion during two-stage carcinogenesis in SENCAR mouse skin, and also suppressed TPA-induced COX activity (Katijyar, et al., 1992). Green tea catechins inhibited DMBA-induced mammary gland carcinogenesis in female Sprague-Dawley rats (Tanaka, et al., 1997a). Fujiki et al. introduced a new theory in cancer prevention with regard to its mechanism of action: green tea catechins acting as a new class of chemical chaperones (Kuzuhara,et al., 2008). In a pilot study, green tea extract was shown to be an effective supplement for the chemoprevention of metachronous colorectal adenomas (Shimizu, et al., 2008).

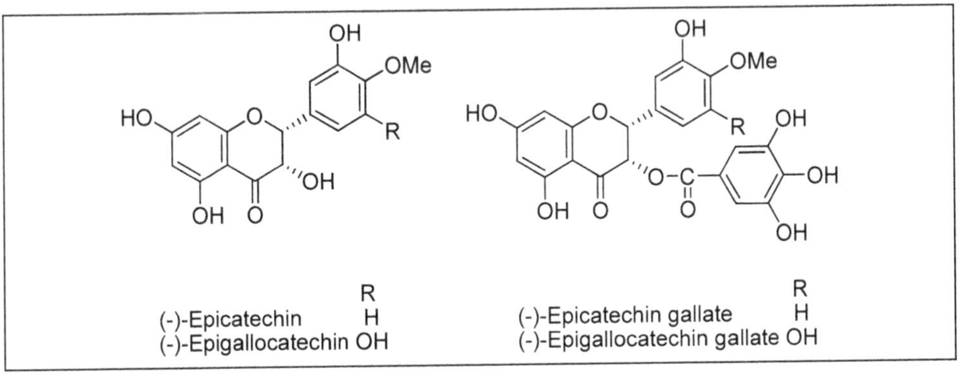

	R			R
(-)-Epicatechin	H		(-)-Epicatechin gallate	H
(-)-Epigallocatechin	OH		(-)-Epigallocatechin gallate	OH

Fig. 8. The chemical structures of polyphenolics from green tea.

4.1.8 Beetroot

The beetroot, also known as table beet, garden beet, red beet or informally simply as beet, is one of the many cultivated varieties of beets (*Beta vulgaris* L., *Chenopodiaceae*) and arguably the most commonly encountered variety in North America, Central America and Britain. The usually deep-red roots are eaten boiled, either as a warm vegetable or as a cold salad with added oil and vinegar, or raw and shredded, either alone or in combination with any salad vegetable. Beetroots are a rich source of potent antioxidants and nutrients, including magnesium, sodium, potassium and vitamin C, as well as betaine, which is important for cardiovascular health. Oral administration of a beetroot extract inhibited tumor promotion by DMBA/TPA in mouse skin, and tumor promotion by 4-nitroquinoline 1-oxide (4NQO)/glycerol in lung carcinogenesis in mice (Kapadia, et al., 1996). In addition, orally administered beetroot extract inhibited mouse skin two-stage carcinogenesis, DMBA/ultraviolet B, and (±)-(E)-4-methyl-2-[(E)-hydroxyamino]-5-nitro-6-methoxy-3-hexanamide (NOR-1)/TPA, as well as liver carcinogenesis by *N*-nitrosodiethylamine (DEN) plus phenobarbital (Kapadia, et al., 2003).

4.1.9 Ginger and its components

Ginger is the rhizome of *Zingiber officinale* Rosc. (*Zingiberaceae*), and is consumed as a delicacy, medicine, or spice. The characteristic odor and flavor of ginger is caused by a mixture of zingerone, shogaols and gingerols, volatile oils that compose one to three percent of the weight of fresh ginger. Topical application of an ethanol extract of ginger inhibited TPA-induced tumor promotion during two-stage carcinogenesis in mouse skin (Katiyar, et al., 1996). Pre-application of an ethanol extract of ginger onto the skin of SENCAR mice resulted in significant inhibition of TPA-induced epidermal ODC, COX and lipoxygenase activities as well as ODC mRNA expression in a dose-dependent manner. Topical application of [6]-gingerol inhibited tumor promotion by DMBA/TPA in mouse skin, and also suppressed TPA-induced epidermal ODC activity and inflammation (Park, et al., 1998).

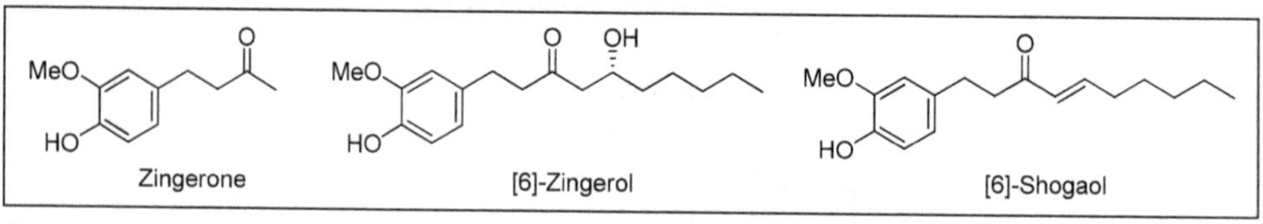

Fig. 9. The chemical structures of phenolics from *Zingiber officinale*.

4.1.10 *Allium* plants

Allium sativum L. (*Liliaceae*) is commonly known as garlic, its close relatives include the onion, shallot, leek, chive, and rakkyo. Garlic is native to central Asia, and has long been a staple in the Mediterranean region, and is a popular seasoning in Asia, Africa, and Europe. It was known to Ancient Egyptians, and has been used throughout its history for both culinary and medicinal purposes. Garlic extract inhibited tumor promotion by DMBA/TPA in mouse skin (Nishino, et al., 1989).

Rakkyo (the bulbs of *Allium chinense* G.Don) is used in folk medicine as tonic to the intestines and a stomach. A 20% ethanol extract of rakkyo bulbs suppressed two-stage carcinogenesis by DMBA/TPA in mouse skin (Okuyama, et al., 1995).

4.1.11 Edible mushrooms and their components

In Japan, mushrooms are a very important food. The beneficial effects of edible and medicinal mushrooms are now being recognized. Studies on mushrooms have been developed within the life sciences discipline worldwide. They have become increasingly popular in Japan as an ordinary food or supplement with the mounting scientific evidence of its useful functions. I believe edible mushrooms contribute to the prevention or treatment of life-style related diseases and can be classified as a functional food. Topical application of methanol extracts from *Mycoleptodonoides aitchisonii* (Berk.) Maas G. (*Steccherinaceae*) and *Hypsizygus marmoreus* (Peck.) Bigelow (*Tricholomataceae*) inhibited tumor promotion by DMBA/TPA in female ICR mouse skin (Yasukawa, et al., 1994a, 1996e). Its active components, ergosterol and its peroxide were isolated from *H. marmorus* (Yasukawa, et al., 1994a) and showed inhibition same carcinogenic test (Yasukawa, et al., 1994a). On the other hand, these sterols were isolated from *Chlorella vulgaris* Beij. (*Chlorophyceae*), a green alga, for anti-inflammatory agents, and ergosterol peroxide inhibited tumor promotion by DMBA/TPA in mouse skin (Yasukawa, et al., 1996a).

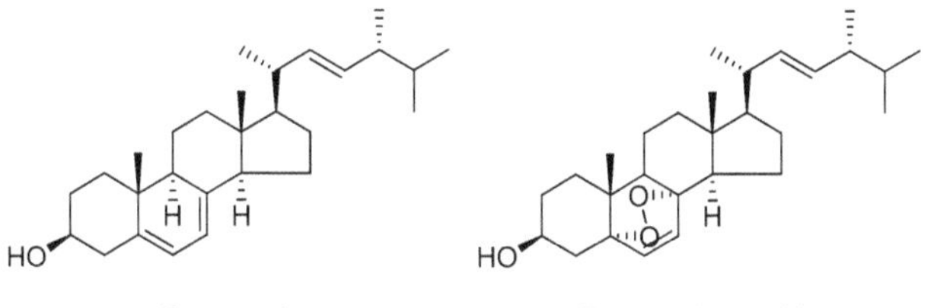

Ergosterol   Ergosterol peroxide

Fig. 10. The chemical structures of sterols from *Hypsizygus marmoreus*.

4.1.12 Red malt molds and their components

Monascus spp. (*M. Purpureus* Went. and *M. Anka* K. Satô, *Monascaceae*) are molds purplish-red in color. Species of *Monascus* have been utilized for hundreds of years for making fermented foods and preserving meat. This fungus is of importance because of its use in the form of red yeast rice in the production of certain fermented foods in Japan. However, the discovery of cholesterol-lowering statins produced by the mold has prompted research into its possible medical uses. The naturally occurring lovastatin and analogs are called monacolin K, L, J, and also occur in their hydroxy acid forms along with dehydroxymonacolin and compactin (mevastatin). The prescription drug lovastatin, identical to monacolin K, is the principal statin produced by *M. purpureus*. Topical application of Monascus Pigment (an ethanol extract of *M. anka*) and monascorubrin, one of the components from *M. anka*, inhibited tumor promotion by DMBA/TPA in mouse skin (Yasukawa, et al., 1994b). Furthermore, oral administration of Monascus pigment inhibited DMBA/TPA two-stage carcinogenesis in mouse skin (Yasukawa, et al., 1996f).

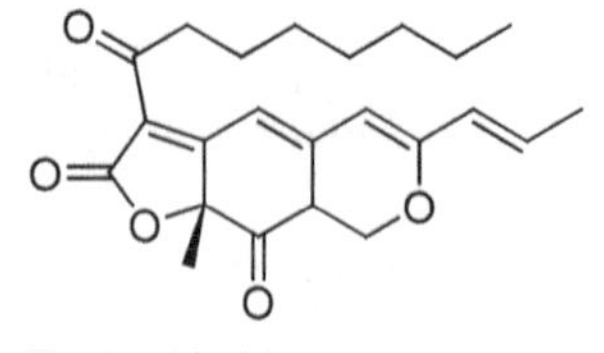

Monascorubrin

Fig. 11. The chemical structure of monascorubrin from the red malt mold.

4.2 Supplemental plants

With the increase in life expectancy comes a greater focus on health. Supplements are a popular part of health maintenance, and are typically taken separately from the diet. Dietary supplements, also known as food supplements or nutritional supplements, are intended to supplement the diet and provide nutrients, such as vitamins, minerals, fiber, fatty acids, or amino acids, that may be missing or not be consumed in sufficient quantities in the diet. The European Union's Food Supplements Directive of 2002 requires that the safety of supplements be demonstrated, both in dosages and purity. In Japan, many people use supplement because of life-style related diseases and cancer, and I discuss the study of the plant supplements from the viewpoint of cancer prevention.

4.2.1 Ginseng and its components

Oral administration of white and red ginseng (*Panax ginseng* C.A. Mayer, *Araliaceae*) suppressed colon carcinogenesis by 1,2-dimethylhydrazine (DMH) in rat (Fukushima, et al., 2001). In benzo[*a*]pyrene (BP)-induced lung carcinogenesis in mice, 5- or 6- year old ginseng root was more effective than 1.5- to 4-year old ginseng root. The ginsenosides Rg_3, Rg_5 and Rh_2 are active components in ginseng, and act either singularly or synergistically in cancer prevention (Yun, et al., 2001). The methanol extract of san-chi ginseng (the roots of *Panax notoginseng* (Burk.) F.H. Chen) suppressed skin carcinogenesis by DMBA/TPA, liver carcinogenesis by DEN/Phenobarbital, lung carcinogenesis by 4NQO/glycerol in mice (Konoshima, et al., 1996). Moreover, the methanol extract of san-chi inhibited skin carcinogenesis by NOR-1/TPA, as well as DMBA/fumonisin B1 in mice (Konoshima, et al., 1999). The ginsenoside Rg_1 slightly suppressed tumor promotion by DMBA/TPA in mouse skin (Konoshima, et al., 1996).

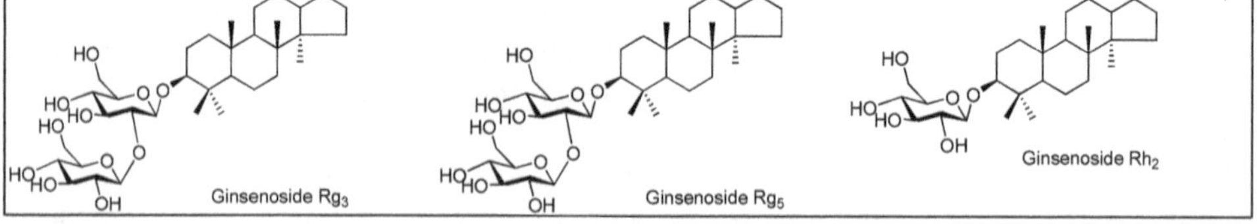

Ginsenoside Rg_3 Ginsenoside Rg_5 Ginsenoside Rh_2

Fig. 12. The chemical structure of ginsenosides from ginseng.

4.2.2 Seabuckthorn and its components

The fruit of seabuckthorn (*Hippophae rhamnoides* L., *Elaeagnaceae*) is dense in carotenoids, vitamin C, vitamin E, amino acids, dietary minerals and polyphenols. The nutrient and phytochemical constituents of seabuckthorn berries have potential value in the treatment of inflammatory disorders, cancer or other diseases. Seabuckthorn is a herbal remedy reputedly used over centuries to relieve cough, aid in digestion, invigorate blood circulation and alleviate pain.

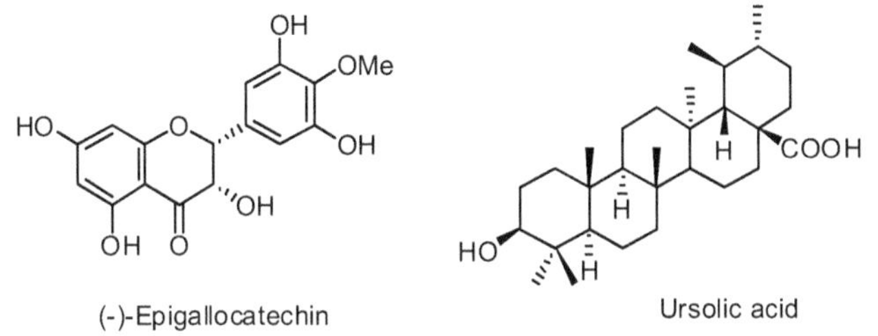

(-)-Epigallocatechin   Ursolic acid

Fig. 13. The chemical structures of (–)-epigallocatechin and ursolic acid from the branches of seabuckthorn.

Its bark and leaves have been used for treating diarrhea and dermatological disorders. The methanol extract of seabuckthorn branches suppressed tumor promotion in two-stage carcinogenesis by DMBA/TPA in mouse skin, and the active components ursolic acid and (–)-epigallocatechin were isolated from the active fractions of the methanol extract (Yasukawa, et al., 2009).

4.2.3 Neem

Azadirachta indica A. Juss. (Neem) is a tree in the mahogany family *Meliaceae*. It is one of two species in the genus *Azadirachta*, and is native to the Indian Subcontinent, growing in tropical and semi-tropical regions. Neem products have been observed to be anthelmintic, antifungal, antidiabetic, antibacterial, antiviral, contraceptive and sedative. It is a major component of Ayurvedic and Unani medicine and is particularly prescribed for skin disease. All parts of the tree are said to have medicinal properties (seeds, leaves, flowers and bark) and are used for preparing many different medical preparations. Neem leaves were found to inhibit tumor promotion by DMBA/TPA in mouse skin (Arora, et al., 2011). Inhibition of carcinogenesis in response to neem treatment was accompanied by an overexpression of signal transducer and activator of transcription 1 (STAT1) and activator protein 1 (AP-1) and decrease in nuclear factor-kappa B (NF-κB) expression (Arora, et al., 2011).

4.2.4 Supplemental mushrooms and their components

Chaga (the sclerotia of *Inonotus obliquus* (Pers. Fr.) Pil., *Hymenochaetaceae*) has been widely used as a folk medicine in the treatment of cancer, cardiovascular disease and diabetes in Russia, Poland, and several Baltic countries. In Japan and Korea, chaga is used as a supplement during cancer treatment. More recently, this herb has been assessed for its cancer-preventing activity. Oral administration of chaga was found to inhibit tumor promotion by DMBA/TPA in mouse skin (Akita & Yasukawa, 2011). Other researchers have isolated triterpene derivatives from chaga. Of these triterpenes, inotodiol and 3β-hydroxylanosta-8,24-dien-21-al were reported to restrain a cancer-causing promotion process (Nakata, et al., 2007; Taji, et al.,2008).

In Korea, meshima (*Phellinus linteus* (Berk et Curt) Teng, *Hymenochactaceae*) is also the most popular herb used by cancer patients. Oral administration of an aqueous extract of meshima suppressed tumor promotion by DMBA/TPA in mouse skin (Yasukawa, et al., 2007).

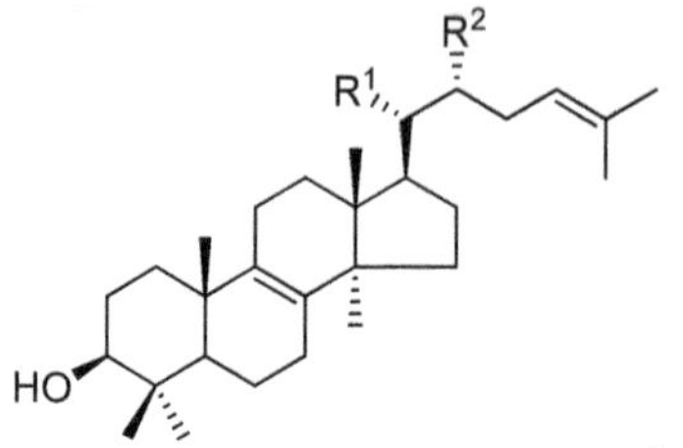

	R^1	R^2
Inotodiol	CH_3	OH
3β-Hydroxylanosta-8,24-dien-21-al	CHO	H

Fig. 14. The chemical structures of triterpenoids from Chaga (*Inonotus obliquus*).

4.3 Crude drugs

A crude drug is any naturally occurring, unrefined substance derived from organic or inorganic sources such as plants, animals, bacteria, organs or whole organisms, and is intended for use in the diagnosis, cure, mitigation, treatment, or prevention of disease in man or other animals. Crude drugs are primary used in disease, but are also used in health maintenance. These medicinal plants are typically taken in the form of spices and as additives. Below, I describe various medicinal plants and mushrooms.

4.3.1 *Compositae* plants and their active components

Several species and subspecies of *Taraxacum* are widely distributed in Japan, and the roots of these plants (*T. Platycarpum* Dahlst., *T. Japonicum* Koidz., etc.) have been used as bitter stomachic, diuretic, anti-mastopathy and anti-inflammatory folk medicines in China and Japan. Interestingly, dandelion (*T. officinale* F.H. Wigg) leaves have been regarded as a vegetable in Europe. The methanol and water extracts of *T. japonicum* inhibited tumor promotion by TPA or fumonisin B1 in DMBA-initiated mice (Takasaki, et al., 1999a). Several triterpenoids have been isolated from the flowers of *T. officinale* and *T. platycarpum* (Akihisa, et al., 1996; Yasukawa, et al., 1996d), taraxasterol and faradiol inhibited tumor promotion by DMBA/TPA in mouse skin (Yasukawa, et al., 1996c). Furthermore, taraxasterol and taraxerol inhibited same experiment (Takasaki, et al., 1999b).

Atractylodis Rhizoma, the rhizome of *Atractylodes japonica* Koidzumi, is traditionally used in Kampo medicine. The methanol extract of Atractylodis Rhizoma inhibited two-stage carcinogenesis by DMBA/TPA in mouse skin (Yu, et al., 1994). The active component, atractylon, was isolated from the active fraction of the methanol extract of Atractylodis Rhizoma (Yu, et al., 1994).

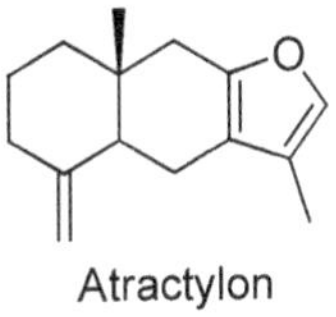

Atractylon

Fig. 15. The chemical structure of atractylon from Atractylodis Rhizoma.

Safflower (*Carthamus tinctorius* L.) is a highly branched, herbaceous, thistle-like annual. It is commercially cultivated for the vegetable oil extracted from its seeds. The pigment in safflower is benzoquinone-based carthamin, and is a quinone-type natural dye. Dried safflower flowers are used in traditional Chinese medicine to alleviate pain, increase circulation, and reduce bruising. Topical application of the methanol extract of safflower inhibited tumor promotion by DMBA/TPA in mouse skin. The active agents, stigmasterol and other phytosterols were isolated from the active fraction of safflower, and stigmasterol inhibited tumor promotion by DMBA/TPA in mouse skin (Kasahara, et al., 1994). Subsequently, alkane-6,8-diols were isolated from other active safflower fractions (Akihisa, et al., 1994, 1997). Alkanediol from safflower and synthetic C29-alkane-6,8-diol inhibited tumor promotion by DMBA/TPA in mouse skin (Motohashi, et al., 1995; Yasukawa, et al., 1996b).

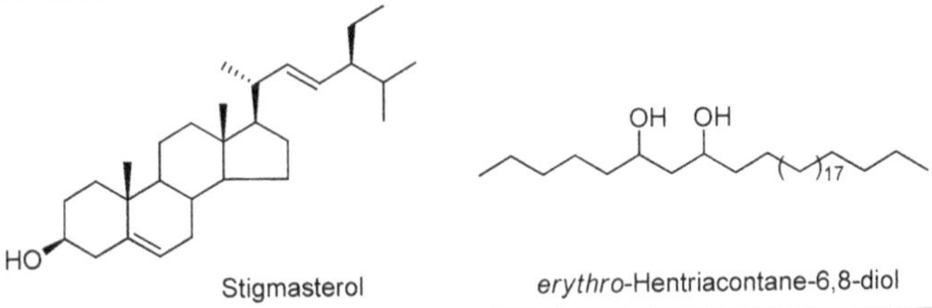

Stigmasterol   *erythro*-Hentriacontane-6,8-diol

Fig. 16. The chemical structures of stigmasterol and alkane-6,8-diol from safflower.

4.3.2 Pruni Cortex and its active components

Cherry blossoms are the flowers of any of several trees of the genus *Prunus*, including the Japanese cherry (*Prunus serrulata* Franch, *Rosaceae*), which is sometimes called sakura in Japanese. Edible cherries generally come from cultivars of the related species *Prunus avium* L. and *Prunus cerasus* L. Pruni Cortex (the bark of *Prunus jamasakura* Sieb. ex Koidz.) is used for infectious diarrhea, food poisoning and catarrhal gastritis. The methanol extract of Pruni Cortex inhibited two-stage carcinogenesis by DMBA/TPA in mouse skin (Yasukawa, et al., 1998c). The active agent, octacosyl ferulate was isolated from the active fraction of Pruni Cortex, and inhibited tumor promotion by DMBA/TPA in mouse skin (Yasukawa, et al., 1998c). Octacosyl ferulate inhibited the phosphorylation of histone by protein kinase C (PK-C) in a concentration-dependent manner.

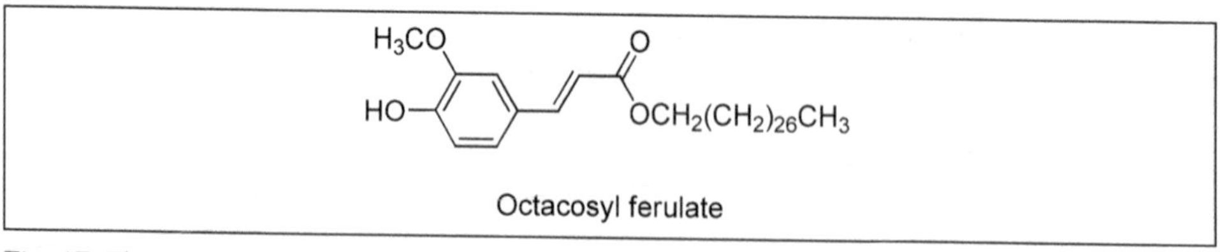

Octacosyl ferulate

Fig. 17. The chemical structures of octacosyl ferulate from Pruni Cortex.

4.3.3 Achyranthes aspera

Achyranthes aspera L. (*Amaranthaceae*) is an indigenous medicinal plant of Asia, South America and Africa, and its leaves are commonly used by traditional healers in the treatment of fever (especially malarial fever), dysentery, asthma, hypertension and diabetes. The dried herb is used to treat colicky children and also as an astringent in gonorrhea treatment. The topical application of a methanol extract of *A. aspera* leaves suppressed two-stage carcinogenesis by DMBA/TPA in mouse skin (Chakraborty, et al., 2002).

4.3.4 Galangal and its active components

Galangal (the rhizome of *Alpinia officinarum* Hance, *Zingiberaceae*) is a perennial herbaceous plant native to southeastern Asia. Galangal has been used externally for skin infections, skin cancer and gum diseases, and internally for digestive upsets, chronic gastritis, gastric ulceration and epigastric and rheumatic pain. A methanol extract of galangal inhibited TPA-induced tumor promotion DMBA/TPA in mouse skin. Seven diarylheptanoids were isolated from the methanol extract for inhibitory activity against TPA-induced inflammatory ear edema in mice (Yasukawa, et al., 2008).

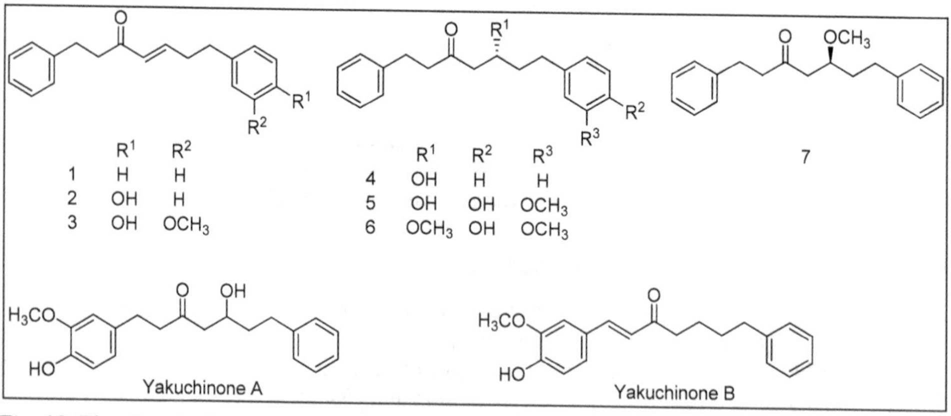

Fig. 18. The chemical structures of diarylheptanoids from *Alpinia* plants.

Lee et al. reported that a methanol extract *Alpinia oxyphylla* Miquel (*Zingiberaceae*) fruits suppressed tumor promotion by DMBA/TPA in mouse skin (Lee, et al., 1998). Yakuchinones A and B were isolated from the active fraction of the methanol extract as active components.

4.3.5 Medicinal mushrooms and their active components

The sclerotium of *Poria cocos* Wolf (*Polyporaceae*) is traditionally used in Kampo medicine as a diuretic and as a sedative. Many lanostane-type and 3,4-secolanostane-type triterpene acids have been isolated from *P. cocos*. The methanol extract of *P. cocos* inhibited tumor promotion by DMBA/TPA in mouse skin (Kaminaga, et al., 1996b). Of these triterpene acids, pachymic acid, 3-*O*-acetyl-16α-hydroxytrametenolic acid, and poricoic acid B inhibited tumor promotion by DMBA/TPA in mouse skin (Kaminaga, et al.,1996a). The activity of these triterpene acids was ten times greater than other lanostane-type triterpenes against TPA-induced tumor promotion in mouse skin.

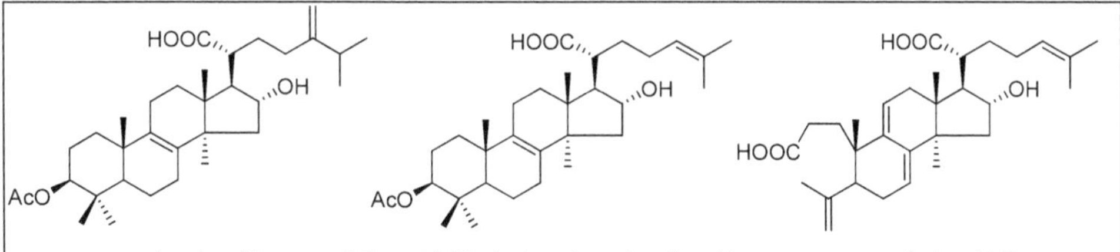

pachymic acid   3-*O*-acetyl-16α-hydroxytrametenolic acid   poricoic acid B

Fig. 19. The chemical structures of triterpenoids from Poria (*Poria cocos*).

4.4 Kampo medicines

The fundamentals of Chinese medicine came to Japan between the 7th and 9th centuries. Currently, herbal medicines in Japan are regulated as pharmaceutical preparations; their ingredients are exactly measured and standardized, unlike other places such as the U.S.A., Europe, and China. Both industry and government conduct extensive monitoring of agricultural and manufacturing processes as well as post-marketing surveillance to guarantee the safety of these preparations. Kampo prescriptions follow the Standard Kampo formula nomenclature ver. 1.0, March 5th, 2005.

4.4.1 Shoseiryuto (Xiao-Qing-Long-Tang)

Shoseiryuto is a mixture of eight herbal components (Pinellia tuber, Glycyrrhiza, Cinnamon bark, Schisandra fruit, Asiasarum root, Paeony root, Ephedra herb and Ginger), and has been used in Japan for the treatment of pulmonary diseases such as asthma, and bronchitis as well as allergic diseases. Oral administration of Shoseiryuto suppressed skin tumors induced by DMBA/TPA, pulmonary tumors induced by 4NQO/glycerol, liver tumors induced by DEN/phenobarbital in mice (Konoshima, et al., 1994).

4.4.2 Juzentaihoto (Shi-Quan-Da-Bu-Tang)

Juzentaihoto has been used as a nourishing agent, a so-called "Hozai" (in Japanese), for improving disturbances and imbalances in the homeostatic condition of the body. This drug is composed of ten components (Glycyrrhiza, Atractylodes rhizome, Ginseng, Astragalus root, Cinnamon bark, Rehmannia root, Paeony root, Cnidium Rhizome, Japanese Angelica root and Poria sclerotium) and has been used effectively for plausible complaints of consumption of vital energy, lack of appetite, night sweats, circulatory problem and anemia. Oral administration of Juzentaihoto suppressed endometrial carcinogenesis by MNU/estradiol-17β in mice (Lian, et al., 2002; Niwa, et al., 2001). Moreover, Juzentaihoto orally suppressed tumor promotion by DMBA/TPA in mouse skin (Haranaka, et al., 1987).

4.4.3 Rikkunshito (Liu-Jun-Zi-Tang)

Rikkunshito consist of eight components (Glycyrrhiza, Ginger, Atractylodes rhizome, Jujube, Citrus unshiu peel, Ginseng, Pinellia tuber, and Poria sclerotium). In Japan, Rikkunshito has been used to treat functional dyspepsia and dyspepsia associated with organic disease. Topical application of a methanol extract of Rikkunshito inhibited tumor promotion by DMBA/TPA in mouse skin (Yasukawa, et al., 1995). Furthermore, oral administration of Rikkunshito suppressed skin tumors induced by DMBA/TPA in mice (Yasukawa, et al., 1996g). It was also observed that treatment with Rikkunshito reversed immunosuppression during DMBA/TPA-induced carcinogenesis (Yasukawa, et al., 1996g).

4.4.4 Shousaikoto (Xiao-Chai-Hu-Tang)

The Kampo medicine Shousaikoto has been used clinically to treat various inflammatory diseases including chronic hepatitis. Shousaikoto contains seven components (Glycyrrhiza, Ginger, Bupleurum root, Jujube, Scutellaria root, Ginseng and Pinellia tuber). This prescription has been used in the treatment of pneumonia and pulmonary tuberculosis since ancient times and is frequently used in the treatment of inflammatory respiratory diseases. In animal experiments, oral administration of Shousaikoto suppressed DMH-induced colonic carcinogenesis in rats (Sakamoto, et al., 1993).

4.4.5 Choreito (Zhu-Ling-Tang)

Choreito has been used for urinary frequency, feeling of residual urine, hematuria. Choreito consist of five components (Asini corii colla, Talc stone, Alisma rhizome, Polyporus sclerotium, Poria sclerotium), and is used as a diuresis of the kidney, and bladder, as well as in the treatment of uropathy. Oral administration of Choreito suppressed urinary bladder carcinogenesis induced by N-butyl-N-(4-hydroxybutyl)-nitrosamine (BHBN)/sodium saccharin (SS) in rats (Sugiyama, et al., 1994). Of the components of Choreito, Polyporus sclerotium seems to be a key component in its inhibitory activity in the bladder tumor promotion test.

4.5 Essential oils

An essential oil is a concentrated hydrophobic liquid containing volatile aromatic compounds derived from plants. Essential oils are generally extracted by distillation, and other processes include expression, or solvent extraction. Various essential oils have been used medicinally at different periods in history, while many common essential oils have medicinal properties that have been applied in folk medicine since ancient times and are still widely used today (Burt, 2004; Prabuseenivasan, et al., 2006).

4.5.1 Sage (*Salvia libanotica*) oil

Salvia libanotica Boiss. & Gaill. (*Labiatae*) is a strongly aromatic perennial shrub. Its healing properties are well known and it is widely used by herbalists for the treatment of headache, stomachache and respiratory problems. The oil extract contains ketones such as camphor and α- and β-thujone, terpenes such as limonene and α- and β-pinene, and alcohols such as borneol and linalool. Moreover, oxides such as 1,8-cineol and esters such as linalyl acetate are also found in sage oil. Sage oil was observed to inhibit tumor promotion by DMBA/TPA in mouse skin (Gali-Muhtasib, & Affara, 2000).

4.5.2 Garlic (*Allium sativum*) oil

Garlic oil from *Allium sativum* L. (*Liliaceae*) is rich in sulfur compounds, and a major component is diallyl disulphide, and is a suspected irritant. It was found that garlic oil inhibited tumor promotion by DMBA/TPA in mouse skin (Belman, 1983; Perchellt, et al., 1990).

4.5.3 Onion (*Allium cepa*) oil

Onion oil from the seeds of *Allium cepa* L. (*Liliaceae*) may present a risk of skin irritation and/or sensitization similar to garlic oil. Onion oil inhibited tumor promotion by DMBA/TPA (Belman, 1983; Perchellt, et al., 1990) and by BP/croton oil (Sadhana, et al., 1988) in mouse skin.

4.5.4 Sandalwood (*Santalum album*) oil

Sandalwood (*Santalum album* L., *Santalaceae*) comes from medium-sized fragrant trees and its oil has found wide use in the cosmetics industry. Sandalwood oil inhibited tumor promotion by DMBA/TPA in mouse skin (Dwivedi & Abu-Ghazaleh, 1997; Dwivedi & Zhang, 1999). The mechanism of its activity is due, in part, to the inhibition of TPA-induced epidermal ODC activity (Dwivedi & Zhang, 1999).

5. Conclusion

Humans have used plants as foods and natural medicines since ancient times. Crude drugs, typically safer than synthetic drugs, have been used as both spices and supplements. Natural medicines have been used as anti-cancer agents by inhibiting the promotion process, and it is important that these are consumed in small quantities for extended periods of time. The study of cancer prevention using plants is generating vast amounts of information regarding their benefits. This paper provides, an outline of studies focusing on plant extracts. Several active components have been isolated, and their chemical structures have been and continue to be determined. In addition, structure-activity relationships, elucidation of physiological activities at the molecular level, and development of strategies that allow for the production of sufficient supplies of these agents are issues for further investigation. The continued search for natural medicines is necessary for finding additional sources of active components that are suitable for clinical application. For this purpose, we will harness the strength of researchers from various fields with the goal for cancer prevention.

6. References

Akihisa, T.; Nozaki, A.; Inoue, Y. ; Yasukawa, K.; Kasahara, Y.; Motohashi, S.; Kumaki, K.; Tokutake, N.; Takido, M. & Tamura, T. (1997). Alkanediol from flower petals of *Carthamus tinctorius, Phytochemistry*, Vol.45, No. 4, pp. 725-728, ISSN 0031-9422

Akihisa, T.; Oinuma, H.; Tamura, T.; Kasahara, Y.; Kumaki, K.; Yasukawa, K. & Takido, M. (1994). *erythro*-Hentriacontane-6,8-diol and 11 other alkane-6,8-diols from *Carthamus tinctorius, Phytochemistry*, Vol.36, No. 1, pp. 105-108, ISSN 0031-9422

Akihisa, T. & Yasukawa, K. (2001). Antitumor-Promoting and Anti-inflammatory Activities of triterpenoids and Sterols from Plants and Fungi, In: *Studies in Natural Products Chemistry (Vol.25), Bioactive Natural Products (Part F)*, Atta-ur-Rahman, (ed.), pp. 43-87, Elsevier Science B.N., ISBN 9780080440019, Amsterdam, The Netherlands

Akihisa, T., Yasukawa, K.; Oinuma, H.; Kasahara, Y.; Yamanouchi, S.; Takido, M.; Kumaki, K. & Tamura, T. (1996). Triterpene alcohols from the flowers of Compositae and their anti-inflammatory effects., *Phytochemistry*, Vol.43, No.6, pp. 1255-1260, ISSN 0031-9422

Akihisa, T.; Yasukawa, K. & Tokuda, H. (2003). Potentially cancer chemopreventive and anti-inflammatory terpenoids from natural sources, In: *Studies in Natural Products Chemistry (Vol.29), Bioactive Natural Products (Part J)*, Atta-ur-Rahman, (ed.), pp. 73-126, Elsevier Science B.N., ISBN 9780444515100, Amsterdam, The Netherlands

Akita, A. & Yasukawa, K. (2011). Inhibitory effect of chaga (*Inonotus obliquus*) on tumor promotion in two-stage mouse skin carcinogenesis, *Japanese Journal of Complementary and Alternative Medicine*, Vol.8, No.1, pp. 29-32, ISSN 1348-7922

Alam, A.; Khan, N.; Sharma, S.; Saleem, M. & Sultana, S. (2002). Chemopreventive effect of *Vitis vinifera* extract on 12-O-tetradecanoyl-13-phorbol acetate-induced cutaneous oxidative stress and tumor promotion in murine skin, *Pharmacological Research*, Vol.46, No.6, pp. 557-564, ISSN 1043-6618

Arora, N.; Bansal, M.P. & Koul, A. (2011). *Azadirachta indica* exerts chemopreventive action against murine skin cancer: studies on histopathological, ultrastructural changes and modulation of NF-kappaB, AP-1, and STAT1, *Oncology Research*, Vol.19, No.5, pp. 179-191, ISSN 0965-0407

Banning, M. (2005). The carcinogenic and protective effects of food, *British Journal of Nursing*, Vol.14, No.20, pp. 1070-1074, ISSN 0966-0461

Belman, S. (1983). Onion and garlic oils inhibit tumor promotion, *Carcinogenesis*, Vol.4, No.8, pp. 1063-1065, ISSN 0143-3334

Birt, D.F.; Pelling, J.C.; Pour, P.M.; Tibbels, M.G.; Schweickert, J. & Bresnick, E. (1987). Enhanced pancreatic and skin tumorigenesis in cabbage-fed hamsters and mice, *Carcinogenesis*, Vol.8, No.7, pp. 913-917, ISSN 0143-3334

Bishayee, A. & Dhir, N. (2009). Resveratrol-mediated chemoprevention of diethylnitrosamine-initiated hepatocercinogenesis: inhibition of cell proliferation and induction of apoptosis, *Chemico-Biological Interactions*, Vol.179, No.2-3, pp. 131-144, ISSN 0009-2797

Bomser, J.A.; Singletary, K.W.; Wallig, M.A. & Smith, M.A.L. (1999). Inhibition of TPA-induced tumor promotion in CD-1 mouse epidermis by a polyphenolic fraction from grape seeds, *Cancer Letters*, Vol.135, No.2, pp. 151-157, ISSN 0304-3835

Bresnick, E.; Birt, D.F.; Woltermen, K.; Wheeler, M. & Markin, R.S. (1990). Reduction in mammary tumorigenesis in the rat by cabbage and cabbage residue, *Carcinogenesis*, Vol.11, No.7, pp. 1159-1163, ISSN 0143-3334

Burt, S. (2004). Essential oils: their antibacterial properties and potential applications in foods – a review, *International Lournal of Food Microbiology*, Vol.94, No.3, pp. 223-253, ISSN 0168-1605

Chakraborty, A.; Brantner, A.; Mukainaka, T.; Nobukuni, Y.; Kuchide, M.; Konoshima, T.; Tokuda, H. & Nishino, H. (2002). Cancer chemopreventive activity of *Achyranthes aspera* leaves on Etpstein-Barr virus activation and two-stage mouse skin carcinogenesis, *Cancer Letters*, Vol.177, No.1, pp. 1-5, ISSN 0304-3835

Dwivedi, C. & Abu-Ghazaleh, A. (1997). Chemopreventive effects of sandalwood oil on skin pappilomas in mice, *European Journal of Cancer Prevention*, Vol.6, No.4, pp. 399-401, ISSN 0959-8278

Dwivedi, C. & Zhang, Y. (1999). Sandalwood oil prevents skin tumour development in CD-1 mice, *European Journal of Cancer Prevention*, Vol.8, No.5, pp. 449-455, ISSN 0959-8278

Fukushima, S.; Wanibuchi, H. & Li, W. (2001). Inhibition by ginseng of colon carcinogenesis in rats, *Journal of Korean Medical Science*, Vol.16(Supple), pp. S75-S80, ISSN 1011-8934

Gali-Muhtasib, H.U. & Affara, N.I. (2000). Chemopreventive effects of sage oil on skin papillomas in mice, *Phytomedicine*, Vol.7, No.2, pp. 129-136, ISSN 0944-7113

Grubbs, C.J.; Steele, V.E.; Casebolt, T.; Juliana, M.M.; Eto, I.; Whitaker, L.M.; Dragnev, K.H.; Kelloff, G.J. & Lubet, R.L. (1995). Chemoprevention of chemically-induced mammary carcinogenesis by indole-3-carbinol, *Anticancer Research*, Vol.15, No.3, pp. 709-716, ISSN 0250-7005

Haranaka, R.; Kosoto, H.; Hirama, N.; Hanawa, T.; Hasegawa, R.; Hyun, S.-J.; Nakagawa, S.; Haranaka, K.; Satomi, N.; Sakurai, A.; Yasukawa, K. & Takido, M. (1987). Antitumor activities of Zyuzen-taiho-to and Cinnamomi Cortex, *Journal of Medical and Pharmaceutical Society for Wakan-Yaku* Vol.4, No.1, pp. 49–58, ISSN 0289-730X

Hirayama, T. (1984). Epidemiology of stomach cancer in Japan. With special reference to the strategy for the primary prevention, *Japanese Journal of Clinical Oncology*, Vol.14, No.2, pp. 159-168, ISSN 0368-2811

Huang, M.-T.; Ho, C.-T.; Wang, Z.Y.; Ferraro, T.; Lou, Y.-R.; Stauber, K.; Ma, W.; Georgiadis, C.; Laskin, J.D. & Conney, A.H. (1994). Inhibition of skin tumorigenesis by rosemary and its constituents carnosol and ursolic acid, *Cancer Research*, Vol.54, No. 3, pp. 701-708, ISSN 0008-5472

Kapadia, G.J.; Azuine, M.A.; Sridhar, R.; Okuda, Y.; Tsuruta, A.; Ichiishi, E.; Mukainake, T.; Takasaki, M.; Konoshima, T.; Nishino, H. & Tokuda, H. (2003). Chemoprevention of DMBA-induced UV-B promoted, NOR-1-induced TPA promoted skin carcinogenesis, and DEN-induced Phenobarbital promoted liver tumors in mice by extract of beetroot, *Pharmacological Research*, Vol.47, No.2, pp. 141-148, ISSN 1043-6618

Kapadia, G.J.; Tokuda, H.; Konoshima, T. & Nishino, H. (1996). Chemoprevention of lung and skin cancer by *Beta vulgaris* (beet) root extract, *Cancer Letters*, Vol.100, No.1-2, pp. 211-214, ISSN 0304-3835

Kaminaga, T.; Yasukawa, K.; Kanno, H.; Tai, T.; Nunoura, Y. & Takido M. (1996a). Inhibitory effect of lanostane-type triterpene acids, the components of *Poria cocos*, on tumor promotion by 12-O-tetradecanoylphorbol-13-acetate in two-stage carcinogenesis in mouse skin, *Oncology*, Vol.53, No.5, pp. 382–385, ISSN 0030-2414

Kaminaga, T.; Yasukawa, K.; Takido, M.; Tai, T. & Nunoura Y. (1996b). Inhibitory effect of *Poria cocos* on 12-O-tetradecanoylphorbol-13-acetate-induced ear oedema and tumour promotion in mouse skin, *Phytotherapy Research*, Vol.10, No.7, pp. 581–584, ISSN 0951-418X

Kasahara, Y.; Kumaki, K.; Katagiri, S.; Yasukawa, K.; Yamanouchi, S.; Takido, M.; Akihisa, T.; Tamura, T. (1994). Carthami Flos extract and its component, stigmasterol, inhibit tumor promotion in mouse skin two-stage carcinogenesis, *Phytotherapy Research*, Vol.8, No.6, pp. 327–331, ISSN 0951-418X

Katiyar, S.K.; Agarwal, R. & Mukhtar, H. (1996). Inhibition of tumor promotion in SENCAR mouse skin by ethanol extract of *Zingiber officinale* rhizome, *Cancer Research*, Vol.56, No.5, pp. 1023-1030, ISSN 0008-5472

Katiyar, S.K.; Agarwal, R., Wood, G.S. & Mukhtar, H. (1992). Inhibition of 12-O-tetradecanoylphorbol-13-acetate-caused tumor promotion in 7,12-dimethylbenz[a]- anthracene-initiated SENCAR mouse skin by a polyphenolic fraction isolated from green tea, *Cancer Research*, Vol.52, No.24, pp. 6890-6897, ISSN 0008-5472

Kim, D.J.; Han, B.S.; Ahn, B.; Hasegawa, R.; Shirai, T.; Ito, N. & Tsuda, H. (1997). Enhancement by indole-3-carbinol of liver and thyroid gland neoplastic development in a rat medium-term multiorgan carcinogenesis model, *Carcinogenesis*, Vol.18, No.2, 377-381, ISSN 0143-3334

Kohno, H.; Taima, M.; Sumida, T.; Azuma, Y.; Ogawa, H. & Tanaka, T. (2001). Inhibitory effect of mandarin juice rich in β-ceyptoxanthin and hesperidin on 4-(methylnitrosamino)-1-(3-pyridyl)-1-butanone-induced pulmonary tumorigenesis in mice, *Cancer Letters*, Vol.174, No.2, pp. 141-150, ISSN 0304-3835

Konoshima, T.; Takasaki, M.; Kozuka, M. & Tokuda, H. (1994). Anti-tumor promoting activities of Kampo prescriptions. II. Inhibitory effects of Shouseiryu-to on two-stage carcinogenesis of mouse skin tumors and mouse pulmonary tumors, *Yakugaku Zasshi*, Vol.114, No.4, pp. 248-256, ISSN 0031-6903

Konoshima, T.; Takasaki, M. & Tokuda, H. (1996). Anti-tumor-promoting activity of the roots of *Panax notoginseng* (1), *Natural medicines*, Vol.50, No.2, pp. 158-162, ISSN 1340-3443

Konoshima, T.; Takasaki, M. & Tokuda, H. (1999). Anti-carcinogenesis activity of the roots of *Panax notoginseng*. II, *Biological & Pharmaceutical Bulletin*, Vol.22, No.10, pp. 1150-1152, ISSN 0918-6158

Konoshima, T.; Tokuda, H.; Kozuka, M.; Okamoto, E. & Tanabe, M. (1987). Inhibitory effects on Epstein-Barr virus activation and antitumor promoting effects of crude drugs (I), *Shoyakugaku Zasshi*, Vol.41, No.4, pp. 344-348, ISSN 1340-3443

Kuzuhara, T.; Suganuma, M. & Fujiki, H. (2008). Green tea catechin as a chemical chaperone in cancer prevention, *Cancer Letters*, Vol.261, No.1, pp. 12-20, ISSN 0304-3835

Lee, E.; Park, K.-K.; Lee, J.-M.; Chun, K.-S.; Kang, J.Y.; Lee, S.-S. & Surh, Y.-J. (1998). Suppression of mouse skin tumor promotion and induction of apoptosis in HL-60 cells by *Alpinia oxyphylla* Miquel (Zingiberaceae), *Carcinogenesis*, Vol.19, No.8, pp. 1377-1381, ISSN 0143-3334

Lian, Z.; Niwa, K.; Gao, J.; Tagami, K.; Hashimoto, M.; Yokoyama, Y.; Mori, H. & Tamaya, T. (2002). Shimotsu-to is the agent in Juzen-taiho-to responsible for the prevention of endometrial carcinogenesis in mice, *Cancer Letters*, Vol.182, No.1, pp. 19-26, ISSN 0304-3835

Manson, M.M.; Hudson, E.A.; Ball, H.W.L.; Barrett, M.C.; Clark, H.L.; Judah, D.J.; Verschoyle, R.D. & Neal, G.E. (1998). Chemoprevention of aflatoxin B_1-induced carcinogenesis by indole-3-carbinol in rat liver — predicting the outcome using early biomarkers, *Carcinogenesis*, Vol.19, No.10, pp. 1829-1836, ISSN 0143-3334

Molteni, A.; Brizio-Molteni, L. & Persky, V. (1995). In vitro hormonal effects of soybean isoflavones, *The journal of Nutrition*, Vol.125, No.3, pp. 751S-756S, ISSN 0022-3166

Morse, M.A. & Stoner, G.D. (1993). Cancer chemoprevention: principles and prospects, *Carcinogenesis*, Vol.14, No.9, pp. 1737-1746, ISSN 0143-3334

Motohashi, S.; Akihisa, T.; Tamura, T.; Tokutake, N.; Takido, M. & Yasukawa, K. (1995). Alkane-6,8-diols: Inhibitor of tumor promotion in two-stage carcinogenesis in mouse skin, *Journal of Medicinal Chemistry*, Vol.38, No.21, pp. 4155-4156, ISSN 0022-2623

Murakami, A.; Ohigashi, H. & Koshimizu, K. (1996). Anti-tumor promotion with food phytochemicals: a strategy for cancer chemoprevention, *Bioscience, Biotechonolgy, and Biochemistry*, Vol.60, No.1, pp. 1-8, ISSN 0916-8451

Nakata, T.; Yamada, T.; Taji, S.; Ohishi, H.; Wada, S.; Tokuda, H.; Sakuma, K. & Tanaka, R. (2007). Structure determination of inonotsuoxides A and B and in vivo anti-tumor promoting activity of inotodiol from the sclerotia of *Inonotus obliquus*, *Bioorganic & Medicinal Chemistry*, Vol.15, No.1, pp. 257-264, ISSN 09680896

Narisawa, T.; Fukaura, Y.; Oshima, S.; Inakuma, T.; Yano, M. & Nishino, H. (1999). Chemoprevention by the oxygenated carotenoid beta-cryptoxanthin of N-methylnitrosourea-induced colon carcinogenesis in F344 rats, *Japanese Journal of Cancer Research*, Vol.90, No.10, pp. 1061-1065, ISSN 0910-5050

Narisawa, T.; Takahashi, M.; Kotanagi, H.; Kusaka, H.; Yamazaki, Y.; Koyama, H.; Fukaura, Y.; Nishizawa, Y.; Kotsugai, M.; Isoda, Y.; Hirano, J. & Tanida, N. (1991). Inhibitory effect of dietary Perilla oil rich in the n-3 polyunsaturated fatty acid α–linolenic acid on colon carcinogenesis in rats, *Japanese Journal of Cancer Research*, Vol.82, No.10, pp. 1089-1096, ISSN 0910-5050

Narisawa, T.; Fukaura, Y.; Yazawa, K.; Ishikawa, C.; Isoda, Y. & Nishizawa, Y. (1994). Colon cancer prevention with a small amount of dietary perilla oil high in alpha-linolenic acid in an animal model, *Cancer*, Vol.73, No.8, pp. 2069-2075, ISSN 0008-543X

Nishino, H.; Iwashima, A.; Itakura, Y.; Matsuura, H. & Fuwa, T. (1989). Antitumor-promoting activity of garlic extracts, *Oncology*, Vol.46, No.4, pp. 277-280, ISSN 0030-2414

Niwa,K.; Hashimoto, M.; Morishita, S.; Lian, Z.; Tagami, K.; Mori, H. & Tamaya, T. (2001). Preventive effects of Juzen-taiho-to on N-methyl-N-nitrosourea and estadiol-17β-induced endometrial carcinogenesis in mice, *Carcinogenesis*, Vol.22, No.4, pp. 587-591, ISSN 0143-3334

Oganesian, A.; Hendricks, J.D. & Williams, D.E. (1997). Long term dietary indole-3-carbinol inhibits diethylnitrosamine-induced hepatocarcinogenesis in the infant mouse model. *Cancer Letters*, Vol.118, No.1, pp. 87-94, ISSN 0304-3835

Ohigashi, H.; Takamura, H.; Koshimizu, K.;Tokuda, H. & Ito, Y. (1986). Search for possible antitumor promoters by inhibition of 12-O-tetradecanoylphorbol-13-acetate-induced Epstein-Barr virus activation; ursolic acid and oleanolic acid from anti-inflammatory Chinese medicinal plant, *Glechoma hederaceae* L., *Cancer Letters*, Vol.30, No.2, pp. 143-151, ISSN 0304-3835

Ohta, T.; Nakatsugi, S.; Watanabe, K.; Kawamori, T.; Ishikawa, F.; Morotomi, M.; Sugie, S.; Toda, T.; Sugimura, T. & Wakabayashi, K. (2000). Inhibitory effects of *Bifidobacterium*-fermented soy milk on 2-amino-1-methyl-6-phenylimidazol[4,5-*b*]-pyridine-induced rat mammary carcinogenesis, with a partial contribution of its component isoflavones, *Carcinogenesis*, Vol.21, No.5, pp. 937-941, ISSN 0143-3334

Okuyama, T.; Matsuda, M.; Kishi, N.; Lee, S.-N.; Baba, M.; Okada, Y. & Nishina, H. (1995). Studies on the cancer chemoprevention of natural resourcens. XI Anti-tumor promoting activities of the crude drug "Xiebai" and kampo prescriptions composed of "Xiebai", *Natural Medicines*, Vol.49, No.3, pp. 261-265, ISSN 1340-3443

Park, K.-K.; Chun, K.-S.; Lee, J.-M.; Lee, S.S. & Surh, Y.-J. (1998). Inhibitory effects of [6]-gingerol, a major pungent principle of ginger, on phorbol ester-induced inflammation, epidermal ornithine decarboxylase activity and skin tumor promotion in ICR mice, *Cancer Letters*, Vol.129, No.2, pp. 139-144, ISSN 0304-3835

Perchellet, J.P.; Perchellet, E.M. & Belman, S. (1990). Inhibition of DMBA-induced mouse skin tumorigenesis by garlic oil and inhibition of two tumor-promotion stage by garlic and onion oils, *Nutrition and Cancer*, Vol.14, No.3-4, pp. 183-193, ISSN 0163-5581

Pitot, H.C. & Dragan, Y.P. (1991). Facts and theories concerning the mechanisms of carcinogenesis, *The FASEB Journal*, Vol.5, No.9, pp. 2280-2286, ISSN 0892-6638

Prabuseenivasan, S.; Jayakumar, M. & Ignacimuthu, S. (2006). In vitro antibacterial activity of some plant essential oils, BMC Complementary and Alternative Medicine, Vol.6, pp. 1-8, ISSN 1472-6882

Sadhana, A.S.; Rao, A.R.; Kucheria, K. & Bijani, V. (1988). Inhibitory action of garlic oil on the initiation of benz[*a*]pyrene-induced skin carcinogenesis in mice, *Cancer Letters*, Vol.40, No.2, pp. 193-197, ISSN 0304-3835

Sakamoto, S.; Mori, T.; Sawaki, K.; Kawachi, Y.; Kuwa, K.; Kudo, H.; Suzuki, S.; Sugiura, Y.; Kasahara, N. & Nagasawa, H. (1993). Effects of Kampo (Japanese Herbal) medicine "Sho-Saiko-To" on DNA-synthesizing enzyme activity in 1,2-dimethlhydrazine-induced colonic carcinomas in rats, *Planta Medica*, Vol.59, No.2, pp. 152-154, ISSN 0032-0943

Shimizu, Fukutomi, Y.; Ninomiya, M.; Nagura, K.; Kato, T.; Araki, H.; Suganuma, M.; Fujiki,

H. & Moriwaki, H. (2008). Green tea extracts for the prevention of metachronous colorectal adenomas: a pilot study, *Cancer Epidemiology, Biomarkers & Prevention*, Vol.17, No.11, pp. 3020-3025, ISSN 1055-9965

Slaga, T.J.; Fischer, S.M.; Nelson, K. & Gleason, G.L. (1980). Studies of the mechanism of skin tumor promotion: evidence for several stages in promotion, *Proceedings of the National Academy of Sciences of the United States of America*, Vol.77, No.6, pp. 3659-3663, ISSN 0027-8424

Sporn, M.B. (1976). Approaches to prevention of epithelial cancer during the preneoplastic period, *Cancer Research*, Vol.36, No.7, pp. 2699-2702, ISSN 0008-5472

Srivastava, B. & Shukla, Y. (1998). Antitumour promoting activity of indole-3-carbinol in mouse skin carcinogenesis, *Cancer Letters*, Vol.134, No.1, pp. 91-95, ISSN 0304-3835

Sugiyama, K.; Azuhata, Y. & Matsuura, D. (1994). Antitumor promoting effect of components of Chorei-to on rat urinary bladder carcinogenesis in a short-term test with concanavalin A, *Journal of Traditional Medicine*, Vol.11, No.3, pp. 214-219, ISSN 1340-6302

Takasaki, M.; Konoshima, T.; Tokuda, H.; Masuda, K.; Arai, Y.; Shiojima, K. & Ageta, H. (1999a). Anti-carcinogenesis activity of *Taraxacum* Plant. I, *Biological & Pharmaceutical Bulletin*, Vol.22, No.6, pp. 602-605, ISSN 0918-6158

Takasaki, M.; Konoshima, T.; Tokuda, H.; Masuda, K.; Arai, Y.; Shiojima, K. & Ageta, H. (1999b). Anti-carcinogenesis activity of *Taraxacum* Plant. II, *Biological & Pharmaceutical Bulletin*, Vol.22, No.6, pp. 606-610, ISSN 0918-6158

Taji, S.; Yamada, T.; Wada, S.; Tokuda, H.; Sakuma, K. & Tanaka, R. (2008). Lanostane-type triterpenoids from the sclerotia of *Inonotus obliquus* possessing anti-tumor promoting activity, *European Journal of Medicinal Chemistry*, Vol.43, No.11, pp. 2373-2379, ISSN 0223-5234

Tanaka, H.; Hirose, M.; Kawabe, M.; Sano, M.; Takesada, Y.; Hagiwara, A. & Shirai, T. (1997a). Post-initiation inhibitory effects of green tea catechin on 7,12-dimethylbenz[*a*]-anthracene-induced mammary gland carcinogenesis in female Sprague-Dawley rats, *Cancer Letters*, Vol.116, No.1, pp. 47-52, ISSN 0304-3835

Tanaka, H.; Makita, H.; Kawabata, K.; Mori, H.; Kakumoto, M.; Satoh, K.; Hara, A.; Sumida, T.; Tanaka, T. & Ogawa, H. (1997b). Chemoprevention of azoxymethan-induced rat colon carcinogenesis by the naturally occurring flavonoids, diosmin and hesperidin, *Carcinogenesis*, Vol.18, No.5, pp. 957-965, ISSN 0143-3334

Tanaka, T.; Kojima, T.; Morishita, Y. & Mori, H. (1992). Inhibitory effects of the natural products indole-3-carbinol and sinigrin during initiation and promotion phases of 4-nitroquinoline 1-oxide-induced rat tongue carcinogenesis, *Japanese Journal of Cancer research (Gann)*, Vol.83, No.8, pp. 835-842, ISSN 0910-5050

Tanaka, T.; Kohno, H.; Murakami, M.; Shimada, R.; Kagami, S.; Sumida, T.; Azuma, Y. & Ogawa, H. (2000). Suppression of azoxymethane-induced colon carcinogenesis in male F344 rats by mandarin juices rich in β-cryptoxanthin and hesperidin, *International Journal of Cancer*, Vol.88, No.,1, pp. 146-150, ISSN 0020-7136

Vanamala, J.; Leonardi, T.; Patil, B.S.; Taddeo, S.S.; Murphy, M.E.; Pike, L.M.; Chapkin, R.S.; Lupton, J.R. & Turner, N.D. (2006). Suppression of colon carcinogenesis by bioactive compounds in grapefruit, *Carcinogenesis*, Vol.27, No.6, pp. 1257-1265, ISSN ISSN 0143-3334

Yasukawa, K. (2010). Cancer Chemopreventive Agents: Natural Pentacyclic Triterpenoids, In: *Pentacyclic Triterpenes as Promising Agents in Cancer*, J.A.R. Salvador, (ed.), pp. 127-157, Nova Publisher ISBN 978-1-60876-973-5, New York, U.S.A.

Yasukawa, K.; Akihisa, T.; Inoue, Y.; Tamura, T.; Yamanouchi, S. & Takido, M. (1998a). Inhibitory effects of the methanol extracts from Compositae plants on 12-*O*-tetradecanoylphorbol-13-acetate-induced ear oedema in mice, *Phytotherapy Research*, Vol.12, No.6, pp. 484–487, ISSN 0951-418X

Yasukawa, K.; Akihisa, T.; Kanno, H.; Kaminaga, T.; Izumida, M.; Sakoh, T.; Tamura, T. & Takido M. (1996a). Inhibitory effects of sterols isolated from *Chlorella vulgaris* on 12-*O*-tetradecanoyl- phorbol-13-acetate-induced inflammtion and tumor promotion in mouse skin, *Biological & Pharmaceutical Bulletin*, Vol.19, No.4, pp. 573–576, ISSN 0918-6158

Yasukawa, K.; Akihisa, T.; Kasahara, Y.; Kaminaga, T.; Kanno, H.; Kumaki, K.; Tamura, T. & Takido, M. (1996b). Inhibitory effect of alkane-6,8-diols, the components in safflower, on tumor promotion by 12-*O*-tetradecanoylphorbol-13-acetate in two-stage carcinogenesis in mouse skin, *Oncology*, Vol.53, No.2, pp. 133–136 ISSN 0030-2414

Yasukawa, K.; Akihisa, T.; Kasahara, Y.; Ukiya, M.; Kumaki, K.; Tamura, T.; Yamanouchi, S. & Takido, M. (1998b). Inhibitory effect of heliantriol C, the component of the flower of edible chrysanthemum, on tumor promotion by 12-*O*-tetradecanoylphorbol-13-acetate in two-stage carcinogenesis in mouse skin, *Phytomedicine*, Vol.5, No.3, pp. 215–218, ISSN 0944-7113

Yasukawa, K.; Akihisa, T.; Oinuma, H.; Kaminaga, T.; Kanno, H.; Kasahara, Y.; Kumaki, K.; Tamura, T.; Yamanouchi, S. & Takido, M. (1996c). Inhibitory effect of taraxastane-type triterpenes on tumor promotion by 12-*O*-tetradecanoylphorbol-13-acetate in two-stage carcinogenesis in mouse skin, *Oncology*, Vol.53, No.4, pp. 341–344, ISN 0030-2414

Yasukawa, K.; Akihisa, T.; Oinuma, H.; Kasahara, Y.; Kimura, Y. ; Yamanouchi, S.; Kumaki, K.; Tamura, T. & Takido, M. (1996d). Inhibitory effect of di-and trihydroxy triterpenes from the Compositae flowers on 12-*O*-tetradecanoylphorbol-13-acetate induced inflammation in mice, *Biological & Pharmaceutical Bulletin*, Vol.19, No.10, pp. 1329–1331, ISN 0918-6158

Yasukawa, K.; Aoki, T.; Takido, M.; Ikekawa, T.; Saito, H. & Matsuzawa, T. (1994a). Inhibitory effects of ergosterol isolated from the edible mushroom *Hypsizigus marmoreus* on TPA-induced inflammatory ear oedema and tumour promotion in mice, *Phytotherapy Research*, Vol.8, No.1, pp. 10–13, ISSN 0951-418X

Yasukawa, K.; Demitrijevic, S.M., Evans, F.J., Kawabata, S. & Takido M. (1998c). Inhibitory effect of Prunus Cortex extract and its component, octacosyl ferulate, on tumor promotion by 12-*O*-tetradecanoylphorbol-13-acetate in two-stage carcinogenesis in mouse skin, *Phytotherapy Research*, Vol.12, No.4, pp. 261–265, ISSN 0951-418X

Yasukawa, K.; Kanno, H.; Kaminaga, T.; Takido, M.; Kasahara, Y. & Kumaki, K. (1996e). Inhibitory effect of methanol extracts from edible mushroom on TPA-induced ear oedema and tumour promotion in mouse skin, *Phytotherapy Research*, Vol.10, No.4, pp. 367–369, ISSN 0951-418X

Yasukawa, K.; Kitanaka, S.; Kawata, K. & Goto, K. (2009). Anti-tumor promoters phenolics and triterpenoid from *Hippophae rhamnoides*, *Fitoterapia*, Vol.80, No.3, pp. 164–167, ISSN 0367-326X

Yasukawa, K.; Matsubara, H. & Sano Y. (2010). Inhibitory effect of artichoke (*Cynara cardunculus*) on TPA-induced inflammation and tumor promotion in two-stage carcinogenesis in mouse skin, *Journal of Natural Medicines*, Vol.64, No.3, pp. 388–391, ISSN 1340-3443

Yasukawa, K.; Sun, Y.; Kitanaka, S.; Tomizawa, N.; Miura, M. & Motohashi S. (2008). Inhibitory effect of the Rhizomes of *Alpinia officinarum* on TPA-induced inflammation and tumor promotion in two-stage carcinogenesis in mouse skin, *Journal of Natural Medicines*, Vol.62, No.3, pp. 374–378, ISSN 1340-3443

Yasukawa, K.; Takahashi, H.; Kitanaka, S.; Hirayama, H. & Shigemoto K. (2007). Inhibitory effect of an aqueous extract of *Phellinus linteus* on tumor promotion in mouse skin, *Mushroom Science and Biotechnology*, Vol.15, No.2, pp. 97–101, ISSN 1348-7388

Yasukawa, K.; Takahashi, M.; Natori, S.; Kawai, K.; Yamazaki, M.; Takeuchi, M. & Takido, M. (1994b). Azaphilones inhibit tumor promotion by 12-*O*-tetradecanoylphorbol-13-acetate in two-stage carcinogenesis in mice, *Oncology*, Vol.51, No.1, pp. 108–112, ISSN 0030-2414

Yasukawa, K.; Takahashi, M.; Yamanouchi, S. & Takido, M. (1996f). Inhibitory effect of oral administration of Monascus pigment on tumor promotion in two-stage carcinogenesis in mouse skin, *Oncology*, Vol.53, No.3, pp. 247–249, ISN 0030-2414

Yasukawa, K.; Takido, M.; Takeuchi, M. & Nakagawa, S. (1989). Effect of chemical constituents from plants on 12-*O*-tetradecanoylphorbol-13-acetate-induced inflammation in mice, *Chemical & Pharmaceutical Bulletin*, Vol. 37, No.4, pp. 1071-1073, ISSN 0009-2363

Yasukawa, K.; Yu, S.-Y.; Kakinuma, S. & Takido M. (1995). Inhibitory effect of Rikkunshi-to, a traditional Chinese herbal prescription, on tumor promotion in two-stage carcinogenesis in mouse skin, *Biological & Pharmaceutical Bulletin*, Vol.18, No.5, pp.730–733, ISSN 0918-6158

Yasukawa, K.; Yu, S.Y. & Takido M. (1996g). Inhibitory effect of oral administration of Rikkunshi-to on tumor promotion in two-stage carcinogenesis in mouse skin, *Journal of Traditional Medicine*, Vol.13, No.2, pp. 180–184, ISSN 1340-6302

Yoshizawa, S.; Horiuchi, T.; Fujiki, H.; Yoshida, T.; Okuda, T. & Sugimura, T. (1987). Antitumor promoting activity of (–)-epigallocatechin gallate, the main constituent of Tannin in green tea, *Phytotherapy Research*, Vol.1, No.1, pp. 44-47, ISSN 0951-418X

Yu, S.-Y., Yasukawa, K. & Takido, M. (1994). Atractylodis Rhizoma extract and its component, atractylon, inhibit tumor promotion in mouse skin two-stage carcinogenesis, *Phytomedicine*, Vol.1, No.1, pp. 55–58, ISSN 0944-7113

Yun, T.-K.; Lee, Y.-S.; Lee, Y.-H.; Kim, S.I. & Yun, H.Y. (2001). Anticarcinogenic effect of *Panax ginseng* C.A. Meyer and identification of active compounds, *Journal of Korean Medical Science*, Vol.16, Suppl., pp. S6-S18, ISSN 1011-8934

Zhao, J.; Wang, J.; Chen, Y. & Agarwl, R. (1999). Anti-tumor-promoting activity of a polyphenolic fraction isolated from grape seeds in the mouse skin two-stage initiation-promotin protocol and identification of procyanidin B5-3'-gallate as the most effective antioxidant constituent, *Carcinogenesis*, Vol.20, No.9, pp. 1737-1745, ISSN 0143-3334

8

A Comparison Between Lignans from Creosote Bush and Flaxseed and Their Potential to Inhibit Cytochrome P450 Enzyme Activity

Jennifer Billinsky, Katherine Maloney, Ed Krol and Jane Alcorn
Drug Design and Discovery Research Group, College of Pharmacy and Nutrition,
University of Saskatchewan
Canada

1. Introduction

The popularity in natural product use we witness today arose from a growing public skepticism about taking "pharmaceutical chemicals" to treat illness. Such skepticism was supplanted by a public perception that "medications" from natural sources are safer to use and have similar efficacies as their pharmaceutical equivalents. The diverse assortment of natural products on the shelves of pharmacies, health food stores, and grocery stores attest to this enhanced public demand, but has compelled regulatory agencies to question the adequacy of the safety and efficacy data associated with the use of these products (Natural Health Products Directorate 2007). In the current regulatory environment, full realization of the wellness and therapeutic value of these natural products can only come about with more rigorous assessments of their safety and efficacy.

This is particularly true of natural products that contain lignans as the principal bioactive component. Interest in lignans continues to grow due to an increased awareness of their putative health benefits. One such product, Chaparral, contains lignans extracted from creosote bush. Creosote bush had centuries of traditional use by aboriginal peoples of the Southwestern United States as an effective natural medicine and was marketed as an extract of the plant in capsule form based on this historical medicinal value (Clark & Reed 1992). While traditional creosote bush use appears to be quite safe, chronic use of Chaparral led to reports of toxicity (Clark & Reed 1992; Gordon et al., 1995; Batchelor et al., 1995; Grant et al., 1998). Nordihydroguaiaretic acid (NDGA) is the major lignan in creosote bush, which is believed to be responsible for both the efficacious and toxic properties of Chaparral (Grice et al., 1968; Moore 1989; Arteaga et al., 2005; Lambert et al., 2004). Wagner and Lewis 1980 previously reported that NDGA undergoes oxidation to "activated NDGA" (Wagner & Lewis 1980). Billinsky et al. 2008 suggest this "activated NDGA" is the result of an autoxidation process to a stable dibenzocyclooctadiene product of NDGA (Billinsky & Krol 2008). Whether this dibenzocyclooctadiene is present in traditional creosote bush products or is formed *in vivo* is not known.

The recent popularity of lignans from flaxseed, which are currently marketed as concentrated extracts of the principal plant lignan, secoisolariciresinol diglucoside (SDG), in products such as Brevail™ and Beneflax™, arises from recent promising clinical trial evidence of their chemopreventive and therapeutic properties for a variety of chronic diseases (Pan et al., 2007; Hallund et al., 2008; Zhang et al., 2008). Following oral consumption, the glucose groups of SDG are cleaved to form the aglycone, secoisolariciresinol (SECO), which is further metabolized to the mammalian lignans, enterodiol (ED) and enterolactone (EL), by colonic bacteria (Rickard et al., 1996; Borriello et al., 1985a). Flaxseed also contains smaller amounts of other lignans such as mataresinol, and lariciresinol. The presence of anhydrosecoisolariciresinol (ASECO) was reported in flaxseed (Charlet et al., 2002). However, its actual presence is questioned as the acid hydrolysis method used to extract and quantify lignans from flaxseed can convert SECO into ASECO (Mazur et al., 1996). Which lignan form mediates the putative health effects is not known, but little evidence of toxicity exists with their use, and most clinical trial data identifies their relative safety. Interestingly, a comparison of the structure of NDGA from creosote bush with the flaxseed lignan, SDG and its aglycone form, SECO, identifies remarkable structurally similarity, yet with obvious differences in their safety profiles (Figure 1).

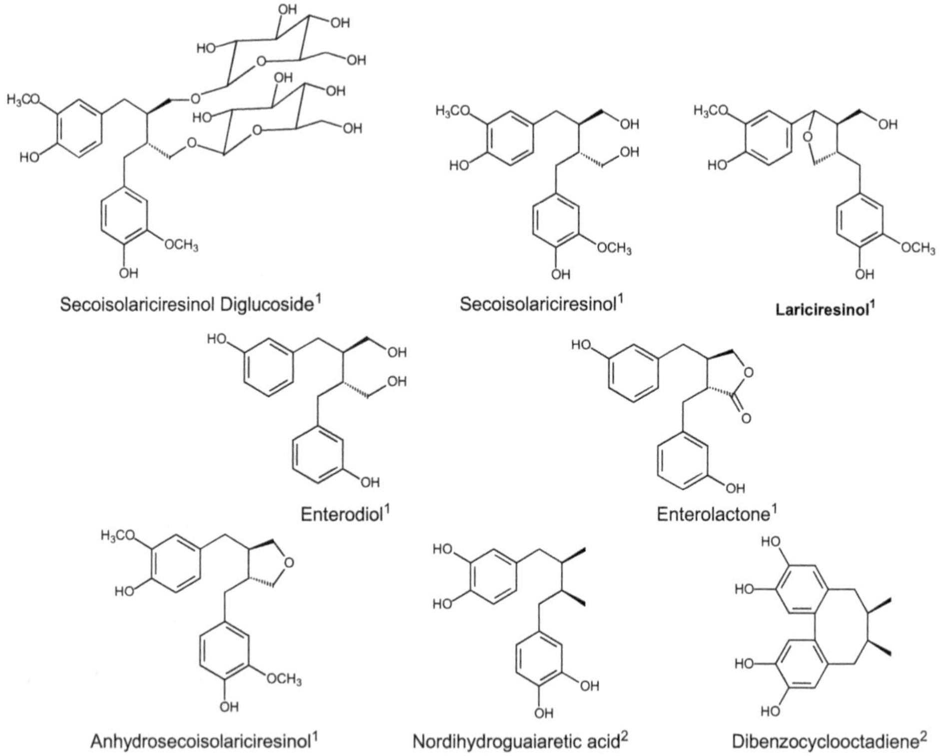

Secoisolariciresinol Diglucoside[1]   Secoisolariciresinol[1]   Lariciresinol[1]

Enterodiol[1]   Enterolactone[1]

Anhydrosecoisolariciresinol[1]   Nordihydroguaiaretic acid[2]   Dibenzocyclooctadiene[2]

Fig. 1. Structures of lignans derived from Flaxseed[1] and Creosote bush[2].

Why lignan in chaparral is associated with toxicity while lignans from flaxseed have limited reported toxicity may relate to differences in their ability to inhibit cytochrome P450 (P450) enzymes. Cytochrome P450 enzymes are the principal detoxification mechanisms of the body and mediate the elimination of a wide variety of drugs, phytochemicals, and environmental toxicants. Consequently, interactions involving P450 enzymes are widely reported in the literature. Such P450 enzyme interactions often involve P450 inhibition, which may proceed either through mechanism-based, irreversible interaction with a P450 enzyme or by a reversible competitive interaction between two substrates for the same P450. Both inhibition mechanisms represent common underlying mechanisms for toxicity associated with pharmaceutical products, phytochemicals and environmental toxicants (Fowler & Zhang 2008).

Mechanism-based, irreversible inhibition of P450 usually follows from bioactivation by P450 to a reactive metabolite that, in turn, covalently binds to the enzyme (heme or apoprotein) and prevents further P450 activity (Kalgutkar et al., 2007). Enzyme function is only restored with synthesis of new enzyme. Alternatively, the reactive metabolite may bind to other macromolecules (i.e. protein, nucleic acid) to inhibit their function or act as a hapten leading to an immune response with toxicological outcomes (Kalgutkar et al., 2007). Hence, P450-mediated bioactivation to reactive metabolites can represent an important mechanism of toxicity associated with natural product use. Reversible competitive interactions at the same P450 can also result in toxicity when natural products are present simultaneously with other chemicals whose metabolic clearance is predominantly dependent upon a particular P450 enzyme (Fowler & Zhang 2008). Competitive interactions, then, may lead to the accumulation of a compound and eventual toxicity. Given the potential for significant adverse outcomes, evaluation of P450 inhibition is commonly investigated during standard safety assessments for drugs, environmental contaminants, and phytochemicals.

Our purpose was to determine whether mechanism-based, irreversible inhibition and/or reversible, competitive P450 inhibition might explain the differences in apparent toxicity between oral consumption of naturally occurring lignans from creosote bush, which have known toxicity, and flaxseed, which show relative safety. Additionally, such information is important to determine whether lignans present a significant concern with respect to their potential for P450-mediated interactions. As a proof-of-concept study, rat hepatic microsomal systems were employed to investigate the hypothesis that lignan from creosote bush undergoes P450-enzyme mediated bioactivation to form reactive metabolites while flaxseed lignans do not. Furthermore, we hypothesized that lignan from creosote bush inhibits P450 enzyme activity via mechanism-based and/or reversible inhibition mechanisms and that glutathione (GSH) can attenuate the inhibition. The use of rat also supports current investigations in our laboratories concerning lignan efficacy and pharmacokinetics in rat models of hyperlipidemia and hyperglycemia (Felmlee et al., 2009). Such investigations will make an invaluable contribution to our understanding of the safety of natural products containing lignan as the principal bioactive component.

2. Cytochrome P450-mediated formation of reactive metabolites

Cytochrome P450 enzyme interactions are commonly touted as a mechanism of toxicity (Fowler & Zhang 2008; Stresser et al., 2000). In particular, bioactivation, or the metabolic activation of a compound to an electrophilic reactive intermediate, which subsequently undergoes covalent binding to critical cellular macromolecules and interferes with their function, has long-standing recognition as a biochemical mechanism of organ toxicity (Miller & Miller 1947; Mitchell et al., 1973; Masubuchi et al., 2007). Several examples exist of natural products undergoing P450-mediated bioactivation and irreversible P450 enzyme inhibition and hepatotoxicity (Johnson et al., 2003; Zhou et al., 2004; Surh & Lee 1995; He et al., 1998; Kent et al., 2002). Furthermore, natural products are known to result in significant interactions with coadministered therapeutic agents resulting in adverse effects or therapeutic failures (Dietz & Bolton 2007; Yuan et al., 2004; Kupiec & Raj 2005). With the growing interest in lignans for their health and wellness or therapeutic values, assessments of their safety are necessary to support their use.

Structural features of the lignans suggest their potential for oxidation to quinone derivatives, a class of compounds known to be electrophilic reactive intermediates (Bolton et al., 1994; Iverson et al., 1995). Since SDG is unlikely absorbed due to the polar nature of the glycosidic groups, it was not investigated for their potential to undergo hepatic P450-mediated bioactivation to a reactive intermediate. Previous studies in our laboratory identified NDGA's (the major lignan of creosote bush) ability to undergo autoxidation to a reactive quinone species (Billinsky et al., 2007; Billinsky & Krol 2008). Billinsky et al., 2007 had previously reported that NDGA underwent autoxidation and conversion via an *ortho*-quinone reactive intermediate to three glutathione (GSH) adducts (Billinsky et al., 2007). Furthermore, in the absence of GSH NDGA autoxidation resulted in the formation of a novel dibenzocyclooctadiene (Billinsky & Krol 2008). The autoxidation of NDGA to a reactive intermediate in rat hepatic microsomes (Billinsky et al., 2007) did not result in the inactivation of P450 enzyme activity. These findings are not unexpected as the literature suggests *ortho*-quinones do not usually undergo adduct formation with cellular macromolecules, instead their damage is usually mediated through an increase in oxidative stress (Chichirau et al., 2005; O'Brien 1991; Monks et al., 1992). Although *ortho*-quinones may isomerize to *para*-quinone methides *in vivo*, a quinone derivative known to form covalent adducts with cellular macromolecules (Powis 1987), this process is unlikely to occur as NDGA is substituted at the benzylic carbon, which severely hinders the isomerization process (Iverson et al., 1995).

Current studies indicate that SECO (the aglycone form of the major flaxseed lignan, SDG) underwent conversion to lariciresinol, both in the presence and absence of GSH, without formation of a stable reactive quinone intermediate. No GSH adducts were observed following microsomal incubations. ASECO was also examined as its structure is intermediate of NDGA and SECO. For ASECO, all control experiments showed no product formation; however, in the presence of GSH a product peak in MS-ESI(-) with a m/z 648.19 [M-H]- was observed. This mass is consistent with the formation of an ASECO-GSH adduct, which is likely derived from an ASECO *para*-quinone methide.

These studies, in conjunction with the growing interest in their use, compelled an investigation into their potential for mechanism-based inhibition and/or reversible inhibition of P450 isoforms. The use of *in vitro* microsomal systems for assessments of cytochrome P450 inhibition potential by drug candidates and natural products is a commonly employed technique to determine the likelihood for pharmacokinetic interactions resulting from P450 enzyme inhibition (Stresser et al., 2000).

3. Mechanism-based inhibition of cytochrome P450 enzymes

We examined the ability of creosote bush and flaxseed lignans to inhibit the activity of CYP3A, CYP2C and CYP1A2 enzymes as these isoforms are principally involved in the metabolism of drugs and other natural products on the market today. To determine whether lignans result in mechanism-based inhibition of P450 enzymes initial experiments examined the extent of inhibition as a function of pre-incubation time and lignan concentration.

SDG did not cause mechanism-based inhibition of any P450 isoform at any concentration tested. The data also suggests that SDG does not cause reversible inhibition of P450 isoforms, as metabolite formation remained the same at pre-incubation time 0 at all SDG concentrations tested. This result was not unexpected given the physicochemical characteristics of SDG. Hydrophilic molecules tend not to be substrates for P450 enzymes and are primarily eliminated from the body via renal elimination mechanisms. Furthermore, studies have failed to detect systemic levels of SDG (Kuijsten et al., 2005b), suggesting that it is not absorbed from the gastrointestinal tract or undergoes extensive first pass metabolism. Studies further suggest that this first-pass metabolism occurs at the gastrointestinal level, where the glucosidic groups of SDG are cleaved to produce the aglycone, SECO (Thompson et al., 1991; Borriello et al., 1985c). SECO is likely the flaxseed lignan form available for absorption following the oral consumption of flaxseed products (Nesbitt et al., 1999; Axelson et al., 1982d).

SECO did not cause significant inhibition of CYP1A2. SECO inhibited CYP3A in a concentration-dependent but not time-dependent manner suggesting that SECO is a reversible inhibitor of the three isoforms. Reversible inhibition is consistent with the lack of GSH adduct formation following microsomal incubation of SECO in the presence of GSH. However, at 2000 µM SECO inhibited 6β-, 16α- and 2α-hydroxytestosterone formation by only 36.2 ± 7.26%, 65.7 ± 8.36% and 64.4 ± 6.36%, respectively.

ASECO caused limited inhibition of CYP1A2, 2B, and 2C11, with moderate inhibition of CYP3A at the highest concentration (100 µM) resulting in 49.2 ± 1.8% inhibition after 20 minutes preincubation. As with SDG and SECO, ASECO showed concentration-dependent but not time-dependant inhibition which suggests P450 inhibition by reversible mechanisms. These results are interesting, as in the presence of GSH, we observed an ASECO adduct that was consistent with *para*-quinone methide formation (Bolton et al., 1994; Awad et al., 2002). Despite this observation, mechanism-based inhibition of P450 activity was not identified in our studies.

Enterodiol (ED) failed to inhibit P450 activity and rather caused activation of CYP1A2, 3A, 2B and 2C11 activity particularly at shorter preincubation times (Figure 2). Although an apparent inhibition of CYP3A activity was observed after a 20 min pre-incubation (Figure 2b), control samples without ED showed a large %CV of 91.8% relative to the samples pre-incubated with ED for 20 min.

EL caused concentration-dependent, but not time-dependent, inhibition of CYP1A2 and only at high concentrations with 500 µM EL inhibiting CYP1A2 to 14.3 ± 23% that of control (data not shown). EL also caused concentration-dependent inhibition of CYP3A.

Interestingly, EL caused activation of 16α-hydroxytestosterone (16α-OH) formation, a metabolite pathway shared by CYP2B and CYP2C11. Given the ability of EL to inhibit 2α-OH formation, a pathway largely catalyzed by CYP2C11, increased 16α-OH formation may be due to activation of CYP2B activity by EL.

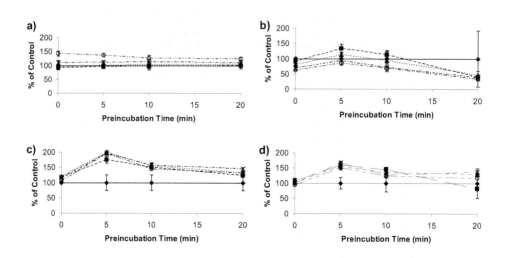

Fig. 2. Cytochrome P450 enzyme activity (as percent of control) as a function of Enterodiol concentration and pre-incubation time. a) CYP1A2, b) CYP3A, c) CYP2B/2C11 and d) CYP2C11. Enterodiol (closed diamond = 0 μM; closed square = 50 μM; closed triangle = 100 μM; symbol 'x' = 250 μM; open circle = 500 μM) was pre-incubated in pooled male rat hepatic microsomes (n=4) for different time periods. At the end of each pre-incubation period, testosterone (50 μM) and methoxyresorufin (0.5 μM) was added and metabolite formation was determined after a 15 min and 8 min reaction time, respectively. Each point is the mean of 3 replicates ± percent coefficient of variation.

NDGA generally caused concentration-dependent but not time-dependent inhibition of all CYP isoforms (data not shown). We anticipated that NDGA could be an irreversible inhibitor given its ability to form a reactive *ortho*-quinone intermediate. Since this is an autoxidation process and not a P450 catalyzed process, it appears that the *ortho*-quinone does not inhibit P450 *in vitro* (Billinsky et al., 2007; Billinsky & Krol 2008). Generally, marked inhibition was not observed until NDGA concentrations reached 100 μM or higher. At a pre-incubation time of 20 minutes and a concentration of 200 μM, NDGA inhibited CYP1A2, 2B/2C11 and 2C11 to 3.55 ± 12.0%, 21.2 ± 8.81% and 21.2 ± 9.37% of control, respectively. NDGA caused complete inhibition of formation of 6β-OH via CYP3A at pre-incubation time of 20 minutes and a concentration of 200 μM.

The NDGA dibenzocyclooctadiene did not cause significant inhibition of CYP2B/2C11 and did not cause time-dependant inhibition of any of the tested isoforms (data not shown). The NDGA dibenzocyclooctadiene significantly inhibited CYP3A and CYP1A2 to 42.9 ± 3.6%, and 13.9 ± 4.3% of control, respectively, at 100 μM.

Our studies provided no evidence of mechanism-based inhibition of the P450 enzymes by either the lignans of creosote bush or flaxseed.

4. Reversible inhibition of cytochrome P450 enzymes

To determine whether lignans inhibit specific P450 enzymes through reversible mechanisms, we monitored the metabolite formation of P450-probe substrates by rat hepatic microsomes in the presence of different concentrations of lignan and probe substrates. Since time- and concentration-dependent experiments indicated that SDG and ED were neither reversible nor irreversible inhibitors of P450 enzyme activity, we excluded SDG and ED from our evaluations for reversible inhibition. We estimated the % inhibition at each lignan concentration and when possible estimated the IC50 values to provide a measure of potency of the inhibition. Lineweaver-Burke plots were constructed to determine the mechanism of inhibition. HPLC results from lignan incubations indicated substrate depletion at a testosterone concentration of 25 μM, representing ½ K_M for the substrate. Consequently, this concentration was not included in any of the graphical representations and analysis. Reversible inhibition of P450 enzyme activity by the flaxseed lignans tended to show more specificity than the creosote bush lignans. Although our studies provide evidence of reversible inhibition of rat P450 enzyme activity by the lignans of creosote bush and flaxseed, such inhibition required rather high lignan concentrations.

Our data suggest SECO is a more specific inhibitor of P450 enzymes and causes a marked reduction in CYP3A activity only at high SECO concentrations. Such concentrations are substantially greater than the levels anticipated under physiological conditions (25-100 μM) (Hu et al., 2007). Our data also show that SECO activates CYP2B activity at lower probe substrate concentrations.

SECO caused a concentration-dependent decrease in 6β-OH formation, which is mediated by CYP3A (Figure 3a). A plot of 6β-OH formation (at K_M) as a function of the logarithmic concentration of SECO yielded an IC50 value of 373 μM (95% CI 266-523). A Lineweaver-Burke plot showed a pattern almost consistent with that of competitive inhibition, but the lines intersected in the upper right hand quadrant near the y-axis (not shown). This suggests SECO inhibits CYP3A activity consistent with atypical Michaelis-Menten kinetics (Folk et al., 1962; Atkins 2005).

The formation of 16α-OH testosterone, representing CYP2B/2C11 activity, was largely unaffected by SECO at testosterone concentrations of 100 and 250 μM (Figure 3b). At 50 μM testosterone, SECO concentrations ≥50 μM increased the formation of 16α-OH testosterone. Since CYP2C11 activity was generally unaffected by SECO (Figure 3c), SECO-mediated activation of CYP2B likely explains the increased formation of 16α-OH testosterone. The percent of control activity of the various CYP isoforms tested at K_M, 2×K_M and V_{Max} testosterone is summarized in Table 1.

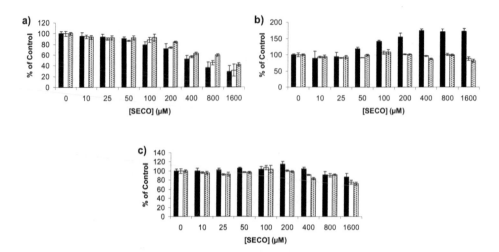

Fig. 3. Secoisolariciresinol (SECO) concentration dependent inhibition of a) CYP3A, b) CYP2B/2C11 and c) CYP2C11 using testosterone (solid bar = 50 μM; open bar = 100 μM; stipled bar = 250 μM) as the probe substrate in incubation reactions (15 min) with pooled (n=4) male, rat liver microsomes. Each point represents the mean of 3 replicates ± percent coefficient of variation.

	6β-OHT (CYP3A)		16α-OHT (CYP2B/2C11)		2α-OHT (CYP2C11)	
	Percent of Control Activity (mean ± % CV)		Percent of Control Activity (mean ± % CV)		Percent of Control Activity (mean ± % CV)	
Testosterone/ Methoxyresorufin	SECO 50 μM	SECO 1600 μM	SECO 50 μM	SECO 1600 μM	SECO 50 μM	SECO 1600 μM
K_M	90.7 ± 5.0	29.0 ± 11	117.5 ± 5.1	172 ± 8.1	106.1 ± 1.7	86.0 ± 7.6
$2K_M$	86.4 ± 1.1	31.8 ± 11	91.0 ± 0.5	87.4 ± 5.2	97.3 ± 0.5	75.0 ± 4.0
V_{Max}	91.9 ± 3.6	42.4 ± 3.1	98.4 ± 2.8	80.9 ± 5.2	97.1 ± 2.3	71.9 ± 3.3

Table 1. The percent of control activity (mean ± % CV) for the formation of 6β-, 16α- and 2α-hydroxytestosterone (OHT) in pooled (n=4) rat liver microsomes by 50 and 1600 μM Secoisolariciresinol (SECO) at the K_M, $2 \times K_M$ and ~V_{Max} of testosterone.

We further examined the ability of an additional flaxseed lignan, ASECO, to inhibit P450 enzyme activity. Whether ASECO is present in flaxseed remains controversial as the identification of ASECO in flaxseed may be an artifact of the analytical techniques employed by Charlet et al. (Charlet et al., 2002). Our lab has produced ASECO by acid hydrolysis of SECO using the same methods as Charlet et al., 2002 (Charlet et al., 2002). Furthermore,

A Comparison Between Lignans from Creosote
Bush and Flaxseed and Their Potential to Inhibit Cytochrome P450 Enzyme Activity

181

ASECO could be formed during the isolation process for lignan enriched flaxseed products such as Beneflax™, and with oral consumption of flaxseed lignan products small amounts of ASECO could form within the acidic environment of the stomach. Such factors warranted an examination of ASECO's ability to inhibit P450 enzyme activity.

Pre-incubation time- and concentration- dependant experiments showed that ASECO was not an inhibitor of CYP2B/2C11. Due to overlapping and unresolvable HPLC peaks, the inhibition of CYP2C11, measured by 2α-OH testosterone formation could not be assessed. ASECO maximally inhibited CYP1A2 when methoxyresorufin concentration was at the K_M of the enzyme, with the greatest extent of inhibition occurring at 100 μM ASECO (70.8 $\pm$ 3.9% of control) (Figure 4a). Further increases in the extent of inhibition at higher ASECO concentrations was not observed, but this may be due to an inability to completely solubilize ASECO. Therefore, data for 150 and 200μM are not shown. ASECO generally caused a concentration-dependent inhibition of CYP3A at all testosterone concentrations, although the pattern of inhibition became inconsistent at ASECO concentrations beyond 100 μM, which is likely due to solubility issues (Figure 4b). The percent of control activity of the formation of resorufin and 6β-OH tested at K_M, 2$\times K_M$ and V_{Max} of methoxyresorufin and testosterone is summarized in Table 2. A plot of the 6β-OH formation (at K_M) as a function of the logarithmic concentration of ASECO yielded an IC50 value of 36.4 μM (95% CI 21.9-60.3). The IC50 value for CYP1A2 inhibition was greater than 200 μM. A Lineweaver-Burke plot gave parallel lines, a pattern consistent with uncompetitive inhibition (not shown).

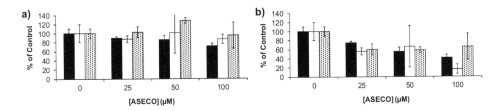

Fig. 4. Anhydrosecoisolariciresinol (ASECO) concentration dependent inhibition of a) CYP1A2 and b) CYP3A using methoxyresorufin (solid bar = 0.5 μM; open bar = 1 μM; stipled bar = 2.5 μM) and testosterone (solid bar = 50 μM; open bar = 100 μM; stipled bar = 250 μM) as the probe substrates, respectively, in incubation reactions (8 min and 15 min, respectively) with pooled (n=4) male, rat liver microsomes. Each point represents the mean of 3 replicates $\pm$ percent coefficient of variation.

SDG (and SECO) is often referred to as the precursor for the enterolignans, ED and EL (Thompson et al., 1991; Borriello et al., 1985a; Kuijsten et al., 2005; Axelson et al., 1982c; Bambagiotti-Alberti et al., 1994). Much of the putative health benefits of flaxseed lignans are ascribed to the enterolignan forms, although definitive data for such assertions is lacking. Following oral consumption, SDG is converted to SECO, which further undergoes metabolism to ED and then to EL by colonic bacterial activity (Axelson et al., 1982b). The literature reports significant systemic and urinary levels of EL and its conjugated forms

(Jacobs et al., 1999; Axelson et al., 1982a) and much lower levels of ED suggesting that EL and ED are absorbed following their conversion within the gastrointestinal tract. This warranted an investigation of their potential to inhibit P450 enzyme activity.

Testosterone/ Methoxyresorufin	Resorufin (CYP1A2)		6β-OHT (CYP3A)	
	Percent of Control Activity (mean ± % CV)		Percent of Control Activity (mean ± % CV)	
	ASECO 25 µM	ASECO 100 µM	ASECO 25 µM	ASECO 100 µM
K_M	89.6 ± 19.5	70.8 ± 3.9	74.0 ±3.5	40.9 ± 6.5
$2K_M$	87.5 ± 14.1	86.4 ± 14.0	55.5 ± 7.8	15.6 ± 10.2
V_{Max}	102.6 ± 3.8	94.7 ± 12.5	59.7 ± 12.2	65.2 ± 28.7

Table 2. The percent of control activity (mean ± % CV) for the formation of 6β-hydroxytestosterone (OHT) and resorufin in pooled (n=4) rat liver microsomes by 25 and 100 µM Anhydrosecosiolariciresinol (ASECO) at the K_M, $2 \times K_M$ and ~V_{Max} of testosterone or methoxyresorufin.

Enterodiol caused CYP2B/2C11 activation in time- and concentration-dependent experiments and thus was not examined for reversible inhibition of these enzymes. EL maximally inhibited CYP1A2 when methoxyresorufin concentration was at the K_M of the enzyme (Figure 5a). EL also caused a concentration-dependent decrease in resorufin formation at $2 \times K_M$ and V_{Max} methoxyresorufin concentrations (Figure 5a). At the K_M of testosterone, EL did not inhibit CYP3A activity and at 500 µM EL, a 3-fold increase in metabolite formation was observed (Figure 5b). However, at $2 \times K_M$ and V_{Max} testosterone concentrations, EL generally caused a concentration-dependent decrease in CYP3A-mediated 6β-OH formation (Figure 5b). For CYP2C11, at the K_M of testosterone, EL generally increased the rate of 2α-OH formation at all EL concentrations. However, EL caused pronounced inhibition at $2 \times K_M$ and V_{Max} testosterone concentrations for the enzyme (Figure 5c). Plots of metabolite formation (at K_M) as a function of the logarithmic concentration of EL yielded IC50 values of 441 µM (95% CI 115-1695), 72.9 µM (95% CI 54.0-98.2) (determined at the V_{Max} due to activation at K_M) and 104 µM (95% CI 85.7-127) (determined at the V_{Max} due to activation at K_M) for CYP1A2, CYP3A and CYP2C11, respectively. The percent of control activity of the various CYP isoforms tested at K_M, $2 \times K_M$ and V_{Max} of methoxyresorufin or testosterone is summarized in Table 3.

Lineweaver-Burke plots were difficult to interpret for EL inhibition of CYP1A2, although the pattern was somewhat consistent with that of competitive inhibition, with the lines intersecting in the upper right hand quadrant (not shown). However, the pattern of the plots for CYP2C11 and CYP3A were consistent with noncompetitive inhibition by EL.

A Comparison Between Lignans from Creosote
Bush and Flaxseed and Their Potential to Inhibit Cytochrome P450 Enzyme Activity

183

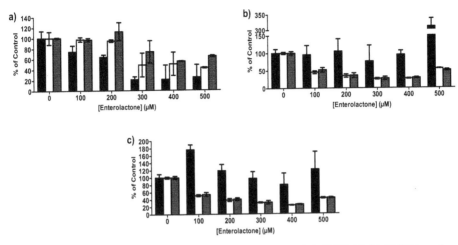

Fig. 5. Enterolactone concentration dependent inhibition of a) CYP1A2, b) CYP3A and
c) CYP2C11 using methoxyresorufin (solid bar = 0.5 µM; open bar = 1 µM; stipled bar = 2.5
µM) and testosterone (solid bar = 50 µM; open bar = 100 µM; stipled bar = 250 µM) as the
probe substrates, respectively, in incubation reactions (8 min and 15 min, respectively) with
pooled (n=4) male, rat liver microsomes. Each point represents the mean of 3 replicates ±
percent coefficient of variation.

	Resorufin (CYP1A2)		6β-OHT (CYP3A)		16α-OHT (CYP2B/2C11)		2α-OHT (CYP2C11)	
	Percent of Control Activity (mean ± % CV)		Percent of Control Activity (mean ± % CV)		Percent of Control Activity (mean ± % CV)		Percent of Control Activity (mean ± % CV)	
Testosterone/ Methoxy- resorufin	EL 100 µM	EL 500 µM	EL 100 µM	EL 500 µM	EL 100 µM	EL 500 µM	EL 100 µM	EL 500 µM
K_M	74.2 ± 13.8	24.7 ± 23.7	95.1 ± 26.8	309.9 ± 26.0	262.7 ± 17.1	302.5 ± 11.4	176.2 ± 13.2	120.2 ± 48.1
$2K_M$	97.4 ± 12.2	42.6 ±1.0	45.5 ± 4.2	55.0 ± 0.7	86.9 ± 1.8	61.9 ± 2.1	51.0 ± 2.9	42.4 ± 1.9
V_{Max}	96.7 ± 1.1	64.7 ± 1.6	52.0 ± 6.4	50.2 ± 2.3	75.4 ± 5.4	60.1 ± 2.7	53.9 ± 5.5	43.0 ± 1.7

Table 3. The percent of control activity (mean ± % CV) for the formation of resorufin, and
6β-, 16α- and 2α-hydroxytestosterone (OHT) in pooled (n=4) rat liver microsomes by 100
and 500 µM Enterolactone (EL) at the K_M, 2×K_M and ~V_{Max} of methoxyresorufin or
testosterone.

In general, NDGA caused a concentration-dependent decrease in CYP1A2, CYP3A, CYP2B and CYP2C11 activity (Figure 6). For CYP1A2, NDGA caused more prominent inhibition at the K_M of methoxyresorufin (Figure 6a), but for the CYP3A, CYP2B/2C11, and CYP2C11, NDGA caused most pronounced inhibition of testosterone metabolite formation at the V_{Max} for testosterone (Figure 6b, 6c, 6d). Furthermore, at the K_M of testosterone, NDGA increased the 16α- and 2α-hydroxylation of testosterone, index pathways for CYP2B/2C11 and CYP2C11, respectively. Activation of metabolism was more pronounced for 16α-OH formation. The IC50 values were calculated at the K_M of the substrate for CYP1A2 and CYP3A and at V_{Max} for testosterone for CYP2B/2C11 and CYP2C11, as activation was observed at the K_M for CYP2B/2C11 and CYP2C11. Plots of metabolite formation as a function of the logarithmic concentration of NDGA yielded IC50 values of 63.5 µM (95% CI 11.8-341), 97.3 µM (95% CI 49.6-191), 68.7 µM (95% CI 46.4-102) and 96.6 µM (95% CI 55.3-169) for CYP1A2, CYP3A, CYP2B/2C11 and CYP2C11, respectively. The percent of control activity of the various CYP isoforms tested at K_M, $2 \times K_M$ and V_{Max} of methoxyresorufin or testosterone is summarized in Table 4.

	Resorufin (CYP1A2)		6β-OHT (CYP3A)		16α-OHT (CYP2B/2C11)		2α-OHT (CYP2C11)	
	Percent of Control Activity (mean ± % CV)		Percent of Control Activity (mean ± % CV)		Percent of Control Activity (mean ± % CV)		Percent of Control Activity (mean ± % CV)	
Testosterone/ Methoxy- resorufin	NDGA 25 µM	NDGA 200 µM	NDGA 25 µM	NDGA 200 µM	NDGA 25 µM	NDGA 200 µM	NDGA 25 µM	NDGA 200 µM
K_M	84.1 ± 16.2	6.7 ± 13.5	81.8 ± 6.4	17.6 ± 11.7	158.3 ± 6.2	123.2 ± 8.8	118.0 ± 3.9	57.3 ± 8.6
$2K_M$	100.6 ± 1.7	17.9 ± 4.2	66.6 ± 1.8	12.4 ± 30.7	88.7 ± 4.5	42.2 ± 26.0	93.0 ± 2.9	37.5 ± 26.1
V_{Max}	109.1 ± 1.1	40.2 ± 7.9	63.6 ± 3.9	11.1 ± 3.5	79.8 ± 3.4	27.6 ± 0.3	88.7 ± 3.8	29.7 ± 0.1

Table 4. The percent of control activity (mean ± % CV) for the formation of resorufin, and 6β-, 16α- and 2α-hydroxytestosterone (OHT) in pooled (n=4) rat liver microsomes by 25 and 200 µM Nordihydroguaiaretic acid (NDGA) at the K_M, $2 \times K_M$ and $\sim V_{Max}$ of methoxyresorufin or testosterone.

Lineweaver-Burke plots for NDGA inhibition of CYP1A2 showed a pattern consistent with competitive inhibition, but with the lines intersecting in the upper right hand quadrant near the y-axis (not shown). For CYP3A the pattern was consistent with noncompetitive inhibition. For the CYP2B/2C11 and CYP2C11 pathways, the Lineweaver-Burke plots were more difficult to interpret. At higher NDGA concentrations, parallel lines suggested uncompetitive inhibition. However, activation of these pathways at the K_M of testosterone (Figure 6c and 6d) likely affected the overall pattern observed in these plots (not shown).

A Comparison Between Lignans from Creosote
Bush and Flaxseed and Their Potential to Inhibit Cytochrome P450 Enzyme Activity

185

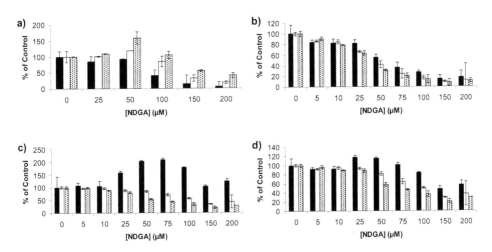

Fig. 6. Nordihydroguaiaretic acid (NDGA) concentration dependent inhibition of a) CYP1A2, b) CYP3A c) CYP2B/2C11, and d) CYP2C11 using methoxyresorufin (solid bar = 0.5 µM; open bar = 1 µM; stipled bar = 2.5 µM) and testosterone (solid bar = 50 µM; open bar = 100 µM; stipled bar = 250 µM) as the probe substrates, respectively, in incubation reactions (8 min and 15 min, respectively) with pooled (n=4) male, rat liver microsomes. Each point represents the mean of 3 replicates ± percent coefficient of variation.

Although previous studies showed that in the presence of GSH NDGA is oxidized to NDGA-GSH adducts and prevents the formation of NDGA dibenzocyclooctadiene (Billinsky & Krol 2008a), inhibition of P450 activity was still observed. For NDGA dibenzocyclooctadiene, the activity of CYP2C11, as monitored by 2α-OH testosterone formation, could not be assessed, as the dibenzocyclooctadiene eluted at the same retention time as 2α-OH testosterone during the HPLC run. There was sufficient peak overlap which could not be separated so we could not accurately achieve reliable data. For CYP1A2, the dibenzocyclooctadiene caused more prominent inhibition at the K_M of methoxyresorufin (Figure 7a), but for CYP3A and CYP2B/2C11 slightly greater inhibition of testosterone metabolite formation at the testosterone V_{Max} was observed (Figure 7b, 7c). At the V_{Max} of testosterone, dibenzocyclooctadiene concentrations of 50 to 150 µM increased the formation of resorufin, an index pathway for CYP1A2 (Figure 7a). Dibenzocyclooctadiene did not cause significant inhibition of CYP2B/2C11 as evidenced by no substantial decrease in 16α-OH formation (Figure 7c). Plots of metabolite formation as a function of the logarithmic concentration of NDGA dibenzocyclooctadiene yielded an IC50 value of 36.8 µM (95% CI 25.3-53.6) for CYP3A. For CYP1A2, the data did not yield an interpretable value due to extensive variation in the data. The percent of control activity of the various CYP isoforms tested at K_M, 2×K_M and V_{Max} of methoxyresorufin or testosterone is summarized in Table 5.

Lineweaver-Burke plots for dibenzocyclooctadiene inhibition of CYP1A2 showed a pattern consistent with competitive inhibition, but with the lines intersecting in the upper right hand quadrant near the y-axis and for CYP3A the pattern was consistent with noncompetitive inhibition (not shown).

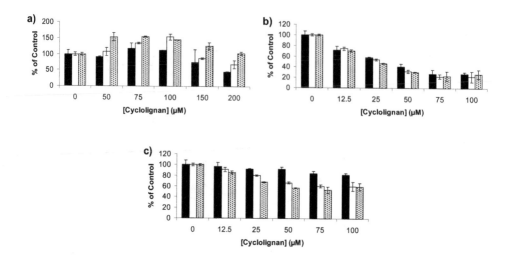

Fig. 7. Dibenzocyclooctadiene (cyclolignan) concentration dependent inhibition of a) CYP1A2, b) CYP3A, and c) CYP2B/2C11 using methoxyresorufin (solid bar = 0.5 µM; open bar = 1 µM; stipled bar = 2.5 µM) and testosterone (solid bar = 50 µM; open bar = 100 µM; stipled bar = 250 µM) as the probe substrates, respectively, in incubation reactions (8 min and 15 min, respectively) with pooled (n=4) male, rat liver microsomes. Each point represents the mean of 3 replicates ± percent coefficient of variation.

	Resorufin (CYP1A2)		6β-OHT (CYP3A)		16α-OHT (CYP2B/2C11)	
	Percent of Control Activity (mean ± % CV)		Percent of Control Activity (mean ± % CV)		Percent of Control Activity (mean ± % CV)	
Testosterone/ Methoxyresorufin	DIB 50 µM	DIB 200 µM	DIB 12.5 µM	DIB 100 µM	DIB 12.5 µM	DIB 100 µM
K_M	90.3 ± 2.5	45.3 ± 1.0	71.5 ± 7.4	26.9 ± 3.5	96.8 ± 7.0	82.0 ± 2.5
$2K_M$	107.4 ± 12.4	68.6 ± 12.1	74.0 ± 3.5	21.8 ± 10.0	91.3 ± 4.1	60.4 ± 8.2
V_{Max}	153.8 ± 12.7	103.4 ± 4.8	70.0 ± 2.2	26.4 ± 8.0	85.4 ± 2.9	59.6 ± 7.0

Table 5. The percent of control activity (mean ± % CV) for the formation of resorufin, and 6β-, 16α- and 2α-hydroxytestosterone (OHT) in pooled (n=4) rat liver microsomes by 12.5, 50, 100 and 200 µM Dibenzocyclooctadiene (DIB) at the K_M, $2 \times K_M$ and $\sim V_{Max}$ of methoxyresorufin or testosterone.

A Comparison Between Lignans from Creosote
Bush and Flaxseed and Their Potential to Inhibit Cytochrome P450 Enzyme Activity

187

5. Inhibition of CYP1A2 by nordihydroguaiaretic acid in the presence of glutathione

The effect of adding GSH to microsomal incubations before the addition of NDGA was studied to determine whether GSH could attenuate inhibition at various time and inhibitor concentrations. GSH had little impact on NDGA inhibition of CYP1A2 activity (data not shown). The calculated IC50 for NDGA in the presence and absence of GSH was 63.5 µM (95% CI 11.8-341) and 80.1 µM (95% CI 22.6-284), respectively, for CYP1A2. These observations suggest that GSH *in vitro* does not protect against reversible P450 inhibition by the creosote bush lignan, NDGA.

Interestingly, at lower probe substrate concentrations (50 µM) for NDGA, GSH attenuated inhibition, and appeared to cause activation of CYP1A2 (not shown), while dibenzocyclooctadiene increased the metabolite formation of the index pathway for CYP2B/2C11. Although P450 enzyme activation has been observed for other compounds (Stresser et al., 2000c; Lasker et al., 1984), the relevance of this phenomenon on *in vivo* metabolism is not known (Stresser et al., 2000b; Houston & Kenworthy 2000).

6. Summary of inhibition of rat CYP3A, CYP2B, CYP2C11 and CYP1A2 by lignans

Lineweaver-Burke plots of the inhibition data suggest that lignans largely caused reversible inhibition via a combination of competitive, noncompetitive, and uncompetitive mechanisms. The lignans EL, NDGA and its dibenzocyclooctadiene autoxidation product, inhibited a combination of CYP3A, CYP2B/2C11 and CYP1A2 activity suggesting that these lignans act as general reversible inhibitors of P450 activity. Interestingly, EL also activated the CYP2B/2C11 index pathway, the relevance of which is not known.

The ability of lignans to activate P450 enzyme activity in the presence of low probe substrate concentrations for the P450 index pathways may account for the mixed type inhibition we observed (Stresser et al., 2000). Nonetheless, our *in vitro* results suggest that potential for pharmacokinetic interactions via inhibition of P450-mediated elimination by flaxseed lignans is extremely limited. Concentration at the P450 active site is a principal determinant of the potential for clinically relevant interactions (Bjornsson et al., 2003). Systemic levels reported in the literature suggest that lignan concentrations achieved at the P450 active site would be insufficient to cause significant inhibition. Even following oral consumption, when portal vein concentrations and hence, hepatic concentrations, of lignans are expected to be much greater than systemic levels, the competing phase II reactions (i.e. glucuronidation, sulfation) (Axelson & Setchell 1980; Dean et al., 2004) would diminish the availability of lignans at the P450 enzyme active sites. The clinical use of lignans should not be associated with adverse outcomes resulting from inhibition of P450-mediated metabolism.

Table 6 summarizes the estimated IC50 values for lignan-mediated reversible inhibition different P450 isoforms. For lignans that failed to inhibit specific P450 isoforms the value reported represents the solubility limit for the respective lignan. Table 7 summarizes the type of reversible inhibition mechanism exhibited by each lignan for a particular P450 isoform.

	CYP1A2	CYP3A	CYP2B/ CYP2C11	CYP2C11
Secoisolariciresinol	ND[a]	373 (266-523)	> 1600	> 1600
Anhydrosecoisolariciresinol	> 200	36.4 (21.9-60.3)	> 200	ND[b]
Enterolactone	441 (115-1695)	72.9[c] (54.0-98.2)	> 500	104[c] (85.7-127)
Nordihydroguaiaretic acid	63.5 (11.8-341)	97.3 (49.6-191)	68.7[c] (46.4-102)	96.6[c] (55.3-169)
Dibenzocyclooctadiene	ND[a]	36.8 (25.3-53.6)	ND[a]	ND[b]

ND = not determined
[a]No inhibition was observed at any lignan concentration
[b]Could not assess due to overlapping peak on high performance liquid chromatography
[c]IC50 assessed at V_{Max}

Table 6. Summary of estimated lignan IC50 values (μM) (with 95% confidence intervals displayed in brackets) for CYP1A2, CYP 3A, CYP2B/2C11 and CYP2C11. IC50 values were determined at probe substrate K_M, except where noted.

	CYP1A2	CYP3A	CYP2B/ CYP2C11	CYP2C11
Secoisolariciresinol	NO	Competitive	NO[a]	NO
Anhydro- secoisolariciresinol	Uncompetitive	Uncompetitive	NO	NO
Enterolactone	Competitive	Noncompetitive[a]	NO[a]	Noncompetitive[a]
Nordihydroguaiaretic acid	Competitive	Noncompetitive	Uncompetitive[a]	Uncompetitive[a]
Dibenzocyclooctadiene	Competitive	Noncompetitive	NO	Could not assess

NO = No inhibition was observed
[a]Activation of P450 activity was observed.

Table 7. Summary of the type of P450 enzyme inhibition caused by lignans of creosote bush and flaxseed.

7. Conclusions

In conclusion, our data does not support the hypothesis that the differential toxicity between lignans of creosote bush and flaxseed may be due to differences in their capacity to undergo P450-mediated bioactivation to electrophilic reactive intermediates or reversible P450 enzyme inhibition. NDGA's autoxidation to a reactive quinone intermediate warrants further investigation as a possible mechanism associated with its known toxicity. Nonetheless, our *in vitro* data suggests the potential for inhibition of P450-mediated elimination of compounds by the lignans of creosote bush and flaxseed is limited. Their use for promotion of health and wellness or for therapeutic reasons should not be associated with adverse outcomes resulting from inhibition of P450-mediated metabolism. For the flaxseed lignans, our *in vitro* metabolism data is supported by the emerging clinical data on

A Comparison Between Lignans from Creosote
Bush and Flaxseed and Their Potential to Inhibit Cytochrome P450 Enzyme Activity

189

flaxseed lignan administration where no adverse effects have been reported as of yet. Such promising clinical trial data associated with the flaxseed lignans warrants further evaluations of their safety and efficacy, which remains a focus in our laboratory.

8. Acknowledgements

This study was performed with the assistance of Natural Sciences and Engineering Research Council of Canada (NSERC) and Canada Foundation for Innovation grants. J.B. was the recipient of an NSERC Postgraduate Scholarship. The authors would like to thank Alister Muir from Agriculture and Agrifood Canada, Saskatoon, SK for the kind gifts of SDG and SECO. In addition we thank Krista Thompson for running the UPLC-MS experiments.

9. References

Arteaga, S., Andrade-Cetto, A., and Cardenas, R. (2005). Larrea tridentata (Creosote bush), an abundant plant of Mexican and US-American deserts and its metabolite nordihydroguaiaretic acid. *J.Ethnopharmacol.*, Vol.98, No.3, pp. 231-239.

Atkins, W. M. (2005). Non-Michaelis-Menten kinetics in cytochrome P450-catalyzed reactions. *Annu.Rev.Pharmacol.Toxicol.*, Vol.45, pp. 291-310.

Awad, H. M., Boersma, M. G., Boeren, S., van Bladeren, P. J., Vervoort, J., and Rietjens, I. M. (2002). The regioselectivity of glutathione adduct formation with flavonoid quinone/quinone methides is pH-dependent. *Chem.Res.Toxicol.*, Vol.15, No.3, pp. 343-351.

Axelson, M. and Setchell, K. D. (1980). Conjugation of lignans in human urine. *FEBS Lett.*, Vol.122, No.1, pp. 49-53.

Axelson, M., Sjovall, J., Gustafsson, B. E., and Setchell, K. D. (1982). Origin of lignans in mammals and identification of a precursor from plants. *Nature,* Vol.298, No.5875, pp. 659-660.

Bambagiotti-Alberti, M., Coran, S. A., Ghiara, C., Giannellini, V., and Raffaelli, A. (1994). Revealing the mammalian lignan precursor secoisolariciresinol diglucoside in flax seed by ionspray mass spectrometry. *Rapid Commun.Mass Spectrom.*, Vol.8, No.8, pp. 595-598.

Batchelor, W. B., Heathcote, J., and Wanless, I. R. (1995). Chaparral-induced hepatic injury. *Am.J.Gastroenterol.*, Vol.90, No.5, pp. 831-833.

Billinsky, J. L. and Krol, E. S. (2008). Nordihydroguaiaretic acid autoxidation produces a schisandrin-like dibenzocyclooctadiene lignan. *J.Nat.Prod.*, Vol.71, No.9, pp. 1612-1615.

Billinsky, J. L., Marcoux, M. R., and Krol, E. S. (2007). Oxidation of the lignan nordihydroguaiaretic acid. *Chem.Res.Toxicol.*, Vol.20, No.9, pp. 1352-1358.

Bjornsson, T. D., Callaghan, J. T., Einolf, H. J., Fischer, V., Gan, L., Grimm, S., Kao, J., King, S. P., Miwa, G., Ni, L., Kumar, G., McLeod, J., Obach, R. S., Roberts, S., Roe, A., Shah, A., Snikeris, F., Sullivan, J. T., Tweedie, D., Vega, J. M., Walsh, J., and Wrighton, S. A. (2003). The conduct of *in vitro* and *in vivo* drug-drug interaction studies: a Pharmaceutical Research and Manufacturers of America (PhRMA) perspective. *Drug Metab Dispos.*, Vol.31, No.7, pp. 815-832.

Bolton, J. L., Acay, N. M., and Vukomanovic, V. (1994). Evidence that 4-allyl-o-quinones spontaneously rearrange to their more electrophilic quinone methides: potential bioactivation mechanism for the hepatocarcinogen safrole. *Chem.Res.Toxicol.*, Vol.7, No.3, pp. 443-450.

Borriello, S. P., Setchell, K. D., Axelson, M., and Lawson, A. M. (1985a). Production and metabolism of lignans by the human faecal flora. *J.Appl.Bacteriol.*, Vol.58, No.1, pp. 37-43.

Borriello, S. P., Setchell, K. D., Axelson, M., and Lawson, A. M. (1985b). Production and metabolism of lignans by the human faecal flora. *J.Appl.Bacteriol.*, Vol.58, No.1, pp. 37-43.

Charlet, S., Bensaddek, L., Raynaud, S., Gillet, F., Mesnard, F., and Fliniaux, M. (2002). An HPLC procedure for the quantification of anhydrosecoisolariciresinol. Application to the evaluation of flax lignan content. *Plant Physiology and Biochemistry*, Vol.40, pp. 225-229.

Chichirau, A., Flueraru, M., Chepelev, L. L., Wright, J. S., Willmore, W. G., Durst, T., Hussain, H. H., and Charron, M. (2005). Mechanism of cytotoxicity of catechols and a naphthalenediol in PC12-AC cells: the connection between extracellular autoxidation and molecular electronic structure. *Free Radic.Biol.Med.*, Vol.38, No.3, pp. 344-355.

Clark, F. and Reed, R. (1992). Chaparral-Induced Toxic Hepatitis- California and Texas, 1992. *JAMA*, Vol.268, No.23, pp. 3295-3298.

Dean, B., Chang, S., Doss, G. A., King, C., and Thomas, P. E. (2004). Glucuronidation, oxidative metabolism, and bioactivation of enterolactone in rhesus monkeys. *Arch.Biochem.Biophys.*, Vol.429, No.2, pp. 244-251.

Dietz, B. and Bolton, J. L. (2007). Botanical dietary supplements gone bad. *Chem.Res.Toxicol.*, Vol.20, No.4, pp. 586-590.

Elbarbry, F. A., McNamara, P. J., and Alcorn, J. (2007). Ontogeny of hepatic CYP1A2 and CYP2E1 expression in rat. *J.Biochem.Mol.Toxicol.*, Vol.21, No.1, pp. 41-50.

Felmlee, M. A., Woo, G., Simko, E., Krol, E. S., Muir, A. D., and Alcorn, J. (2009). Effects of the flaxseed lignans secoisolariciresinol diglucoside and its aglycone on serum and hepatic lipids in hyperlipidaemic rats. *Br.J.Nutr.*, pp. 1-9.

Folk, J. E., Wolff, E. C., Schirmer, E. W., and Ornfield, J. (1962). The kinetics of carboxypeptidase B activity. III. Effects of alcohol on the peptidase and esterase activities; kinetic models. *J.Biol.Chem.*, Vol.237, pp. 3105-3109.

Fowler, S. and Zhang, H. (2008). *In vitro* evaluation of reversible and irreversible cytochrome P450 inhibition: current status on methodologies and their utility for predicting drug-drug interactions. *AAPS.J.*, Vol.10, No.2, pp. 410-424.

Gordon, D. W., Rosenthal, G., Hart, J., Sirota, R., and Baker, A. L. (1995). Chaparral ingestion. The broadening spectrum of liver injury caused by herbal medications. *JAMA*, Vol.273, No.6, pp. 489-490.

Grant, K. L., Boyer, L. V., and Erdman, B. E. (1998). Case Report- Chaparral-Induced Hepatotoxicity. *Integrative Medicine*, Vol.1, No.2, pp. 83-87.

Grice, H. C., Becking, G., and Goodman, T. (1968). Toxic properties of nordihydroguaiaretic acid. *Food Cosmet.Toxicol.*, Vol.6, No.2, pp. 155-161.

Hallund, J., Tetens, I., Bugel, S., Tholstrup, T., and Bruun, J. M. (2008). The effect of a lignan complex isolated from flaxseed on inflammation markers in healthy postmenopausal women. *Nutr.Metab Cardiovasc.Dis.*, Vol.18, No.7, pp. 497-502.

He, K., Iyer, K. R., Hayes, R. N., Sinz, M. W., Woolf, T. F., and Hollenberg, P. F. (1998). Inactivation of cytochrome P450 3A4 by bergamottin, a component of grapefruit juice. *Chem.Res.Toxicol.*, Vol.11, No.4, pp. 252-259.

A Comparison Between Lignans from Creosote
Bush and Flaxseed and Their Potential to Inhibit Cytochrome P450 Enzyme Activity

191

Houston, J. B. and Kenworthy, K. E. (2000). *In vitro-in vivo* scaling of CYP kinetic data not consistent with the classical Michaelis-Menten model. *Drug Metab Dispos.*, Vol.28, No.3, pp. 246-254.

Hu, C., Yuan, Y. V., and Kitts, D. D. (2007). Antioxidant activities of the flaxseed lignan secoisolariciresinol diglucoside, its aglycone secoisolariciresinol and the mammalian lignans enterodiol and enterolactone *in vitro*. *Food Chem.Toxicol.*, Vol.45, No.11, pp. 2219-2227.

Iba, M. M., Soyka, L. F., and Schulman, M. P. (1977). Characteristics of the liver microsomal drug-metabolizing enzyme system of newborn rats. *Mol.Pharmacol.*, Vol.13, No.6, pp. 1092-1104.

Iverson, S. L., Hu, L. Q., Vukomanovic, V., and Bolton, J. L. (1995). The influence of the p-alkyl substituent on the isomerization of o- quinones to p-quinone methides: potential bioactivation mechanism for catechols. *Chem.Res.Toxicol.*, Vol.8, No.4, pp. 537-544.

Jacobs, E., Kulling, S. E., and Metzler, M. (1999). Novel metabolites of the mammalian lignans enterolactone and enterodiol in human urine. *J.Steroid Biochem.Mol.Biol.*, Vol.68, No.5-6, pp. 211-218.

Johnson, B. M., Qiu, S. X., Zhang, S., Zhang, F., Burdette, J. E., Yu, L., Bolton, J. L., and van Breemen, R. B. (2003). Identification of novel electrophilic metabolites of piper methysticum Forst (Kava). *Chem.Res.Toxicol.*, Vol.16, No.6, pp. 733-740.

Kalgutkar, A. S., Obach, R. S., and Maurer, T. S. (2007). Mechanism-based inactivation of cytochrome P450 enzymes: chemical mechanisms, structure-activity relationships and relationship to clinical drug-drug interactions and idiosyncratic adverse drug reactions. *Curr.Drug Metab,* Vol.8, No.5, pp. 407-447.

Kent, U. M., Aviram, M., Rosenblat, M., and Hollenberg, P. F. (2002). The licorice root derived isoflavan glabridin inhibits the activities of human cytochrome P450S 3A4, 2B6, and 2C9. *Drug Metab Dispos.*, Vol.30, No.6, pp. 709-715.

Kuijsten, A., Arts, I. C., Vree, T. B., and Hollman, P. C. (2005). Pharmacokinetics of enterolignans in healthy men and women consuming a single dose of secoisolariciresinol diglucoside. *J.Nutr.*, Vol.135, No.4, pp. 795-801.

Kupiec, T. and Raj, V. (2005). Fatal seizures due to potential herb-drug interactions with Ginkgo biloba. *J.Anal.Toxicol.*, Vol.29, No.7, pp. 755-758.

Lambert, J. D., Dorr, R. T., and Timmermann, B. N. (2004). Nordihydroguaiaretic Acid: A Review of Its Numerous and Varied Biological Activities. *Pharmaceutical Biology,* Vol.42, No.2, pp. 149-158.

Lasker, J. M., Huang, M. T., and Conney, A. H. (1984). *In vitro* and *in vivo* activation of oxidative drug metabolism by flavonoids. *J.Pharmacol.Exp.Ther.*, Vol.229, No.1, pp. 162-170.

Lowry, O. H., ROSEBROUGH, N. J., FARR, A. L., and RANDALL, R. J. (1951). Protein measurement with the Folin phenol reagent. *J.Biol.Chem.*, Vol.193, No.1, pp. 265-275.

Masubuchi, N., Makino, C., and Murayama, N. (2007). Prediction of *in vivo* potential for metabolic activation of drugs into chemically reactive intermediate: correlation of *in vitro* and *in vivo* generation of reactive intermediates and *in vitro* glutathione conjugate formation in rats and humans. *Chem.Res.Toxicol.*, Vol.20, No.3, pp. 455-464.

Mazur, W., Fotsis, T., Wahala, K., Ojala, S., Salakka, A., and Adlercreutz, H. (1996). Isotope dilution gas chromatographic-mass spectrometric method for the determination of isoflavonoids, coumestrol, and lignans in food samples. *Anal.Biochem.*, Vol.233, No.2, pp. 169-180.

Miller, E. C. and Miller, J. A. (1947). The Presence and Significance of Bound Aminoazo Dyes in the Livers of Rats Fed p-Dimethylaminoazobenzene. *Cancer Research,* No.7, pp. 468-480.

Mitchell, J. R., Jollow, D. J., Potter, W. Z., Davis, D. C., Gillette, J. R., and Brodie, B. B. (1973). Acetaminophen-induced hepatic necrosis. I. Role of drug metabolism. *J.Pharmacol.Exp.Ther.,* Vol.187, No.1, pp. 185-194.

Monks, T. J., Hanzlik, R. P., Cohen, G. M., Ross, D., and Graham, D. G. (1992). Quinone chemistry and toxicity. *Toxicol.Appl.Pharmacol.,* Vol.112, No.1, pp. 2-16.

Moore, Michael. (1989). Medicinal Plants of the Desert and Canyon West. pp. 27-29.

Natural Health Products Directorate. (2007). Natural Health Products Compliance Guide Version 2.1.

Nesbitt, P. D., Lam, Y., and Thompson, L. U. (1999). Human metabolism of mammalian lignan precursors in raw and processed flaxseed. *Am.J.Clin.Nutr.,* Vol.69, No.3, pp. 549-555.

O'Brien, P. J. (1991). Molecular mechanisms of quinone cytotoxicity. *Chem.Biol.Interact.,* Vol.80, No.1, pp. 1-41.

Pan, A., Sun, J., Chen, Y., Ye, X., Li, H., Yu, Z., Wang, Y., Gu, W., Zhang, X., Chen, X., Demark-Wahnefried, W., Liu, Y., and Lin, X. (2007). Effects of a flaxseed-derived lignan supplement in type 2 diabetic patients: a randomized, double-blind, cross-over trial. *PLoS.ONE.,* Vol.2, No.11, pp. e1148.

Powis, G. (1987). Metabolism and reactions of quinoid anticancer agents. *Pharmacol.Ther.,* Vol.35, No.1-2, pp. 57-162.

Rickard, S. E., Orcheson, L. J., Seidl, M. M., Luyengi, L., Fong, H. H., and Thompson, L. U. (1996). Dose-dependent production of mammalian lignans in rats and *in vitro* from the purified precursor secoisolariciresinol diglycoside in flaxseed. *J.Nutr.,* Vol.126, No.8, pp. 2012-2019.

Stresser, D. M., Blanchard, A. P., Turner, S. D., Erve, J. C., Dandeneau, A. A., Miller, V. P., and Crespi, C. L. (2000). Substrate-dependent modulation of CYP3A4 catalytic activity: analysis of 27 test compounds with four fluorometric substrates. *Drug Metab Dispos.,* Vol.28, No.12, pp. 1440-1448.

Surh, Y. J. and Lee, S. S. (1995). Capsaicin, a double-edged sword: toxicity, metabolism, and chemopreventive potential. *Life Sci.,* Vol.56, No.22, pp. 1845-1855.

Thompson, L. U., Robb, P., Serraino, M., and Cheung, F. (1991). Mammalian lignan production from various foods. *Nutr.Cancer,* Vol.16, No.1, pp. 43-52.

Vuppugalla, R. and Mehvar, R. (2005). Enzyme-selective effects of nitric oxide on affinity and maximum velocity of various rat cytochromes P450. *Drug Metab Dispos.,* Vol.33, No.6, pp. 829-836.

Wagner, P. and Lewis, R. A. (1980). Interaction between activated nordihydroguaiaretic acid and deoxyribonucleic acid. *Biochem.Pharmacol.,* Vol.29, No.24, pp. 3299-3306.

Yuan, C. S., Wei, G., Dey, L., Karrison, T., Nahlik, L., Maleckar, S., Kasza, K., Ang-Lee, M., and Moss, J. (2004). Brief communication: American ginseng reduces warfarin's effect in healthy patients: a randomized, controlled Trial. *Ann.Intern.Med.,* Vol.141, No.1, pp. 23-27.

Zhang, W., Wang, X., Liu, Y., Tian, H., Flickinger, B., Empie, M. W., and Sun, S. Z. (2008). Dietary flaxseed lignan extract lowers plasma cholesterol and glucose concentrations in hypercholesterolaemic subjects. *Br.J.Nutr.,* Vol.99, No.6, pp. 1301-1309.

Zhou, S., Koh, H. L., Gao, Y., Gong, Z. Y., and Lee, E. J. (2004). Herbal bioactivation: the good, the bad and the ugly. *Life Sci.,* Vol.74, No.8, pp. 935-968.

9

Potential Applications of
Euphorbia hirta in Pharmacology

Mei Fen Shih[1] and Jong Yuh Cherng[2]*
[1]Department of Pharmacy, Chia-Nan University of Pharmacy & Science, Tainan,
[2]Department of Chemistry & Biochemistry, National Chung Cheng University, Chia-Yi,
Taiwan

1. Introduction

Euphorbia is a genus of plants belonging to the family Euphorbiaceae. Botanist and taxonomist Carl Linnaeus assigned the name *Euphorbia* to the entire genus in the physician's honor. *Euphorbia hirta* is a very popular herb amongst practitioners of traditional herb medicine, widely used as a decoction or infusion to treat various ailments including intestinal parasites, diarrhoea, peptic ulcers, heartburn, vomiting, amoebic dysentery, asthma, bronchitis, hay fever, laryngeal spasms, emphysema, coughs, colds, kidney stones, menstrual problems, sterility and venereal diseases. Moreover, the plant is also used to treat affections of the skin. In this chapter we explore those investigations related to their pharmacological activities (see the section 2.2).

2. *Euphorbia hirta*

2.1 Chemical Composition of *Euphorbia hirta*

Phytochemical analysis of *Euphorbia hirta* (*E. hirta*) revealed the presence of reducing sugar, alkaloids, flavonoids, sterols, tannins and triterpenoids in the whole plant. Some of them are well known to possess biological activities (as shown in table 1).

2.1.1 Flavonoids

Epidemiological studies have revealed that polyphenols, including flavonoids, provide a significant protection against development of several chronic diseases such as cardiovascular diseases, cancer, diabetes, infections, aging, and asthma. Two flavonoids have been isolated from *E. hirta*, namely quercitrin and myricitrin (Johnson et al, 1999; Chen, 1991). In general, flavonoids have been reported to possess several proven medicinal properties including antioxidant (Kandaswami & Middleton, 1994), anti-allergic (Singh et al, 2006), antiinflammatory component of asthma (Miller, 2001) and antidiarrheal activity (Galvez et al, 1993; Mallavadhani et al, 2002). Many of the biological actions of flavonoids have been shown to attribute to their antioxidant properties, either through their reducing capacities or as a result of their possible influence on intracellular redox status (Williams et al, 2004). Flavonoids can also interact selectively within the mitogen-activated protein

(MAP) kinase signalling pathway, thereby existing antiinflammation (Lee, 2011) and anti-cancer activity (Ding et al, 2010).

2.1.2 Sterols

Sterols were isolated from E. *hirta* and chemically characterized as cycloarternol, 24-methylene-cycloarternol, β-sitosterol, euphorbol hexacozonate, 1-hexacosanol, tinyaloxin, campesterol and stigmasterol (Atallah and Nicholas, 1972; Galvez et al, 1993; Johnson et al, 1999). The compounds 24-methylene-cycloartenol and β-sitosterol have also been found to exert significant and dose-dependent anti-inflammatory effects, when treating acetate-induced ear inflammation (Martinez-Vazquez et al, 1999).

2.1.3 Tannins

Tannins are not widely known for their anti-inflammatory potential. E. *hirta* possesses a few such chemicals. Phytochemicals work synergistically, however, and therefore these tannins may assist in the anti-inflammatory action of the plant. E. *hirta* presents three hydrolysable tannins, namely, dimeric hydrolysable tannin, euphorbin E and the dimeric dehydroellagitannins, euphorbin A and euphorbin B (Yoshida et al, 1990). The following tannins from the leaves of E. *hirta* were also isolated by using physicochemical and spectroscopic methods: gallic acid, 2,4, 6-tri-O-galloyl-D-glucose and 1,2,3,4, 6-penta-O-galloyl-β-D-glucose as well as the quinic acid ester, 3,4-di-O-galloylquinic acid (Chen 1991).

2.1.4 Triterpenoids

Research has shown that triterpenoids possess anti-inflammatory properties. The triterpenes α-amyrin, β-amyrin, taraxerone (EH-1), taxerol as well as β-amyrin acetate have been identified from E. *hirta* (Martinez-Vazquez et al, 1999; Pinn, 2001; Mukherjee et al, 2004). Extracts of the plant were found to contain β-amyrin, which displayed a significant and dose dependent anti-inflammatory activity against acetate-induced ear inflammation (Martinez-Vazquez et al, 1999) or LPS-induced inflammatory model (Shih et al, 2010). Two additional triterpenoids, namely, taraxerone and 11α, 12α-oxidotaraxerol, have also been found in E. *hirta*. These compounds induce both antibacterial and antifungal effects, as tested against fourteen pathogenic bacteria (Abu-Sayeed et al, 2005).

2.2 Pharmacological effects of Euphorbia hirta

2.2.1 Effects of E. hirta on GI system

Protective effect of E. *hirta* against antitubercular drug-induced cytotoxicity was observed in freshly isolated hepatocytes. Antitubercular drug intoxication alters liver function by affecting aspartate aminotransferase, alanine aminotransferase, alkaline phosphatase, lactate dehydrogenase, triacylglycerol, cholesterol, total protein, albumin, total and direct bilirubin. A dose-dependent increase in percent viability was obtained when antitubercular drug exposed HepG2 cells were treated with different concentrations of alcoholic extract of E. *hirta* (125, 250, 500 and 1000 mg/mL). The effectiveness of liver protection was comparable to a standard hepatoprotective drug silymarin (Brindha et al, 2010). The antihepatotoxic effect of *E. hirta* extracts were also evaluated in experimental models of liver injury in rats induced by CCL4 or paracetamol (Tiwari et al, 2011). Carbon tetrachloride and paracetamol are known to cause liver damage (Recknagel, 1983; James et al., 2003). When administered to rats, they act by inducing oxidative damages to liver cells which leads to cellular necrosis. *E. hirta* exhibited a 70 and 80% hepatoprotection compared to the 80 and 90% one exhibited by silymarin in CCL4 or paracetamol-injured rats, respectively. The extract *E. hirta* was demonstrated effectively in protecting the liver from toxic hepatitis.

Components	Chemicals	Possible biological function	References
Flavonoids	Quercitrin; Myricitrin	Antioxidation; Anti-allergy; Antibacterial activity; Molluscicidal activity; anti-diarrheal activity	Galvez et al, 1993; Kandaswami & Middleton, 1994; Mallavadhani et al, 2002; Singh et al, 2005; Singh et al, 2006; Park & Lee, 2006; Sudhakar et al, 2006; Rajeh et al, 2010; Ding et al, 2010; Lee, 2011
Sterols	Cycloarternol; 24-methylene-cycloarternol; β-sitosterol; euphorbol hexacozonate; 1-hexacosanol; tinyaloxin; campesterol; stigmasterol	anti-inflammatory effects	Martinez-Vazquez et al, 1999
Tannin	euphorbin E; euphorbin A; euphorbin B; gallic acid; 2,4, 6-tri-O-galloyl-D-glucose; 1,2,3,4, 6-penta-O-galloyl-β-D-glucose; 3,4-di-O-galloylquinic acid	anti-inflammatory activity	Yoshida et al, 1990; Chen 1991
Triterpenoids	α-amyrin; β-amyrin; taraxerone; taxerol; β-amyrin acetate; taraxerone; 11α, 12α-oxidotaraxerol	anti-inflammatory activity; anti-pruritic activity; antidiabetic activity; antimicrobial activity	Martinez-Vazquez et al, 1999; Pinn, 2001; Mukherjee et al, 2004; Abu-Sayeed et al, 2005; Park & Lee, 2006; Shih et al, 2010

Table 1. Chemical compounds isolated from *Euphorbia hirta*.

Aqueous leaf extract of *E. hirta* was shown to decrease the gastrointestinal motility in normal rats and decreased the effect of castor oil-induced diarrhoea in mice (Hore et al, 2006; Galvez et al, 1993). The anti-diarrheal activity of *E. hirta* was also effective in arachidonic acid- and prostaglandin E2-induced diarrhoea (Galvez et al, 1993). Quercetin-3-O-β-D-rhamnoside, a flavonoid, was found to be the active component with anti-diarrheal activity (Galvez et al, 1993; Mallavadhani et al, 2002).

2.2.2 Effects of *E. hirta* on analgesic, antipyretic and anti-inflammatory actions

E. hirta exists a dose-dependent analgesic action against chemical (writhing test) and thermic (hot plate test) stimuli from the doses of 20 and 25 mg/kg. This analgesic action was inhibited by pretreatment of naloxone, a specific morphinic antagonist compound. Therefore, it exerts central analgesic properties. In addition, *E. hirta* was effectively against acute pain in carrageenan-induced edema model (Lanhers et al, 1991). An antipyretic activity was obtained at the sedative doses of 100 and 400 mg/kg, on the yeast-induced hyperthermia (Lanhers et al, 1991).

Antiinflammatory effects of *E. hirta* were shown in 12-o-tetradecanoyl phorbol acetate-induced ear edema (Martinez-Vazquez et al, 1999; Lanhers et al, 1991). Although *E. hirta* was ineffective in Freund's adjuvant-induced rheumatoid arthritis model, it reduced the inflammatory hyperalgia of rheumatoid arthritis (Lanhers et al, 1991). The molecular pharmacology basis of this anti-inflammatory effect is revealed in an established inflammation model in lipopolysaccharide (LPS)-activated macrophages (fig 1). In the concentration range without showing cytotoxicity, *E. hirta* produced a remarkable anti-inflammatory effect via its active component of beta-amyrin and showed a dose-related inhibition against LPS-induced NO production (Camuesco et al, 2004; Comalada et al, 2005; Shih et al, 2010). The extract of *E. hirta* and beta-amyrin are able to block most of the iNOS protein functions and NO induction (fig 2). The extract of *E. hirta* and beta-amyrin were not as potent as Indomethacin in preventing LPS-induced PGE2 production (Shih et al, 2010). This indicated that the extract of *E. hirta* and its active component, beta-amyrin, may have less gastrointestinal adverse effect than indomethacin does. The extract of *E. hirta* and its component beta-amyrin could therefore be new selective NO inhibitors with great potential in treating endotoxin-induced inflammation.

2.2.3 Inhibition of allergic reactions and asthma by *E. hirta*

E. hirta has been used to treated asthma as a folk medicine (Watanabe et al, 2005). *E. hirta* functions for the treatment of asthma is probably through synergistic anti-inflammatory and antioxidant activities of especially the flavonoids, sterols and triterpenoids (Park & Lee, 2006). Asthma has long been associated with chronic inflammation and an overall increase in reactive groups and oxidative stress (Nadeem et al, 2003). *E. hirta* also existed significant activity to prevent early and late phase allergic reactions and thereby asthma. *E. hirta* reduced asthma attack has been shown as effective as corticosteroid did in the BALB/c asthmatic mouse mode (Ekpo & Pretorius, 2008). The possible active component of *E. hirta* is thought to be Quercitrin. *E. hirta* ethanol extract significantly prevented eosinophil accumulation and eosinophil peroxidase activity and reduced the protein content in bronchoalveolar lavage fluid in a 'mild' model of asthma (Singh et al, 2006). Taken together, *E. hirta* is a very potent herb medicine in treatment of asthma. Ethanol extract of *E. hirta* has also been shown to inhibit polysorbate 80-induced degranulation of isolated peritoneal mast cells *in vitro*. Thus anti-inflammatory activity of *E. hirta* could be attributed to mast cell membrane stabilization, thereby inhibiting the release of inflammatory mediators (Ramesh & Padmavathi, 2010). *E. hirta* ethanol extract also significantly inhibited dextran-induced rat paw edema, attenuated the release of interleukin-4 (IL-4) and augmented IFN-gamma in ovalbumin-sensitized mouse splenocytes (Singh et al, 2006). Anaphylactic allergic reaction is a life-threatening syndrome induced by the sudden systemic release of inflammatory mediators such as histamine and pro-inflammatory cytokines and can be elicited by various stimulators including compound 48/80 (N-methyl-p-methoxy-phenethylamine) and anti-IgE (Paul et al, 1993). Compound 48/80-induced mortality could also be reduced by *E. hirta* ethanol extract administration in Wistar rats (Youssouf et al, 2007).

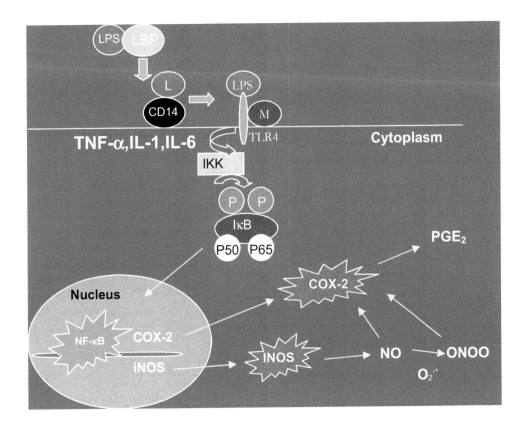

Fig. 1. Inflammatory model in LPS-activated Macrophage.

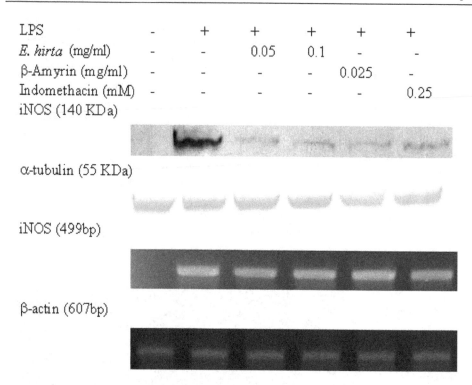

LPS	-	+	+	+	+	+
E. hirta (mg/ml)	-	-	0.05	0.1	-	-
β-Amyrin (mg/ml)	-	-	-	-	0.025	-
Indomethacin (mM)	-	-	-	-	-	0.25
iNOS (140 KDa)						
α-tubulin (55 KDa)						
iNOS (499bp)						
β-actin (607bp)						

Fig. 2. Inhibition of *E. hirta* and β-amyrin on LPS-induced iNOS gene and protein expression.

2.2.4 Burn wound healing of *E. hirta*

Tissue damage from excessive heat, electricity, radioactivity or corrosive chemicals that destroy (denature) protein in the exposed cells is called a burn. Burns disrupt haemostasis because they destroy the protection afforded by the skin. They permit microbial invasion and infection, loss of body fluid and loss of thermoregulation. Various extracts of *E. hirta* exhibited antimicrobial activity against various microbes including those causing burn and wound infections like Pseudomonas aeruginosa and Staphylococcus aureus (Sudhakar et al, 2006; Rajeh et al, 2010). Hence, *E. hirta* could be beneficial in the management of burn wounds. The ethanol extract of whole plant of *E. hirta* was screened for burn wound healing activity in rats as 2% W/W cream. The study was carried out based on the assessment of percentage reduction in original wound. *E. hirta* was showed significant burn wound healing activity (Jaiprakash et al, 2006).

2.2.5 Effects of *E. hirta* on anti-oxidation

Free radicals have been claimed to play an important role in affecting human health by causing several chronic diseases, such as cancer, diabetes, aging, atherosclerosis, hypertension, heart attack and other degenerative diseases (Raghuveer et al, 2009). These free radicals are generated during body metabolism. Exogenous intake of antioxidants can help the body scavenge free radicals effectively. There is a noticeable interest in antioxidants, especially in those which can prevent the presumed deleterious effects of free radicals in the human body, and to prevent the deterioration of fats and other constituents of foodstuffs. In both cases, there is a preference for antioxidants from natural rather than from synthetic sources (Molyneux et al, 2004). At present, most of the antioxidants are manufactured synthetically. The main disadvantage with the synthetic antioxidants is the side effects *in vivo* (Ramamoorthy et al, 2007). Previous studies reported that butylated hydroxyanisole (BHA) and butylated hydroxytoluene (BHT) accumulate in the body and result in liver damage and carcinogenesis (Jiangning et al, 2005). Phytochemical screening of *E. hirta* revealed the presence of several chemicals, including flavanoids, which may be responsible for its strong anti-oxidative activity (Basma et al, 2011). The anti-oxidant activity of *E. hirta* was comparable with that of ascorbic acid and found to be dose dependent (Basma et al, 2011).

2.2.6 Antidiabetic and free radicals scavenging potential of *E. hirta*

Diabetes mellitus is a metabolic disease characterized by hyperglycemia resulting from defects in insulin secretion, insulin action, or both. It is well documented that chronic hyperglycemia of diabetes is associated with long-term damage, dysfunction, and eventually the failure of organs, especially the eyes, kidneys, nerves, heart, and blood vessels. Daily treatment of ethanol and petroleum ether flower extracts of *E. hirta* for three weeks significantly reduced alloxan-induced hyperglycemia, triglycerides and cholesterol (Kumar et al, 2010). Other biochemical parameters such as serum creatinine, urea and alkaline phosphatase levels were also found to be decreased whereas total proteins were found to be increased after treatments. Both extracts of *E. hirta* have significant antioxidant activity compared to other well characterized, standard antioxidant systems. Free radical scavenging potential was assessed against DPPH. The reductive capabilities of extract were compared with ascorbic acid and BHA. The extract showed dose dependent reducing power. This additional antioxidative effect of *E. hirta* may provide extract benefit in preventing oxidative-induced complications in diabetic patients.

2.2.7 Effects of *E. hirta* on anti-infection

The antimicrobial activities of the methanol extracts of *E. hirta* leaves, flowers, stems and roots were evaluated against some medically important bacteria and yeast using the agar disc diffusion method (Sudhakar et al, 2006; Rajeh et al, 2010; Singh et al, 2011). Four Gram positive (*Staphylococcus aureus*, *Micrococcus sp.*, *Bacillus subtilis* and *Bacillus thuringensis*), four Gram negative (*Escherichia coli*, *Klebsiella pneumonia*, *Salmonella typhi* and *P. mirabilis*) and one yeast (*Candida albicans*) species were screened. Inhibition zones ranged between 16-29 mm. Leaves extract inhibited the growth of all tested microorganisms with large zones of inhibition, followed by that of flowers, which also inhibited all the bacteria except *C. albicans*. The most susceptible microbes to all extracts were *S. aureus* and *Micrococcus* sp. Root extract displayed larger inhibition zones against Gram positive bacteria than Gram negative bacteria and had larger inhibition zones compared to stem extract. The lowest MIC values were obtained with *E. coli* and *C. albicans*, followed by *S. aureus* and *P. mirabilis*. All the other bacteria had MIC values of

100.00 mg/mL. Scanning Electron Microscopic (SEM) studies revealed that the cells exposed to leaf extract displayed a rough surface with multiple blends and invaginations which increased with increasing time of treatment, and cells exposed to leaf extract for 36 h showed the most damage, with abundant surface cracks which may be related to final cell collapse and loss of function. Time-kill assay of *C. albicans* indicated a primarily fungicidal effect at 1- and 2-fold MIC. Therefore, methanol extract of *E. hirta* possessed a broad spectrum of antimicrobial activity against studied bacterial strains. However, its inhibitory effect on *H. pylori* effects was weak (Ndip et al, 2007). Interestingly, *E. hirta* was not found to be very effective for anti-fungal activity by others (Abu-Sayeed et al, 2005; Singh et al, 2011). Taken together, *E. hirta* can be used to discover new bioactive natural products that may serve as leads in the development of new pharmaceuticals.

The antiretroviral activities of extracts of *E. hirta* were investigated *in vitro* on the MT4 human T lymphocyte cell line. A dose-dependent inhibition activity was observed for HIV-1, HIV-2 and SIV (mac251) all three viruses. Methanol extract was found to exert a higher antiretroviral effect than that of the aqueous extract (Gyuris et al, 2009).

2.2.8 Effects of *E. hirta* on molluscicidal activity and Larvicidal activity

Mosquito-transmitted diseases remain a major cause of the loss of human life worldwide with more than 700 million people suffering from these diseases annually (Taubes 1997). Mosquito-borne diseases have an economic impact, including loss in commercial and labor outputs, particularly in countries with tropical and subtropical climates; however, no part of the world is free from vector-borne diseases (Fradin and Day 2002). Larvicidal activity of *E. hirta* has been found in petroleum ether extract with LC50 value 272.36 ppm (Abdul Rahuman et al, 2008).

Many aquatic snails act as vectors for the larvae of trematodes and thereby, cause a number of diseases (Bali et al., 1986). Two diseases carried by aquatic snails, schistosomiasis and fascioliasis, cause immense harm to man and his domestic animals. The freshwater vector snail *Lymnaea acuminata* is the intermediate hosts of *Fasciola hepatica* and *Fasciola gigantica* (Hyman, 1970). Which caused endemic fascioliasis in sheep, cattle, goat and others herbivorous animal. Aqueous stem bark and leaf extracts of plant *E. hirta* have potent molluscicidal activity. Sub-lethal doses (40% and 80% of LC50) of aqueous stem bark and leaf extracts of this plant also significantly alter the levels of total protein, total free amino acid, nucleic acids (DNA and RNA) and the activity of enzyme protease and acid and alkaline phosphatase in various tissues of the vector snail *Lymnaea acuminata* in time and dose dependent manners (Singh et al, 2005).

2.2.9 Immunostimulant effect of *E. hirta* in aquaculture

E. hirta leaves have been used in aquaculture to protect fish from bacterial infection. Aquaculture is one of the fastest growing food-producing fields in the world, with an annual average growth rate of 6.9% per year since 1970 and this sector contributed about 36% of the total global fisheries production in the year 2006 (FAO, 2009; Mohanty & Sahoo, 2010). Infectious diseases are a major problem in aquaculture, causing heavy loss to fish farmers. Immunostimulants increase resistance to infectious diseases by enhancing both specific and nonspecific defence mechanisms. The use of immunostimulants in fish culture is a promising new development in the field (Logambal et al., 2000; Dügenci et al., 2003; Rairakhwada et al., 2007). *Pseudomonas fluorescens* Flügge (Pseudomonadaceae) is an opportunistic bacterial fish pathogen of the freshwater ecosystem, associated with septic and ulcerative condition, necrosis of internal organs, external lesions, loss of pigmentation, and so on (Saharia & Prasad, 2001). The leaf extracts of *E. hirta* administered through the diet enhanced the nonspecific defence mechanism in terms of increased number of activated neutrophils and enhanced the serum lysozyme activity (secreted from active macrophages) in *Cyprinus carpio* Linn. The immunological competence was developed earlier on the plant leaf extract fed fish (on 5th day) than the control fish (on 10th day) after infection with the pathogen. In addition, the extract also exhibited potent antibacterial activity (Pratheepa1 and Sukumaran, 2011). Immunostimulatory activity of *E. hirta* was also found to enhance *in vitro* phagocytosis of neutrophils and macrophages (Ramesh and Padmavathi, 2010).

2.2.10 Effects of *E. hirta* on anti-anxiety

Stress is increasingly recognized as the precipitant of several psychiatric illnesses including anxiety and depression (McEwen, 2000). When rats subjected to chronic immobilization stress (CIS) or forced swim stress (FSS) showed anxiety in the elevated plus maze (EPM) and the open field test (OFT) (Anuradha et al., 2008; Govindarajan et al., 2006; Vyas et al., 2002). In addition to anxiety, stress is also known to produce learning and memory deficits. For example, chronic stress impaired learning in the T-maze and radial arm maze (Ramkumar et al., 2008; Srikumar et al., 2006, 2007) or in other paradigms such as the Barnes maze and Morris water maze (Bodnoff et al., 1995; McLay et al., 1998). The dopaminergic and cholinergic neurotransmitter systems have been shown to be involved in mediating the stress induced deficits (Srikumar et al., 2006, 2007). CIS increased the acetylcholinesterase (AChE) activity in the frontal cortex, hippocampus, and septum, while *E. hirta* treatment brought it to normal levels. FSS increased the AChE activity only in the septum, and *E. hirta* treatment marginally normalized this change. Chronic stress not only induces impairment of learning and memory but also precipitates several affective disorders including depression and anxiety. Sedative properties of aqueous extract of *E. hirta* have been confirmed at high dose (100 mg of dried plant/kg) by showing a decrease of behavioral parameters measured in non-familiar environment tests (activitest and staircase test). For anti-conflict effects appeared at lower doses (12.5 and 25 mg of dried plant/kg) by revealing an enhancement of behavioral parameters measured in the staircase test and in the light/dark choice situation test (Lanhers et al, 1990). Anxiolytic property of *E. hirta* was also demonstrated in chronically stressed rats subjected to EPM and OFT (Anuradha et al, 2008). *E. hirta* treatment showed marked anti-anxiety activity in CIS rats. Co-treatment of rats with flumazenil, bicuculline or picrotoxin resulted in a significant reduction of anxiolytic effect of *E. hirta* indicating that its actions are mediated through $GABA_A$ receptor-benzodiazepine receptor-Cl channel complex. Acetylcholine and the cholinergic system are also known to involve in anxiety. Further study showed that anxiolytic effects of *E. hirta* in rats subjected to CIS was due to suppression of CIS-induced AChE activity in the frontal cortex, hippocampus, and septum brain regions (Anuradha et al, 2010). Together with GABA-mimic effect and AChE reducing effect may explain the anxiolytic activity of *E. hirta*.

2.2.11 Effects of *E. hirta* on renal system

Dickshit (1934) first reported the presence of a toxic principle in *E. hirta* that depressed the cardiovascular system with a resulting fall in blood pressure. The alcoholic and aqueous extracts of this plant have also been shown to depress the blood pressure of the dog (Hazleton and Hellerman, 1954). *E. hirta* is locally used to treat numerous diseases, including hypertension and edema in Africa (Khan et al., 1980). Diuretic effect of the *E. hirta* leaf extracts were assessed in rats using acetazolamide and furosemide as standard diuretic drugs. The water and ethanol extracts (50 and 100 mg/kg) of the plant produced time-dependent increase in urine output. Regarding the secretion of electrolytes, the ethanol extract of *E. hirta* increased the excretion of HCO_3^-, decreased the loss of K^+ and had little effect on renal removal of Na^+. Whereas, the water extract increased the urine excretion of Na^+, K^+ and HCO_3^- that was similar to acetazolamide (Johnson et al, 1999).

The renin–angiotensin system plays a vital role in the maintenance of vascular tone and peripheral resistance. Renin produced from the juxtaglomerular apparatus of the kidney splits angiotensinogen to produce the inactive decapeptide angiotensin I. The latter is then converted to the powerful octapeptide vasoconstrictor, angiotensin II by the action of angiotensin converting enzyme (ACE). ACE inhibitors are important agents for treating hypertension and congestive heart failure (Opie, 1992). *E. hirta* extract possessed compounds with potent ACE inhibitory activities. A dose of 500 mg crude extract expressed about 90% inhibition of the enzyme action. The study also revealed that the most active ACE inhibitory compounds were present in the medium polar (chloroform extract) and very polar (methanol and water) fractions. Extract of *E. hirta* (10 mg/100 mg body weight) also possessed anti-dipsogenic activities (Williams et al, 1997). Both diuresis and ACE inhibition effects of *E. hirta* may explain its antihypertensive effects.

3. Conclusion

Although *E. hirta* has been used wildly to treat various diseases in many countries, most of the involved molecular mechanisms have not been fully explored. However, the pharmacological mechanisms of *E. hirta* in asthma attacks and hypertension were relatively clear. The former can be due to its potent anti-inflammatory and anti-oxidative activities. The later may work through its actions of diuretic activity and ACE inhibition. For anxiolytic effects of *E. hirta* is thought to be mediated through $GABA_A$-mediated Cl channel as well as AChE reduction. The anti-infection of *E. hirta* is due to its direct bactericidal activity. Antiinflammatory and antioxidative activities of *E. hirta* can also be expected to use in treating scald, preventing sepsis or other chronic inflammatory diseases. In overall, there are still many clinical applications of *E. hirta* remained to be investigated for their molecular mechanisms.

4. References

Abdul Rahuman, A., Geetha Gopalakrishnan, Venkatesan, P. & Kannappan, Geetha (2008) Larvicidal activity of some Euphorbiaceae plant extracts against Aedes aegypti and Culex quinquefasciatus (Diptera: Culicidae). *Parasitolog Research*, Vol.102, No.5, (April 2008), pp. 867–873, ISSN 0932-0113

Abu-Sayeed, M., Ali, M.A., Bhattacharjee, P.K., Islam, A., Astaq, G.R.M., Khan, M. & Yeasmin, S. (2005). Biological evaluation of extracts and triterpenoids of Euphorbia hirta. *Pakistan Journal of Science and Industrial Research*, Vol.48, No.2, pp.122–125, ISSN 0030-9885

Atallah A.M., & Nicholas H.J. (1972). Triterpenoids and steroids of Euphorbia pilulifera. *Phytochemistry*, Vol. 2, pp. 1860–1868, ISSN 0031-9422

Anuradha, H., Srikumar, B.N., Shankaranarayana Rao, B.S. (2008) Lakshmana M. Euphorbia hirta reverses chronic stress-induced anxiety and mediates its action through the GABAA receptor benzodiazepine receptor-Cl2 channel complex. *Journal of Neural Transmission*, Vol.115, No.1, (January 2008), pp. 35–42, ISSN 0300-9564

Anuradha, H., Srikumar, B.N., Deepti, N., Shankaranarayana Rao, B.S., & Lakshmana, M. (2010) Restoration of acetylcholinesterase activity by Euphorbia hirta in discrete brain regions of chronically stressed rats. *Pharmaceutical Biology*, Vol.48, No.5, (May, 2010), pp. 499-503, ISSN: 1388-0209

Bali, H.S., Singh, S. & Sharma, S. (1986) The distribution and ecology of vectors snails of Punjab. *Indian Journal of Ecology*, Vol.13, pp. 31–37, ISSN 0304-5250

Basma, A.A., Zakaria, Z., Latha, L.Y. & Sasidharan, S. (2011) Antioxidant activity and phytochemical screening of the methanol extracts of Euphorbia hirta L. *Asian Pacific Journal of Tropical Medicine*, Vol.4, No.5, (May 2011), ISSN 1995-7645

Bodnoff, S.R., Humphreys, A.G., Lehman, J.C., Diamond, D.M., Rose, G.M. & Meaney, M.J. (1995) Enduring effects of chronic corticosterone treatment on spatial learning, synaptic plasticity, and hippocampal neuropathology in young and mid-aged rats. *The Journal of Neuroscience*, Vol.15, No.1, (January 1995), pp. 61–69, ISSN 0270-6474

Brindha, D., Saroja, S., Jeyanthi, G.P. (2010) Protective potential [correction of potencial] of Euphorbia hirta against cytotoxicity induced in hepatocytes and a HepG2 cell line. *Journal of Basic and Clinical Physiology and Pharmacology*, Vol.21, No.4, pp. 401-413, ISSN 0792-6855

Camuesco, D., Comalada, M., Rodriguez-Cabezas, M.E., Nieto, A., Lorente, M.D., Concha, A., Zarzuelo, A. & Galvez J. (2004) The intestinal anti-inflammatory effect of quercitrin is associated with an inhibition in iNOS expression. *British Journal of Pharmacology*, Vol.143, No.7, (December 2004), pp. 908–918, ISSN 1476-5381

Chen, L. (1991) Polyphenols from leaves of Euphorbia hirta L. *Zhongguo Zhong Yao Za Zhi*, Vol.16, No.1, pp. 38–39, 64, ISSN 1001-5302

Comalada, M., Camuesco, D., Sierra, S., Ballester, I., Xaus, J., Galvez, J. & Zarzuelo, A. (2005) In vivo quercitrin anti-inflammatory effect involves release of quercetin, which inhibits inflammation through down-regulation of the NF-kappa B pathway. *The European Journal of Immunology*, Vol.35, No.2, (Feburary 2005), pp. 584–592, ISSN 0014-2980

Dickshit, R.A.O. (1934) Effect of Euphorbia hiffa on the cardiovascular system. Proceedings of Indian Science Congress; p. 349

Ding, M., Zhao, J., Bowman, L., Lu, Y. & Shi, X. (2010) Inhibition of AP-1 and MAPK signaling and activation of Nrf2/ARE pathway by quercitrin. *International journal of oncology*, Vol.36, No.1, (January 2010), pp. 59-67, ISSN 1019-6439

Dügenci, S.K., Arda, N. & Candan, A. (2003). Some medicinal plants as immunostimulant for fish. *Journal of Ethnopharmacology*, Vol.88, No.1, (September 2003), pp. 99–106, ISSN 0378-8741

Ekpo, O.E. & Pretorius, E. (2008) Using The BALB/c Asthmatic Mouse Model to Investigate the Effects of Hydrocortisone and a Herbal Asthma Medicine on Animal Weight. *Scandinavian Journal of Laboratory Animal Science*, Vol.35, No.4, pp. 265-280, ISSN 0901-3393

FAO. The state of world fisheries and aquaculture 2008. (2009). Rome: Food and Agriculture Organization of the United Nations, ISBN 978-92-5-106029-2

Fradin,, M.S. & Day, J.F. (2002) Comparative efficacy of insect repellents against mosquitoes bites. *The New England journal of medicine*, Vol.347, pp. 13–18, ISSN 0028-4793

Galvez, J., Zarzuelo, A., Crespo, M.E., Lorente, M.D., Ocete, M.A. & Jiménez, J. (1993) Antidiarrhoeic activity of Euphorbia hirta extract and isolation of an active flavonoid onstituent. *Planta Medica*, Vol.59, No.4, (Auguster 1993), pp. 333-336, ISSN 0032-0943

Govindarajan, A., Shankaranarayana Rao, B.S., Nair, D., Trinh, M., Mawjee, N., Tonegawa, S. & Chattarji, S. (2006): Transgenic brainderived neurotrophic factor expression causes both anxiogenic and antidepressant effects. *Proceedings of the National Academy of Sciences USA*, Vol.103, No.35, (Auguster 2006), pp. 13208–13213, ISSN 1091-6490

Gyuris, A., Szlávik, L., Minárovits, J., Vasas, A., Molnár, J. & Hohmann, J. (2009)Antiviral activities of extracts of Euphorbia hirta L. against HIV-1, HIV-2 and SIVmac251. *In Vivo*. Vol.23, No.3, (May-Jun 2009), pp. 429-432, ISSN 0258-851X

Hazleton, L.W., Hellerman, R.C., 1954. Studies on the pharmacology of E. piluliera. *Journal of American Pharmaceutical Association*, Vol.40, pp. 474–476, ISSN 1086-5802

Hore, S.K., Ahuja, V., Mehta, G., Pardeep Kumar, Pandey, S.K. & Ahmad, A.H. (2006)Effect of aqueous Euphorbia hirta leaf extract on gastrointestinal motility. *Fitoterapia* Vol.77, (July 2006), pp. 35– 38, ISSN 0367-326X

Hyman, L.H. (1970) The invertebrate, vol. VI. Mollusca I. Mc Graw Hill, New York. ISSN

Jaiprakash B, Chandramohan, Reddy DN. (2006) Burn wound healing activity of Euphorbia hirta. *Ancient Science of Life*, Vol.15, No.3&4, pp. 01-03, ISSN: 0257-7941

Jiangning, G., Xinchu, W., Hou, W., Qinghua, L. & Kaishun, B. (2005) Antioxidants from a Chinese medicinal herb - Psoralea corylifolia L. *Food Chemistry*, Vol.91, No.2, (June 2005), pp. 287-292, ISSN 0308-8146

James, LP., Mayeux, P.R. & Hinston, J.A. (2003)Acetaminophen-induced hepatotoxicity. *Drug Metabolism and Disposition*, Vol.31, pp. 1499-1506, ISSN: 0090-9556

Johnson, P.B., Abdurahman, E.M., Tiam, E.A., Abdu-Aguye, I. & Hussaini, I.M. (1999) Euphorbia hirta leaf extracts increase urine output and electrolytes in rats. *Journal of Ethnopharmacology*, Vol.65, No., (April 1999), pp. 63–69, ISSN 0378-8741

Kandaswami, C. & Middleton, E. (1994) Free radical scavaging and antioxidant activity of plant flavonoids. *Advances in Experimental Medicine and Biology*, Vol.366, pp. 351–376, ISSN 0065-2598

Khan, M.R., Ndaolio, G., Nkunya, M.H.H., Wevers, H. & Sawhney, A. (1980) Studies on African medicinal plants. Part I. Preliminary screening of medicinal plants for antibacterial activity. *Planta Medica*, Vol.Suppl, pp.91–97, ISSN 0032-0943

Kobuchi, H., Roy, S., Sen, C.K., Nguyen, H.G. & Packer, L. (1999) Quercetin inhibits inducible ICAM-1 expression in human endothelial cells through the JNK pathway. *American Journal of Physiology*, Vol.277, No.3, (September 1999), pp. C403–C411, ISSN 0363-6135

Kong, A.N., Yu, R., Chen, C., Mandlekar, S. & Primiano, T. (2000). Signal transduction events elicited by natural products: role of MAPK and caspase pathways in homeostatic response and induction of apoptosis. *Archives of pharmacal research*, Vol.23, No.1, (Feburary 2000), pp.1–16, ISSN 0253-6269

Kumar, S., Malhotra, R. & Kumar, D. (2010) Antidiabetic and free radicals scavenging potential of Euphorbia hirta flower extract. *Indian journal of Pharmaceutical Sciences*, Vol.72, No.4, (July 2010), pp. 533-537, ISSN 0250-474X

Lanhers, M.C., Fleurentin, J., Cabalion, P., Rolland, A., Dorfman, P., Misslin, R. & Pelt JM. (1990) Behavioral effects of Euphorbia hirta L.: sedative and anxiolytic properties. *Journal Ethnopharmacology*, Vol.29, No.2, (May 1990), pp. 189-198, ISSN 0378-8741

Lanhers, M.C., Fleurentin, J., Dorfman, P., Mortier, F. & Pelt, J.M. (1991) Analgesic, antipyretic and anti-inflammatory properties of Euphorbia hirta. *Planta Medica*, Vol.57, No.3, (June 1991), pp. 225-231, ISSN 0032-0943

Lee JK (2011) Anti-inflammatory effects of eriodictyol in lipopolysaccharide-stimulated raw 264.7 murine macrophages. *Archives Pharmacal Research*, Vol.34, No.4, (April 2011), pp. 671-679, ISSN 0253-6269

Logambal, S.M., Venkatalakshmi, S. & Dinakaran, M.R. (2000). Immunostimulatory effect of leaf extract of Ocimum sanctum Linn. In: Oreochromis mossambicus (Peters). *Hydrobiologia*, Vol.430, pp. 113–120, ISSN 1573-5117

Mallavadhani, U.V., Gayatri Sahu, Narasimhan, K., Muralidhar, J. (2002) Quantitative Estimation of an Antidiarrhoeic Marker in Euphorbia hirta Samples. *Pharmaceutical Biology*, Vol.40, No.2, pp. 103-106, ISSN 1388-0209

Martinez-Vazquez, M., Ramirez Apan, T.O., Lazcano, M.E. & Bye, R. (1999) Antiinflammatory active components from n-Hexane extract of Euphorbia hirta. *The Revista de la Sociedad Química de México*, Vol. 43, pp. 103-105, ISSN 0583-7693

McEwen, B.S. (2000) The neurobiology of stress: From serendipity to clinical relevance. *Brain Research*, Vol.886, No.1-2, (December 2000), pp. 172–189, ISSN 0006-8993

McLay, R.N., Freeman, S.M. & Zadina, J.E. (1998): Chronic corticosterone impairs memory performance in the Barnes maze. *Physiology & Behavior*, Vol.63, No.5, (March 1998), pp. 933–937, ISSN 0031-9384

Miller, A.L. (2001) The etiologies, patho-physiology and alternative/complementary treatment of asthma. *Alternative medicine review*, Vol.6, No.1, (Feburary 2001), pp. 20–47, ISSN 10895159

Mohanty, B.R. & Sahoo, P.K. (2010) Immune responses and expression profiles of some immune-related genes in Indian major carp, Labeo rohita to Edwardsiella tarda infection. *Fish and Shellfish Immunology*, Vol.28, (April 2010), p.p. 613–621, ISSN 1050-4648

Molyneux, P. (2004) The use of the stable free radical diphenylpicrylhydrazyl (DPPH) for estimating antioxidant activity. *Songklanakarin Journal of Science and Technology*, Vol.26, No.2, pp. 211-219, ISSN 0125-3395

Mukherjee, K.S., Mukhopadhyay, B., Mondal, S., Gorai, D. & Brahmachari, G. (2004) Triterpenoid Constituents of Borreria articularis. *Journal of the Chinese Chemical Society*, Vol.51, No.1, pp. 229-231, ISSN 0009-4536

Nadeem, A., Chhabra, S.K., Masood, A. & Raj, H.G. (2003) Increased oxidative stress and altered levels of antioxidants in asthma. The Journal of Allergy and Clinical Immunology, Vol.111, No.1, (January 2003), pp. 72-78, ISSN 0091-6749

Ndip, R.N., Tarkang, A.E.M., Mbullah, S.M., Luma, H.N., Malongue, A., Ndip, L.M., Nyongbela, K., Wirmumd, C. & Efange, S.M.N. (2007) In vitro anti-Helicobacter pylori activity of extracts of selected medicinal plants from North West Cameroon. *Journal of Ethnopharmacology*, Vol.114, No.3, (December 2007), pp. 452–457, ISSN 0378-8741

Opie, L. H. (1992). Angiotensin Converting Enzyme Inhibitors: Scientific Basis for Clinical Use, p. 259. ISBN 8810630033 9788810630037 0471588369 9780471588368 1881063003 9781881063001, John Wiley and Sons, New York.

Park, S.J. & Lee, Y.C. (2006) Antioxidants as Novel Agents for Asthma. *Mini Reviews in Medicinal Chemistry*, Vol.6, No.2, (Feburary 2006), pp. 235-240, ISSN 1389-5575

Paul, W.E., Seder, R.A. & Plaut, M. (1993) Lymphokine and cytokine production by Fc epsilon RI+ cells. *Advances in Immunology*, Vol. 53, pp. 1, ISSN 0065-2776

Pinn, G. (2001). Herbal therapy in respiratory diseases. Australian Family Physician, Vol.30, No.8, (September 2001), pp. 775–779, ISSN 0300-8495

Pratheepa, V. & Sukumaran, N. (2011) Specific and nonspecific immunostimulation study of Euphorbia hirta on Pseudomonas fluorescens-infected Cyprinus carpio *Pharmaceutical Biology*, 2011; Vol.49, No.5, (May 2011), pp. 484–491, ISSN 1388-0209

Raghuveer, C. & Tandon, R.V. (2009) Consumption of functional food and our health concerns. *Pakistan Journal of Physiology*, Vol.5, No.1, (January-June 2009), pp. 76-83, ISSN 1819-270X

Rairakhwada D, Pal AK, Bhathena ZP, Sahu NP, Jha A, Mukherjee SC. (2007). Dietary microbial levan enhances cellular non-specific immunity and survival of common carp (Cyprinus carpio) juveniles. *Fish and Shellfish Immunology*, Vol.22, No.4, (May 2007), pp. 477–486, ISSN : 1050-4648

Rajeh, M.A., Zuraini, Z., Sasidharan, S., Latha, L.Y., Amutha, S. (2010) Assessment of Euphorbia hirta L. leaf, flower, stem and root extracts for their antibacterial and antifungal activity and brine shrimp lethality. Molecules, Vol.15, No.9, (Auguster 2010), pp. 6008-6018, ISSN : 1420-3049

Ramamoorthy, P.K. & Bono, A. (2007) Antioxidant activity, total phenolic and flavonoid content of Morinda citrifolia fruit extracts from various extraction processes. Journal of Engineering Scuences and Technology, Vol.2, pp. 70-80, ISSN 2141-2820

Ramkumar, K., Srikumar, B.N., Shankaranarayana Rao, B.S. & Raju, T.R. (2008) Self-stimulation rewarding experience restores stressinduced CA3 dendritic atrophy, spatial memory deficits and alterations in the levels of neurotransmitters in the hippocampus. *Neurochemical Research*, Vol.33, No.9, (September 2008), pp. 1651–1662, ISSN : 0364-3190

Ramesh, K.V. & Padmavathi, K. (2010) Assessment of immunomodulatory activity of Euphorbia hirta L. *Indian Journal of Pharmaceutical Sciences*, Vol.72, No.5, (September 2010), pp. 621-625, ISSN : 0250-474X

Recknagel RO. (1983) A new direction in the study of carbon tetrachloride hepatotoxicity. *Life Sciences*. Vol.33, p.p. 401-408, ISSN: 0024-3205

Saharia, P.K. & Prasad, K.P. (2001) Development of co-agglutination kit for the diagnosis of Pseudomonas fluorescens infection in fishes. *Asian Fisheries Sciences*, Vol.14, pp. 293–300, ISSN : 0116-6514

Shih, M.F., Cheng, Y.D., Shen, C.R. & Cherng, J.Y. (2010) A molecular pharmacology study into the anti-inflammatory actions of Euphorbia hirta L. on the LPS-induced RAW 264.7 cells through selective iNOS protein inhibition. *Journal of Natural Medicines*, Vol.64, No.3, (July 2010), pp. 330-335, ISSN 1340-3443

Singh, B., Dutt, N., Kumar, D., Singh, S. & Mahajan, R. (2011) Taxonomy, Ethnobotany and Antimicrobial Activity of Croton bonplandianum, Euphorbia hirta and Phyllanthus fraternus. *Journal of Advances in Developmental Research*, Vol.2, No.1, pp. 21-29, ISSN : 0976-4704

Singh, G.D., Kaiser, P., Youssouf, M.S., Singh, S., Khajuria, A., Koul, A., Bani, S., Kapahi, B.K., Satti, N.K., Suri, K.A. & Johri, R.K. (2006) Inhibition of Early and Late Phase Allergic Reactions by Euphorbia hirta L. *Phytotherapy Research*, Vol.20, No.4, (April 2006), pp. 316–321, ISSN 0951-418X

Singh, S.K., Yadav, R.P., Tiwari, S. & Singh, A. (2005) Toxic effect of stem bark and leaf of Euphorbia hirta plant against freshwater vector snail Lymnaea acuminata. *Chemosphere*, Vol.59, No.11, (June 2005), pp. 263–270, ISSN 0045-6535

Spencer, J.P.E., Kuhnle, G.G.C., Williams, R.J. & Rice-Evans, C. (2003). Intracellular metabolism and bioactivity of quercetin and its in vivo metabolites. *Biochemical Journal*, Vol.372, pp. 173–181, ISSN 0264-6021

Srikumar, B.N., Raju, T.R. & Shankaranarayana Rao, B.S. (2006): The involvement of cholinergic and noradrenergic systems in behavioral recovery following oxotremorine treatment to chronically stressed rats. *Neuroscience*, Vol.143, No.3, (December 2006), pp. 679–688, ISSN 03064522

Srikumar, B.N., Raju, T.R. & Shankaranarayana Rao, B.S. (2007): Contrasting effects of bromocriptine on learning of a partially baited radial arm maze task in the presence and absence of restraint stress. *Psychopharmacology*, Vol.193, No.3, (Auguster 2007), pp. 363–374, ISSN 0033-3158

Sudhakar, M., Rao, Ch.V., Rao, P.M., Raju, D.B. & Venkateswarlu, Y. (2006) Antimicrobial activity of Caesalpinia pulcherrima, Euphorbia hirta and Asystasia gangeticum. *Fitoterapia*, Vol.77, No.5, (July 2006), pp. 378–380, ISSN 0367-326X

Sun, H., Fang, W-S., Wang, W-Z., & Hu, Chun. (2006) Structure-activity relationships of oleanane- and ursanetype triterpenoids. *Botanical Studies*, Vol.47, pp. 339-368, ISSN 1817-406X

Taubes, G. (1997) A mosquito bites back. New York Times Magazine 24 August, pp 40–46, ISBN 978-0-8070-4402-5

Tiwari1, P., Kumar, K. Ashish Kumar Pandey, A.K., Pandey, A. & Sahu, P.K. (2011) Antihepatotoxic Activity of Euphorbia hirta and by using the combination of Euphorbia hirta and Boerhaavia diffusa Extracts on Some Experimental Models of Liver Injury in Rats. International Journal of Innovative Pharmaceutical Research. Vol.2, No.2, pp. 126-130, ISSN 0976-4607

VanWyk, B-E., Van Oudtshoorn, B. & Gericke, N. (2000). Medicinal Plants of South Africa, 2nd edn. Briza, Pretoria. ISBN 3-8047-2246-6

Vyas, A., Mitra, R., Shankaranarayana Rao, B.S., Chattarji, S. (2002) Chronic stress induces contrasting patterns of dendritic remodeling in hippocampal and amygdaloid neurons. The Journal of Neuroscience, Vol.22, pp. 6810–6818, ISSN 0270-6474

Watanabe T, Rajbhandari KR, Malla KJ, Yahara S: A handbook of medicinal plants of Nepal Ayur Seed Life Environmental Institute, Japan; 2005, 262. ISBN 0395467225

Williams, R.J., Spencer, J.P.E. & Rice-Evans ,C. (2004). Flavonoids: antioxidants or signaling molecules? Free Radical Biology & Medicine, Vol.36, No.7, (April 2004), pp. 838–849, ISSN 0891-5849

Williams, L.A.D., Gossell-Williams, M., Sajabi, A., Barton, E.N. & Fleischhacker, R. (1997) Angiotensin Converting Enzyme Inhibiting and Anti-dipsogenic Activities of Euphorbia hirta Extracts. Phytotherapy Research, 11, 401–402, ISSN 0951-418X

Yoshida, T., Namba, O., Chen, L. and Okuda, T. (1990). Euphorbin E: A Hydrolysable tannin dimer of highly oxidized structure from Euphorbia hirta. Chemical & Pharmaceutical Bulletin (Tokyo), Vol.38, pp. 1113–1115, ISSN 0009-2363

Youssouf, M.S., Kaiser, P., Tahir, M., Singh, G.D., Singh, S., Sharma, V.K., Satti, N.K., Haque, S.E. & Johri, R.K. (2007) Anti-anaphylactic effect of Euphorbia hirta. Fitoterapia, Vol.78, No.7-8, (December 2007), pp. 535–539, ISSN 0367-326X

10

The Metabolites of Food Microorganisms

Hirofumi Takigawa and Yusuke Shibuya

Biological Science Laboratories/Kao Corporation

Japan

1. Introduction

Both medicine and one's daily diet are equally important for health. Ingesting healthy foods every day may reduce the risk of diseases. One of the most important diets in Japan are traditional fermented foods, which possess appetizing flavors, nutritional benefits, and desirable biological activities formed during the fermentation process. Epidemiological studies suggest that the consumption of fermented products may be associated with a lower incidence of certain chronic disease, such as coronary heart diseases, atherosclerosis, and certain types of cancers. In recent years, macrobiotics (i.e. a macrobiotic diet) have been considered to be one of the most popular alternative or complementary comprehensive lifestyle approaches to chronic diseases. The longevity of Japanese people is derived from their diet, which is rich in fermented foods.

Research has found that the physiologically active metabolites of fermentation food starters, specifically long-chain terpenes, such as novel C35-terpenols, were found in a culture of *Bacillus subtilis* KSM 6-10 isolated from pickled vegetables (i.e. tsukemono in Japanese). The biological activities of these foods have been previously studied. In this chapter, we review the active components of fermented foods formed by the starter microorganisms, present our research on these active metabolites, and describe the methods by which to increase the yield of these active components.

2. Active components of fermented foods

Fermented foods have been consumed for centuries worldwide. By ingesting these foods, it may be possible to prevent and alleviate certain diseases, such as cancer and hypertension. According to epidemiological studies, many potential benefits have been linked to the intake of fermented foods.

2.1 Epidemiological studies

Some case-control studies were conducted to assess the association between breast cancer risk and fermented milk consumption (Pieter et al., 1989; Pryor et al.; 1989, Ronco et al., 2002). High intakes of whole and chocolate milk were associated with a significantly increased risk of breast cancer, whereas ricotta cheese and skim yoghurt were associated with a significantly decreased risk.

To evaluate whether a fermented dairy drink containing a probiotic strain could reduce the incidence of common infectious diseases (CIDs), as well as behavioral changes resulting from illness, in children, a double-blinded clinical trial was conducted in the Washington, DC metropolitan area. Six-hundred and thirty-eight children, aged 3-6 years old, that attended a daycare/school were enrolled in the study. The rate of behavioral changes resulting from illness was similar among the active and control groups. However, the incidence rate for CIDs in the active group was 19% lower than that of the control group. Thus, the daily intake of a fermented dairy drink containing a probiotic strain showed some promise in reducing the overall incidence of illness (Merenstein et al., 2010).

One of the most popular and traditional foods in Japan are fermented soybeans (i.e. natto in Japanese). In a large representative cohort study, the association between habitual natto intake and bone mineral density (BMD) was assessed in 944 healthy Japanese women. It was found that there was a significant positive association between natto intake and the rate of change in BMD assessed at the femoral neck (P<0.0001) (Ikeda et al., 2006). Interestingly, there were no significant associations observed between the intake of tofu (non-fermented soybean curd) or boiled soybeans and the rate of change in BMD in postmenopausal women. It was suggested that natto intake may prevent postmenopausal bone loss via the effects of menaquinone or bioavailable isoflavones, which were more abundant in natto than in other soybean product.

The Rotterdam research group examined whether the dietary intake of menaquinone (vitamin K-2) was related to aortic calcification and coronary heart disease (CHD). Their findings suggested that an adequate intake of menaquinone may be important in the prevention of CHD (Johanna et al., 2004).

Recently, active components with desirable effects, such as antihypertensive, antioxidative, and platelet aggregation inhibiting activities, have been isolated from fermented foods. In the subsequent section, some of the active metabolites of starter microorganisms are reviewed, and our research on fermentation products is introduced.

2.2 Menaquinones

Vitamin K is one of the fat soluble vitamins, which exists as either vitamin K1 (phylloquinone) in green plants or vitamin K2 (menaquinone) in animals and bacteria. Vitamin K is necessary for the posttranslational modification of certain proteins and blood coagulation. Menaquinones are classified according to the length of their aliphatic side chain, and are designated as MK-n (see Fig. 9). MK-7 is abundant in cheese or fermented soybeans (natto in Japanese). A Natto containing a high amount of MK-7, which is produced by a special starter (i.e. *Bacillus subtilis* 35 OUV 23481), is an approved food product for its specified health use by the National Health and Nutrition Research in Japan.

2.3 Lactotripeptides

Angiotensin I-converting enzyme (ACE) is an important enzyme in the regulation of blood pressure, as it catalyzes the formation of a potent vasopressor, angiotensin II, from angiotensin I. Two peptides (i.e. Val-Pro-Pro [VPP] and Ile-Pro-Pro [IPP]) that possess ACE inhibiting properties have been isolated from a type of sour milk fermented with

Lactobacillus helveticus and *Saccharomyces cerevisiae* (Nakamura et al., 1995). These tripeptides are barely digested by digestive enzymes, suggesting that, despite their oral administration, these tripeptides remain intact within the intestine and retain their antihypertensive activity until absorption (Ohsawa et al., 2008). Indeed, these peptides demonstrated significant antihypertensive effects in clinical studies (Hata et al., 1996). Although these tripeptides were not generated from beta-casein via human gastrointestinal enzymes, they were produced in a fermented soybean paste (miso in Japanese) by adding casein (Inoue et al., 2009). Two proteolytic enzymes, which are capable of releasing the tripeptides from casein, were identified in *Aspergillus oryzae*, one of the starters in fermented foods, such as miso (Gotou et al., 2009).

In sour milk, the production of antihypertensive peptides (VPP and IPP) is limited during *Lactobacillus helveticus* fermentation, as most of the casein remains unprocessed. To improve the production of these peptides, carboxypeptidase was added with *Lactobacillus helveticus* CM4 to process the C-terminal ends of the precursor peptides (i.e. VPP-Xxx and IPP-Xxx) and form VPP and IPP. The amount of tripeptides yielded was 60 mg/L (Ueno et al., 2004).

2.4 Isoflavones

Japanese-style fermented soy sauce (shoyu in Japanese) is a typical traditional fermented food, and its functional effects have also been previously studied (Kataoka 2005). Some active components (i.e. metabolites), which were not present in the original raw materials such as boiled soybean and wheat, were isolated from fermentation products.

2.4.1 Shoyuflavones

Three tartaric isoflavone derivatives were found in soy sauce (Kinoshita et al., 1997). These isoflavones have not been previously found in any other soy products. They demonstrate inhibitory activities against histidine decarboxylase, resulting in the production of histamine from L-histidine (Kinoshita et al., 1998). Histamine is a mediator of inflammation, allergies, gastric acid secretions, and neurotransmission.

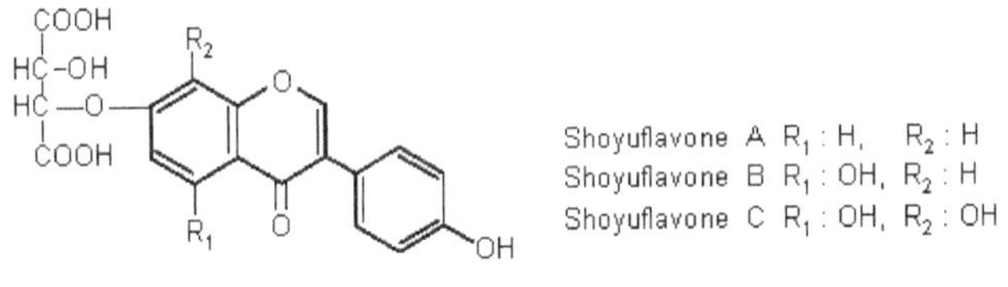

Shoyuflavone A R_1 : H, R_2 : H
Shoyuflavone B R_1 : OH, R_2 : H
Shoyuflavone C R_1 : OH, R_2 : OH

Fig. 1. Structures of shoyuflavones.

2.4.2 Orobol (5,7,3',4'-tetrahydroxyisoflavone)

Tempeh is a fermented soybean product originating from Indonesia, which is also popular outside of Indonesia, as it is odorless. European researchers have isolated several isoflavones, including 5,7,4'-trihydroxyisoflavone (genistein), 7,4'-dihydroxyisoflavone (daidzein), and a novel one, 5,7,3',4'-tetrahydroxyisoflavone (orobol), from a tempeh extract

(Kiriakidis et al., 2005). The effects of these isoflavones on angiogenesis were evaluated using a chicken chorioallantoic membrane assay, and it was found that these isoflavones reduced angiogenesis by 49-75% compared to the negative control (6.3%). It was suggested that these isoflavones should be added to the list of low molecular mass therapeutic agents for the inhibition of angiogenesis.

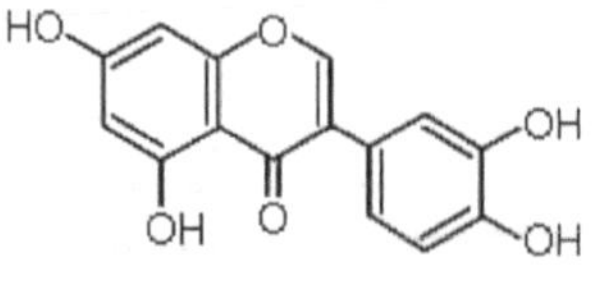

Fig. 2. Structure of orobol (5,7,3',4'-tetrahydroxyisoflavon).

2.4.3 6-hydroxydaidzein and 8-hydroxyglycitein

8-Hydroxyglycitein and 6-hydroxydaidzein were isolated from a soybean paste (miso in Japanese), and were found to act as 1,1-diphenyl-2-picrylhydrazyl (DPPH) radical scavengers (Hirota et al., 2004). These compounds demonstrated DPPH-radical scavenging activity that was as high as that of α-tocopherol, 8-hydroxygenistein, and 8-hydroxydaidzein (Fig. 3). To our best knowledge, this was the first report on the isolation of 8-hydroxyglycitein from a natural source.

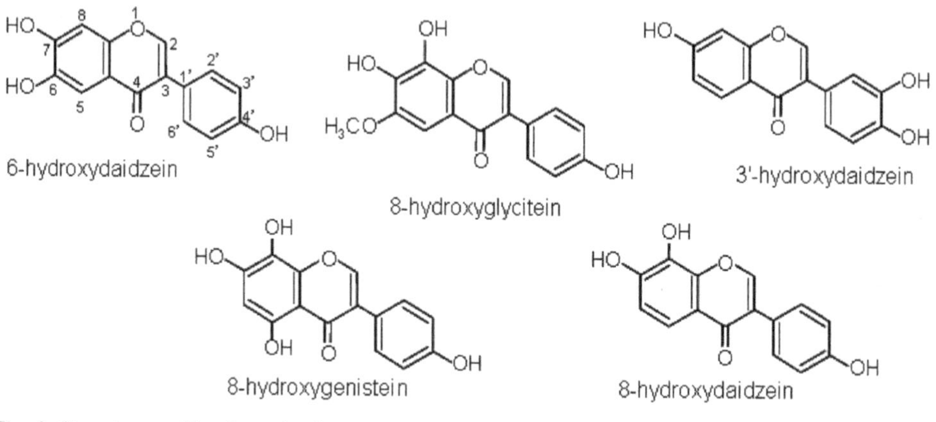

Fig. 3. Structures of hydroxyisoflavones.

2.4.4 3'-hydroxydaidzein

Dou-chi, a traditional soybean food fermented with *Aspergillus* sp., is usually used as a seasoning in Chinese food, and has been also used as a folk medicine in both China and Taiwan. Four phenol compounds, one isoflavanone, eight isoflavones, and one 4-pyrone were isolated from dou-chi (Chen et al., 2005). Among these compounds, 3'-hydroxydaidzein, dihydrodaidzein, and the 4-pyrone compound have not yet been isolated from soybean paste (miso). The structure assigned to the novel 4-pyrone compound was 3-((E)-2-carboxyethenyl)-5-(4-hydroxyphenyl)-4-pyrone-2-carboxylic acid.

2.5 Beta-carbolines

The diethyl ether extract of soy sauce was found to inhibit platelet aggregation induced by collagen and epinephrine. Specifically, the active components were 1-methyl-1,2,3,4-tetrahydro-beta-carboline (MTBC) and 1-methyl-beta-carboline (MBC) (Tsuchiya et al., 1999). The concentrations of MTBC and MBC in commercially available soy sauces are 28-85 ppm and 0.3-4.2 ppm, respectively. MTBC required mean concentrations of 4.6, 4.2, 28.6, 11.6, and 65.8 µg/mL to produce a 50% inhibition of the maximal aggregation response induced by epinephrine, platelet-activating factor, collagen, adenosine 5'-diphosphate, and thrombin, respectively. Thus, soy sauce may be a functional seasoning with a potent preventive effect on thrombi formation.

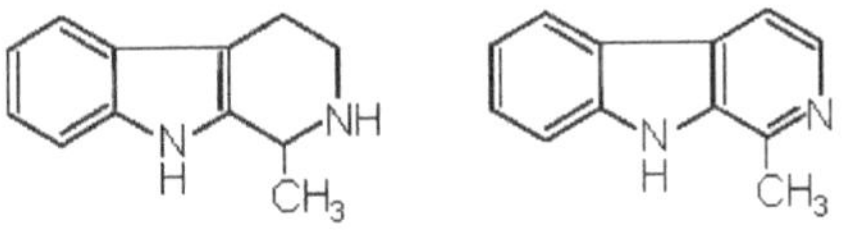

Fig. 4. Structures of beta-carboline derivatives.

2.6 Hydroxy-furanones

4-Hydroxy-2(or 5)-ethyl-5(or 2)-methyl-3(2H)-furanone (HEMF), isolated from the ethyl acetate extract of soy sauce, is a shoyu-like flavor component that is also a potent antioxidant and anticarcinogen (Nagahara et al., 1992). Soy sauce contains other structurally similar flavor components, specifically, 4-hydroxy-5-methyl-3(2H)-furanone (HMF) and 4-hydroxy-2,5-dimethyl-3(2H)-furanone (HDMF) (Fig. 5). HDMF and HMF are thought to form chemically via the Maillard reaction between sugars and amino acids during the heating process. These furanones were investigated for their antioxidative activities. HMF and HDMF, as well as HEMF, were confirmed to have antioxidative properties. The order of potency was as follows: HEMF> HDMF > HMF. Furthermore, HEMF and HDMF are more potent than ascorbic acid.

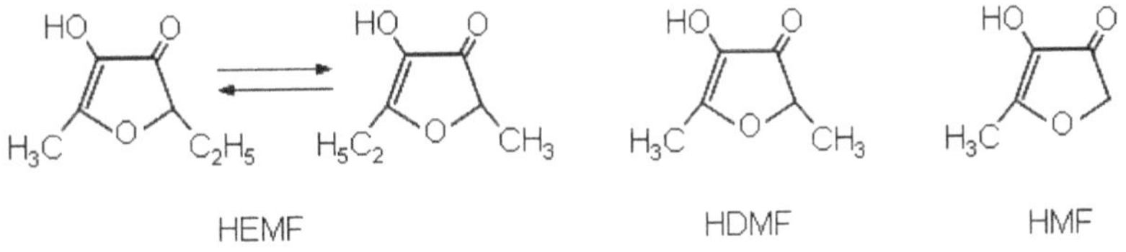

HEMF   HDMF   HMF

Fig. 5. Structures of 4-Hydroxy-2-ethyl-5-methyl-3-furanone and the related compounds.

2.7 Gamma-aminobutyric acid (GABA)

Gamma-aminobutyric acid (GABA) is a non-proteinaceous amino acid formed from the decarboxylation L-glutamate via glutamate decarboxylase (EC 4.1.1.15) (Fig. 6). GABA is a major inhibitory neurotransmitter in the mammalian central nervous system, and has several well-known physiological functions, such as the induction of hypotension and secretion of insulin from the pancreas.

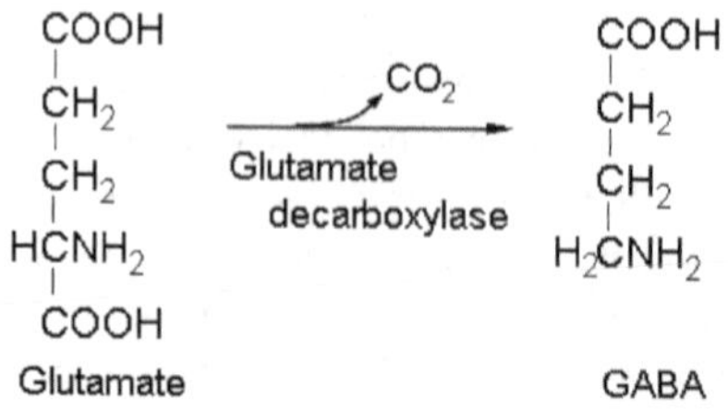

$$\begin{array}{c} \text{COOH} \\ | \\ \text{CH}_2 \\ | \\ \text{CH}_2 \\ | \\ \text{HCNH}_2 \\ | \\ \text{COOH} \\ \text{Glutamate} \end{array} \xrightarrow[\text{decarboxylase}]{\;\;CO_2\;\;\nearrow\;\;} \begin{array}{c} \text{COOH} \\ | \\ \text{CH}_2 \\ | \\ \text{CH}_2 \\ | \\ \text{H}_2\text{CNH}_2 \\ \\ \\ \text{GABA} \end{array}$$

Glutamate decarboxylase

Fig. 6. Structure of γ-aminobutyric acid (GABA).

The blood pressure effects of a fermented milk product containing GABA were evaluated in patients with mild hypertension (Inoue et al., 2003). The study comprised of 39 mildly hypertensive patients (16 women and 23 men), aged 28 to 81 years (mean: 54.2 years). The patients received a daily intake of GABA or placebo for 12 weeks followed by a 2-week treatment-free period (weeks 13 and 14). There was a 17.4 ± 4.3 mmHg decrease in systolic blood pressure and 7.2 ± 5.7 mmHg decrease in diastolic blood pressure in patients receiving GABA. Thus, GABA may be used to lower blood pressure in mildly hypertensive individuals.

Another study evaluated the antihypertensive effects of *Lactobacillus*-fermented milk that was orally administered to spontaneously hypertensive rats (Liu et al., 2011). It was found that eight hours after administrating milk fermented with either *Lactobacillus paracasei* subsp. *paracasei* NTU 101 or *Lactobacillus plantarum* NTU 102 containing GABA, there was a significant decrease in the systolic and diastolic blood pressures of these hypertensive rats.

A simple fermentation process was developed to yield a high amount of GABA (Cock et al., 2010). Specifically, cultivating *Lactobacillus sakei* B2-16 in rice bran extract yields a maximum GABA concentration of 660.0 mM, which is 2.4-fold greater than that achieved without the rice bran extract. Furthermore, a simple and effective fed-batch fermentation process was developed to efficiently convert glutamate into GABA (Li et al., 2010). The GABA concentration obtained with this process was 1005.81 ± 47.88 mM, and the residual glucose and glutamate concentration were 15.28 ± 0.51 g/L and 134.45 ± 24.22 mM after 48 h.

2.8 Polyprenols

Polyprenols are natural long-chain isoprenoid alcohols with a general formula of $H\text{-}(C_5H_8)_n\text{-}OH$, where n is the number of isoprene units. Polyprenols serve as sugar carriers in biosynthetic processes that include protein glycosylation and lipopolysaccharide biogenesis, and are found in small quantities in various plant tissues and microorganism cells. Dolichols, which are found in all living organisms, including humans, are their 2,3-dihydro derivatives (Rezanka et al., 2001). Polyprenols are low molecular natural bioregulators, which are physiologically active, and play a significant modulating role in the cellular process of plants, specifically biosynthesis. The dolichol phosphate cycle facilitates the process of cellular membrane glycosylation, that is, the synthesis of glycoproteins that control cell interactions, support the immune system, and stabilize protein molecules. Out of all these glycoproteins, polyglycoprotein has the capacity to kill cancer cells during chemotherapy, while protecting healthy cells within the body. Polyprenols stimulate the immune system, cellular respiration and spermatogenesis, and possess anti-stress, adaptogenic, anti-ulcerogenic, and wound-healing properties. Dolichols have antioxidative properties, and protect cell membranes from peroxidation. In the subsequent section, our research on polyprenols isolated from food microorganisms will be discussed.

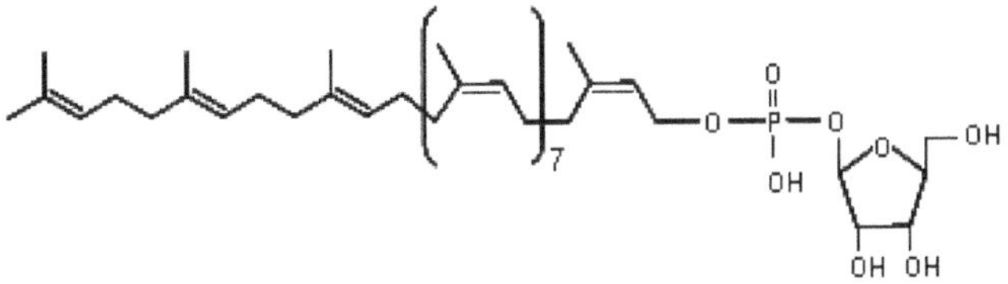

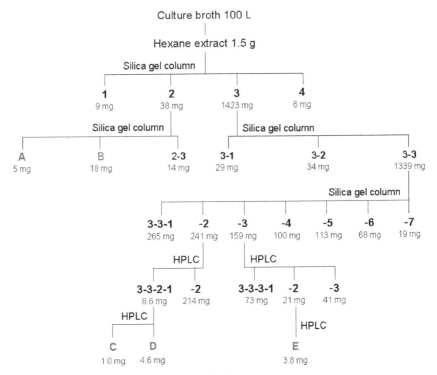

Fig. 7. Structure of a sugar carrier.

2.8.1 Isolation of metabolites from *Bacillus subtilis* KSM6-10

Bacillus subtilis KSM 6-10 was isolated from a traditional pickled vegetable found in Japan (tsukemono in Japanese). Based on its 16S rDNA sequence, which was compared directly to all known sequences within the GenBank databases via the basic local alignment search tool (BLAST), the strain was identified to belong to the genus *Bacillus*.

The procedure for isolating the metabolites of *Bacillus subtilis* KSM 6-10 is presented in Fig. 8. Briefly, without adjusting the pH of the culture broth (pH 7.5-8.0), the entire broth was

Fig. 8. The procedure for isolating terpenes (A-E).

extracted with EtOAc (2 × 5L) to yield 50 mg of a pale brown material. The EtOAc extract was separated by liquid-liquid extraction (50/50; n-hexane/90% aqueous MeOH). Then, the n-hexane extract (1.5 g) was fractioned using a High-Flash column (16 × 60 mm, Yamazen, Osaka, Japan) via a gradient elution from n-hexane to EtOAc, which yielded 4 fractions (20 mL each). Fraction 2 (38 mg) was further fractioned similarly as described above to yield three fractions. Fraction 2-1 produced 5 mg of pure compound **A** and fraction 2-2 produced 18 mg of pure compound **B**. Fraction 3 (1423 mg) was further fractioned in a similar fashion described above to yield three fractions. Then, fraction 3-3 (1339 mg) was further fractioned to yield seven fractions, and fraction 3-3-2 (241 mg) was further fractioned via gradient preparative HPLC (20% to 100% CH_3CN in H_2O) to yield two fractions. Fraction 3-3-2-1 (9 mg) yielded 1 mg of pure compound **C** and 4.6 mg of pure compound **D**. Fraction 3-3-3-2 (21 mg) yielded 3.8 mg of pure compound **E** (Takigawa et al., 2010).

2.8.2 Metabolites of *Bacillus subtilis* KSM6-10

Compounds A and B, tetraprenyl-β-curcumene and tetraprenyl-α-curcumene, respectively, were previously isolated from a spore preparation of the same species (Boroczky et al., 2006), whereas compounds C and D are novel C35-terpenols. Compound E was identified as undecaprenol (C55; bactoprenol) ((Rezanka et al., 2001)).

The proposed biosynthesis pathway of the five terpenes (A-E) is presented in Fig. 9. Mevalonic acid is a key precursor in the pathway, which via the mevalonate pathway produces terpenes

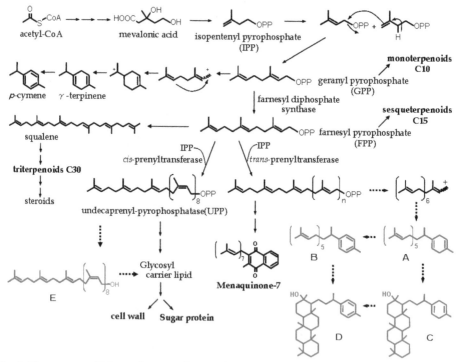

Fig. 9. The proposed biosynthesis pathway of terpenoids.

and steroids. Since the C35-terpenols (C and D) possess polycyclic skeletons, they are thought to be formed via the cyclization of acyclic C35-terpenes (A and B).

Recently, a new terpene cyclase, which is capable of forming pentacyclic C35 terpenols (C and D) from acyclic C35-terpenes (A and B), was purified from a standard strain of *Bacillus subtilis* (Sato et al., 2011). Since our isolate, *Bacillus subtilis* KSM 6-10, showed a 99.8% sequence homology to the standard strain of *Bacillus subtilis*, we are currently studying whether the terpene cyclase of *Bacillus subtilis* KSM 6-10 is homologous to the reported enzyme (Sato et al., 2011).

2.8.2.1 Cell proliferation activity

The cell proliferation activity of the five terpenes (A-E) were assayed in co-cultured hair follicle dermal papilla cells (HFDPC: Cell Applications Inc. USA) and human epidermal keratinocytes (HKC: Invitrogen Corp. USA) (Yuspa et al., 1993). The total amount of bromodeoxyuridine (BrdU) incorporated into the DNA of the monolayer of co-cultured cells was measured with an enzyme-linked immunosorbent assay (ELISA) (Muir et al., 1990). Following a dilution step, compounds A-E (1 mg/ml) were assayed (Fig. 10). Compound E (undecaprenol) was found to be the most active in the co-cultured cells.

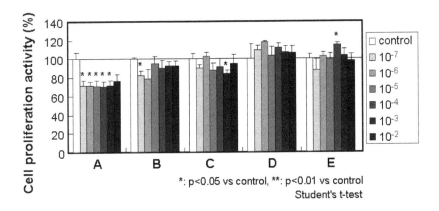

Fig. 10. Cell proliferation activities of various concentrations of compounds A-E.

2.8.2.2 Tyrosinase inhibition

A mushroom tyrosinase inhibition assay was previously conducted using L-dopamine (L-DOPA) as the substrate, and ascorbic acid as the positive control (Lee et al., 2002). Dopacrome formation was measured at 490 nm using a 96-well reader. The assay results are presented in Fig. 11. It was found that, although the C35 terpenes (A, B) did not inhibit tyrosinase, the polyprenols (C, D, E) demonstrated a mild inhibitory effect (Fig. 11).

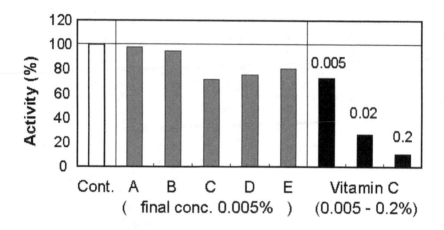

Fig. 11. Tyrosinase inhibition activities of compounds A-E.

2.8.2.3 The production of farnesol

Polyprenols are polyisoprenoid alcohols that contain anywhere from 5 to 25 or more multiprenyl chains with a hydroxyl group at the end (Fig. 12). They are present in all living cells, and referred to as dolichol (C75-C115), bactoprenol (C55), and ficaprenol (C50-C145) (Rezanka et al., 2001). Polyprenyl phosphates are essential intermediates that act as lipid carriers in several biochemical pathways, including N-linked protein glycosylation and cell wall biosynthesis. Certain polyprenols are suggested to be biomarker for aging (Parentini et al., 2005).

Farnesol (C15) is a major fragrance component found in the flowers of many plants, and it is a common intermediate in several essential components, such as sterols and quinones (see Fig. 9). Additionally, it has been utilized as a starting material in synthetic pharmaceuticals. Recently, derivatives of farnesol have become candidates in anti-cancer reagents, as they induce apoptosis in various tumor cell lines (Gibbs et al., 1999; Burke et al., 2002). Thus, recent research efforts are aimed at enhancing the production of polyprenols.

A mutant strain auxotrophic for ergosterol, which blocks farnesyl diphosphate synthase, was reported to produce a low concentration of farnesol (1 mg/L) (Chambon et al., 1990). Although the amount of farnesol produced by the squalene synthase-deficient mutant *Saccharomyces cerevisiae* ATCC 64031 was low (4-6 mg/L), combining glucose with soybean oil results in more than 28 mg/L of farnesol in the soluble fraction of the broth. Thus, this method allows for the over-production of hydrophobic and useful compounds, such as tochopherol and carotenoids. Furthermore, an alkaline pH (7-8) also enhances farnesol production, where it was reported that a concentration of 102.8 mg/L was produced in a jar fermentor (Muramatsu et al., 2008; 2009).

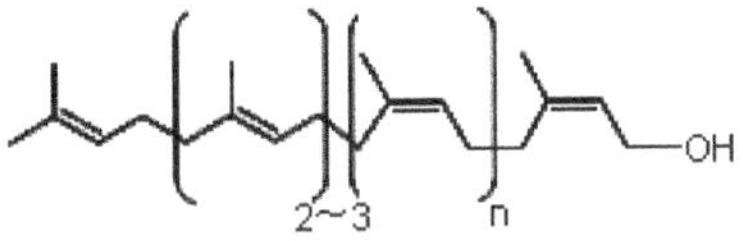

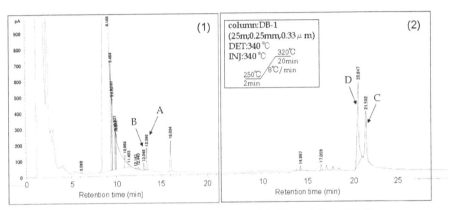

Fig. 12. Structure of a polyprenol.

2.8.2.4 The production of polyprenols from *B. subtilis* KSM6-10 (C-E)

Using a metabolic regulatory fermentation process rather than a genetic modification, we have previously determined a way of increasing the amounts of our isolated polyprenols (C-E). Briefly, *B. subtilis* KSM 6-10 was grown for 2 days at 30°C in a 500-ml flask containing 100 ml of K medium (Takigawa et al., 2010). The whole broth was then extracted with n-hexane, and the extract was analyzed via gas chromatography (GC) (Fig. 13).

Fig. 13. Gas chromatographic analysis of isolate A and B (1), and C and D (2).

Of the additives tested, we found that monoterpenes, such as *p*-cymene and β-myrcene, enhanced the production of C35-terpenes (A and B). Three-hundred ppm of *p*-cymene demonstrated the most prominent effect, which was then further accelerated by the addition of a high concentration of glucose or yeast extract in the medium (Fig. 14).

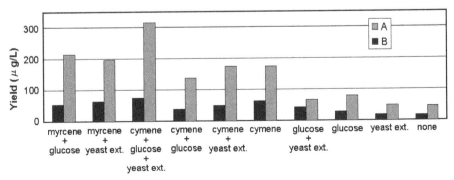

Fig. 14. The effects of additives on the production of compounds A and B.

In our preliminary studies, however, we were not able to enhance the production yields of polyprenols (C-E). Given that prenyltransferase present in *Bacillus subtilis*, which synthesizes undecaprenyl pyrophosphate (see Fig. 9), is stimulated markedly by the addition of monovalent cations, such as K+ and NH4+ (Takahashi et al., 1982), changing the composition of the liquid medium may increase the amount of polyprenols (C-E) produced. In particular, the addition of KH_2PO_4 into the K medium during the mid-log phase of the liquid culture of *B.subtilis* KSM 6-10 may enhance the production of undecaprenyl pyrophosphate synthase, including the amount of polyprenol E produced. This is currently being studied by our research group.

2.9 Sake lees

The traditional Japanese alcoholic beverage (Sake in Japanese) is produced from steamed rice by the simultaneous addition of two microorganisms, *Saccharomyces cerevisiae* and *Aspergillus oryzae* (koji in Japanese). Sake lees (sake kasu in Japanese) is a fine sediment left after the sake filtering process. While a small amount of sake lees is used as a pickling agent for making fermented vegetables (Tsukemono in Japanese), as well as a food material, most of it is considered industrial waste. Recently, the biological activities of sake lees have been investigated. For example, sake less has been shown to inhibit ACE (Saito et al., 1994) and tyrosinase (Jeon et al., 2006). We have recently been assessing whether sake lees has other potential biological activities.

2.9.1 Peroxisome-proliferator activated receptors (PPAR)

Nuclear peroxisome proliferator-activated receptors (PPAR) have been shown to play critical roles in the regulation of energy homeostasis, including lipid and carbohydrate metabolism, inflammatory responses, and cell proliferation, differentiation, and survival. Since PPAR agonists have the potential to prevent or ameliorate diseases, such as hyperlipidemia, diabetes, atherosclerosis, and obesity, we have investigated whether the certain food metabolites can act as natural agonists for PPAR.

2.9.1.1 Peroxisome proliferator-activated receptor luciferase assay

The pBIND-GAL4-PPARαLBD and pBIND-GAL4-PPARδLBD chimeric expression plasmids were prepared, as previously described (Murase et al., 2006). The pG5luc reporter plasmid with the GAL4 binding site was obtained from Promega (Madison, WI). The African green monkey fibroblast cell line CV-1 was obtained from Riken Cell Bank (Tsukuba, Japan). Following a day of cultivation in DMEM, CV-1 cells were transfected using Superfect transfection reagent (QIAGEN, Valencia, CA). The cells were incubated in a transfection mixture containing 6.25 μl of SuperFect, 0.375 μg of pBIND-GAL4-PPAR-LBD expression plasmid, and 0.375 μg of pG5luc reporter plasmid for 3 h at 37°C. They were then incubated for 4 h in fresh DMEM (+5% charcoal-treated FBS). After treatment with or without each sample for 20 h, cells were lysed, and then firefly and *Renilla* luciferase activities were measured using the Dual-Luciferase Reporter Assay System (Promega). Wy-14643 (SIGMA) was used as a positive control for PPARα and GW-501516 (Wako) for PPARδ.

2.9.1.2 The effects of sake lees extracts on PPAR activation

Although both Wy-14643, a PPARα agonist, and GW-501516, a PPARδ agonist, significantly enhanced PPAR-dependent luciferase activities, sake lees extracts (0.02%) also demonstrated a marked effect (Fig. 15). It appears that all of the test samples contained direct ligands for PPARα and PPARδ. Of the sake lees extracts tested, only the water extract demonstrated no activity, suggesting that there are certain hydrophobic components that are related to PPAR activation. Currently, we are in the process of isolating the hydrophobic ligands from sake lees, and hope to report on these active components in the near future.

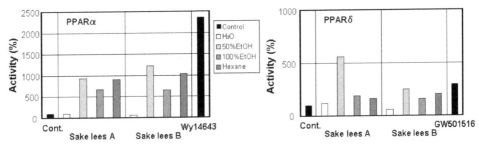

Fig. 15. PPAR activation with sake lees extracts.

2.9.2 Antioxidative effects of sake lees

The antioxidative effects of sake lees extracts were evaluated (Fig. 16). Briefly, the intracellular formation of reactive oxygen species was detected with a fluorescence probe, 5-(and-6)-chloromethyl-2',7'-dichlorodihydrofluorescein diacetate (5,6-CM-H_2DCFDA; Invitrogen). Leukocytes were isolated from male Sprague-Dawley rats (i.e. 10-16 weeks old) and then cultured in the presence of each test samples for 1 h at room temperature. The samples were then loaded with 10 µM 5,6-CM-H_2DCFDA for 20 min, and evaluated via flow cytometry. Of all of the sake lees extracts, the hexane extract demonstrated a significantly decrease in ROS generation, suggesting the presence of antioxidative activity. It is recognized that the antioxidative properties of sake lees result from their hydrophilic compounds, such as ferulic acid and vanillin, which originate from sake. Given that the hydrophobic components with antioxidative properties have not yet been isolated from a sake lees, we are currently attempting to isolate these active components.

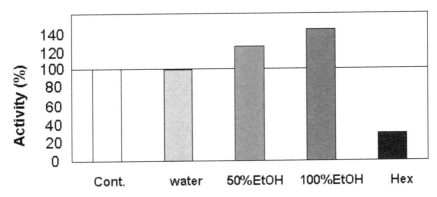

Fig. 16. Antioxidative effects of sake lees extracts.

2.9.3 Antihypertensive activity

The effects of hexane extract of sake lees on blood pressure was investigated in spontaneously hypertensive rats (SHR; 9 weeks old). Specifically, the tail blood pressure was measured using an indirect blood pressure meter (BP-98A, Softron) at 0, 1, 3, 6, and 24 h after a single intravenous injection of the hexane extract of sake lees (100 mg/kg) (Fig. 17). We also confirmed that the hexane extract did not have an effect on the blood pressures of normal Sprague-Dawley rats (data not shown). The active compound appears to be hydrophobic, and different from the other compounds (Saito et al., 1994).

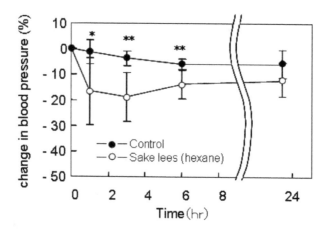

Fig. 17. The antihypertensive effects of the hexane extract containing sake lees.

2.10 Other biological activities

In many Asian countries, there are numerous traditional fermented foods other than tempeh, natto, and dou-chi. For example, kimchi (a fermented vegetable in Korea), fish sauce (Nam pla in Thailand, and Nuoc mam in Vietnam), and fermented tea (Oolong and Pu-erh) all warrant further investigation in regards to their potential biologically active metabolites.

3. Conclusion

Fermented foods contain various metabolites that are produced by their starter microorganisms, and are reported to have many desirable activities, for example antihypertensive (GABA and lactotripeptides), antioxidative (isoflavones), and anticancer (polyprenols) properties. Since they are not digested within the intestine, they may present their biological activities after absorption. By regularly ingesting these foods, it may be possible to prevent and alleviate certain types of diseases.

4. Acknowledgment

We hope that Asian fermented foods will become more popular and contribute to improving the health of individuals worldwide. Finally, we deeply appreciate the editorial board for providing us with the opportunity to discuss the use of fermented foods.

5. References

Boroczky, K.; Lastsch, H.; Wagner-Dobler, I.; Stritzke, K. & Schultz, S. (2006). Cluster analysis as selection and dereplication tool for the identification of new natural compounds from large sample sets. *Chem.Biodiversity*, Vol. 3, No. 6, pp. 622-634

Burke, Y.D.; Ayoubi, A.S.; Werner, S.R.; McFarland, B.C.; Heilman, D.K.; Ruggeri, B.A. & Crowell, P.L. (2002). Effects of the isoprenoids perillyl alcohol and farnesol on apoptosis biomarkers in pancreatic cancer chemoprevention. *Anticancer Res*, Vol. 22, No. 6A, pp. 3127-3134

Chambon, C.; Ladeveze, V.; Oulmouden, A.; Servouse, M. & Karst F. (1990). Isolation and properties of yeast mutants affected in farnesyl diphosphate synthetase. *Curr Genet*, Vol. 18, No. 1, pp. 41-46

Chen, Y.C.; Sugiyama, Y.; Abe, N.; Kuruto-Niwa, R.; Nozawa, R. & Hirota, A. (2005). DPPH radical-scavenging compounds from dou-chi, a soybean fermented food. *Biosci Biotechnol Biochem*, Vol. 69, No. 5, pp. 999-1006

Johanna, M.G.; Cees, V.; Diederick, E.G.; Leon, J.S.; Marjo, H.J.K.; Irene, M.; Albert, H. & Jacqueline, C. M. W. (2004). Dietary intake of menaquinone is associated with a reduced risk of coronary heart disease: The Rotterdam study1. *J. Nutr.Vol.* Vol. 134, pp. 3100-3105

Gibbs, B.S.; Zahn, T.J. Mu, Y.; Sebolt-Leopold, J.S. & Gibbs, RA. (1999). Novel farnesol and geranylgeraniol analogues: A potential new class of anticancer agents directed against protein prenylation. *J Med Chem.* Vol. 42, No. 19, 3800-8

Gotou, T.; Shinoda, T.; Mizuno, S. & Yamamoto, N. (2009). Purification and identification of proteolytic enzymes from *Aspergillus oryzae* capable of producing the antihypertensive peptide Ile-Pro-Pro. *J Biosci Bioeng.* Vol. 107, No. 6, pp. 615-9

Hata, Y.; Yamamoto, M.; Ohni, M.; Nakajima, K.; Nakamura, Y. & Takano, T.(1996). A placebo-controlled study of the effect of sour milk on blood pressure in hypertensive subjects. *Am J Clin Nutr.* Vol. 64, No. 5, pp. 767-71

Hirota, A.; Inaba, M.; Chen, Y.C.; Abe, N.; Taki, S.; Yano, M. & Kawaii, S. (2004). Isolation of 8-hydroxyglycitein and 6-hydroxydaidzein from soybean miso. *Biosci Biotechnol Biochem.* Vol. 68, No. 6, pp. 1372-4

Ikeda, Y.; Iki, M.; Morita, A.; Kajita, E.; Kagamimori, S.; Kagawa, Y. & Yoneshima, H. (2006). Intake of fermented soybeans, natto, is associated with reduced bone loss in postmenopausal women. *J. Nutr.* Vol. 136, pp. 1323-1328

Inoue, K.; Gotou, T.; Kitajima, H.; Mizuno, S.; Nakazawa, T. & Yamamoto, N. (2009). Release of antihypertensive peptides in miso paste during its fermentation, by the addition of casein. *J Biosci Bioeng.* Vol. 108, No. 2, pp. 111-5

Inoue, K.; Shirai, T.; Ochiai, H.; Kasao, M.; Hayakawa, K.; Kimura, M. & Sansawa H. (2003). Blood-pressure-lowering effect of a novel fermented milk containing gamma-aminobutyric acid (GABA) in mild hypertensives. *Eur J Clin Nutr.* Vol. 57, No.3, pp. 490-5

Kataoka, S. (2005) Functional effects of Japanese style fermented soy sauce (shoyu) and its components. *J.Biosci.Bioeng.* Vol. 100, No. 3, pp. 227-234

Kinoshita, E.; Ozawa, Y. & Aishima T. (1997). Novel tartaric acid isoflavone derivatives that play key roles in differentiating Japanese soy sauce. *J.Agric.Food Chem.*, Vol. 45, pp. 3753-3759

Kinoshita, E. & Saito M. (1998). Novel histamine measurement by HPLC analysis used to assay histidine decarboxylase inhibitory activity of shoyuflavones from soy sauce. *Biosci Biotechnol Biochem.* Vol. 62, No. 8, pp. 1488-91

Kiriakidis, S.; Högemeier, O.; Starcke, S.; Dombrowski, F.; Hahne, J.C.; Pepper, M.; Jha, H.C. & Wernert, N. (2005). Novel tempeh (fermented soyabean) isoflavones inhibit *in vivo* angiogenesis in the chicken chorioallantoic membrane assay. *Br J Nutr.* Vol. 93, No. 3, pp. 317-23

Kook, M.C.; Seo, M.J.; Cheigh, C.I.; Pyun, Y.R.; Cho, S.C. & Park H.(2010). Enhanced production of gamma-aminobutyric acid using rice bran extracts by *Lactobacillus sakei* B2-16. *J Microbiol Biotechnol.* Vol. 20, No. 4, pp. 763-6

Lee, S.H.; Choi, S.Y.; Kim, H.; Hwang, J.S.; Lee, B.G.; Gao, J.J. & Kim, S.Y. (2002). Mulberroside F isolated from the leaves of *Morus alba* inhibits melanin biosynthesis. *Biol Pharm Bull.* Vol. 25, No. 8, pp. 1045-8

Li, H.; Qiu, T.; Huang, G. & Cao, Y.(2010). Production of gamma-aminobutyric acid by *Lactobacillus brevis* NCL912 using fed-batch fermentation. *Microb Cell Fact.* Vol. 12, No. 9, pp. 85

Lin, C.H.; Wei, Y.T. & Chou, C.C. (2006). Enhanced antioxidative activity of soybean koji prepared with various filamentous fungi. *Food Microbiology.* Vol. 23, pp. 628-33

Liu, C.F.; Tung, Y.T.; Wu, C.L.; Lee, B.H.; Hsu, W.H. & Pan, T.M. (2011). Antihypertensive effects of *Lactobacillus*-fermented milk orally administered to spontaneously hypertensive rats. *J Agric Food Chem.* Vol. 59, No. 9, pp. 4537-43

Merenstein, D.; Murphy, M.; Fokar, A.; Hernandez, R.K.; Park, H.; Nsouli, H.; Sanders, M.E.; Davis, B.A.; Niborski, V.; Tondu, F. & Shara, NM. (2010). Use of a fermented dairy probiotic drink containing *Lactobacillus casei* (DN-114 001) to decrease the rate of illness in kids: the DRINK study. A patient-oriented, double-blind, cluster-andomized, placebo-controlled, clinical trial. *Eur J Clin Nutr.* Vol. 64, No. 7, pp. 669-77

Machida-Montani, A.; Sasazuki, S.; Inoue, M.; Natsukawa, S.; Shaura, K.; Koizumi, Y.; Kasuga, Y.; Hanaoka, T. & Tsugane, S. (2004). Association of *Helicobacter pylori* infection and environmental factors in non-cardia gastric cancer in Japan. *Gastric Cancer.* Vol. 7, No. 1, pp. 46-53.

Muir, D.; Varon, S. & Manthorpe, M. (1990). An enzyme-linked immunosorbent assay for bromodeoxyuridine incorporation using fixed microcultures. *Anal.Biochem,* Vol. 185, No. 2, pp. 377-82

Muramatsu, M.; Ohto, C.; Obata, S.; Sakuradani, E. & Shimizu, S. (2008). Various oils and detergents enhance the microbial production of farnesol and related prenyl alcohols. *J Biosci Bioeng*. Vol. 106, No. 3, pp. 263-7

Muramatsu, M.; Ohto, C.; Obata, S.; Sakuradani, E. & Shimizu, S. (2009). Alkaline pH enhances farnesol production by *Saccharomyces cerevisiae*. *J Biosci Bioeng*. Vol. 108, No. 1, pp. 52-5

Nagahara, A.; Benjamin. H.; Storkson, J.; Krewson, J.; Sheng, K.; Liu, W. & Pariza, M.W. (1992). Inhibition of benzo[a]pyrene-induced mouse forestomach neoplasia by a principal flavor component of Japanese-style fermented soy sauce. *Cancer Res*. Vol. 52,No. 7, pp. 1754-6

Nakamura Y, Yamamoto N, Sasaki K, Yamazaki S. & Takano T. (1995) Purification and characterization of angiotensin I-converting enzyme inhibitors from sour milk. *J.Dairy Sci*. 78, 777-783

Ohsawa, K.; Satsu, H.; Ohki, K.; Enjoh, M.; Takano, T. & Shimizu, M. (2008) Producibility and digestibility of antihypertensive beta-casein tripeptides, Val-Pro-Pro and Ile-Pro-Pro, in the gastrointestinal tract: analyses using an in vitro model of ammalian gastrointestinal digestion. *J Agric Food Chem*. Vol. 56, No. 3, pp. 854-8

Parentini, I.; Cavallini, G.; Donati, A.; Gori, Z. & Bergamini, E. (2005). Accumulation of dolichol in older tissues satisfies the proposed criteria to be qualified a biomarker of aging. *J Gerontol A Biol Sci Med Sci*. Vol. 60, No. 1, pp. 39-43

Pieter, V.; Jacqueline, M.D.; Jos, W.J.L.; Frans, J.K.; Evert, G.S.; Henny, A.M.B.; Ferd, S. & Rudolph, J.J.Hermus. (1989) Consumption of Fermented Milk Products and Breast Cancer. A Case-Control Study in the Netherlands. *Cancer Res*. Vol. 49, pp. 4020-4023

Pryor, M.; Slattery, M.L.; Robison, L.M. & Egger, M. (1989) Adolescent diet and breast cancer in Utah. *Cancer Res*. Vol. 49, No. 8, pp. 2161-7

Rezanka, T. & Votruba, J. (2001). Chromatography of long chain alcohols (polyprenols) from animal and plant sources. *J Chromatogr A*. Vol. 936, pp. 95-110

Ronco, A.L.; DeStefani, E. & Dattoli, R. (2002) Dairy foods and risk of breast cancer: a case-control study in Montevideo, Uruguay. Eur.J.Cancer Prev. Vol. 11, No. 5, pp. 457-63

Saito, Y.; Wanezaki, K.; Kawato, A. & Imayasu, S. (1994). Structure and activity of angiotensin I converting enzyme inhibitory peptides from sake and sake lees. *Biosci Biotechno.l Biochem*. Vol. 58, No. 10, pp. 1767-71

Sato, T.; Hoshino, H.; Tanno, M.; Nakajima, M. & Hoshino, T.(2011). Sesquarterpenes (C35 terpenes) biosynthesized via the cyclization of a linear C35 isoprenoid by a tetraprenyl-β-curcumene synthase and a tetraprenyl-β-curcumene cyclase: identification of a new terpene cyclase. *J.Am.Chem.Soc*.Vol. 133, No. 25, pp. 9734-7

Takahashi, I. & Ogura K. (1982). Prenyltransferases of *Bacillus subtilis*: undecaprenyl pyrophosphate synthetase and geranylgeranyl pyrophosphate synthetase. *J Biochem*. Vol. 92, No. 5, pp. 1527-37

Takigawa, H.; Sugiyama, M. & Shibuya, Y. (2010). C(35)-terpenes from *Bacillus subtilis* KSM 6-10. *J Nat Prod*. Vol. 73, No. 2, pp. 204-7

Takigawa, H. et al., unpublished data

Tsuchiya, H.; Sato, M. & Watanabe, I. (1999). Antiplatelet activity of soy sauce as functional seasoning. *J Agric Food Chem*. Vol. 47, No. 10, pp. 4167-74

Ueno, K.; Mizuno, S. & Yamamoto, N. (2004). Purification and characterization of an endopeptidase that has an important role in the carboxyl terminal processing of antihypertensive peptides in *Lactobacillus helveticus* CM4. *Lett Appl Microbiol*. Vol. 39, No. 4, pp. 313-8

Yuspa, S.H.; Wang, Q.; Weinberg, W.C.; Goodman, L.; Ledbetter, S.; Dooley, T. & Lichti, U. (1993). Regulation of hair follicle development: an in vitro model for hair follicle invasion of dermis and associated connective tissue remodeling. *J.Invest.Dermatol*. Vol. 101, No. 1, pp. 27S-32S

11

Induction and Activation of Plant Secondary Metabolism by External Stimuli

Fumiya Kurosaki

Laboratory of Plant Resource Sciences, Graduate School of Medicine and Pharmaceutical Sciences for Research, University of Toyama, Sugitani, Toyama
Japan

1. Introduction

It is widely recognized that plant cells are potentially rich sources of commercially important secondary metabolites. The production of secondary metabolites in plants would be mainly controlled by transcriptional activities of a series of genes which encode the specific enzymes in the biosynthetic pathway of desired products. It is likely, however, that the catalytic activities of these enzymes are sometimes repressed or maintained at very low levels, and the mechanism involved in 'switch on' of the genetic information on secondary metabolism in plants is, at present, only very poorly understood. The response of plant cells to 'elicitors' was first studied from the phytopathological point of view to elucidate the regulation mechanism of phytoalexin production. However, extensive investigations clearly indicated (Zhao et al., 2005) that the treatment of plant cells with elicitor-active substances sometimes results in a rapid accumulation of secondary products other than defense-related compounds. Recently, it has been also demonstrated (Gundlach et al., 1992) that the function of elicitors can be sometimes replaced by jasmonic acid and its methyl ester, methyl jasmonate, the plant specific messenger molecules derived from arachidonic acid. Effective application of elicitors and/or jasmonates to the production of useful metabolites in plant cells requires the elucidation of the basic biochemical mechanisms by which these external stimuli regulate the genetic information involved in the biosynthesis of the natural products. Several questions are raised against the external stimuli-induced activation of the secondary metabolites production in plants. 1) How are the external signals recognized by plant cells? 2) How are the signals transduced in the cells? 3) How do the signals alter the expression of biosynthesis-related genes? 4) How are the enzyme activities controlled to produce secondary metabolites? Effective use of elicitors and jasmonates in producing useful metabolites in plants requires the elucidation of these biochemical mechanisms by which these stimuli regulate the genetic information. To answer these questions, we first attempted to elucidate the possible participation of second messengers in the secondary metabolism activation stimulated by exogenous signals.

2. Elicitation and transmembrane signalling mechanisms of phytoalexin production

6-Methoxymellein, an antifungal isocoumarin (Fig. 1), was first isolated as the metabolite that is responsible for the bitter taste in cold-stored carrot roots. It has been shown (Condon

& Kuc, 1960) that this compound accumulates in carrot roots after inoculation with *Ceratocystis fimbriata*, which causes black rot disease in sweet potato but is not pathogenic to carrot. The resulting production of 6-methoxymellein accounted for the resistance of carrot tissue to microbial infection. This compound inhibits the growth of various fungi, yeasts and bacteria in the concentration range of 0.05 - 0.5 mM, *in vitro*, strongly suggesting that the accumulation of this compound in response to fungal invasion is one of the important induced defense mechanisms of the host plant, carrot (Kurosaki & Nishi, 1983).

2.1 Liberation of elicitors during host-pathogen interaction

Preliminary studies indicate that heat-stable and water-soluble substances which show elicitor activity are released during interaction of carrot cells and the fungus. The elicitor was found to lose its activity after digestion with pectinase or proteases, suggesting that oligogalacturonides and/or peptides are essential for the inducing activity. Also, partial hydrolysates of pectic fractions of carrot cell walls prepared with these enzymes showed strong elicitor activity. These results suggest (Kurosaki & Nishi, 1984) that extracellular hydrolases secreted from fungi, including pectinase and proteases, function to liberate oligosaccharides and peptides from carrot cell walls, and the fragments of the extracellular matrix of carrot trigger 6-methoxymellein production (Fig. 1). This was confirmed by an experiment in which filter-sterilized pectinase and trypsin were directly added to carrot cell culture. Biosynthetic activity of 6-methoxymellein was induced in the carrot cells, implying that eliciting substances are released from live carrot cells by the enzymatic action of these hydrolases.

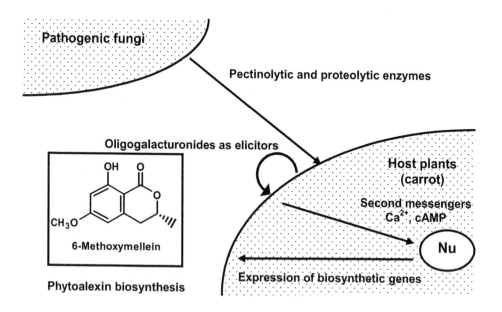

Fig. 1. Elicitation of phytoalexin production in carrot.

2.2 Participation of Ca^{2+} as a second messenger

When elicitor-active pectic fragments were analyzed by ion exchange and gel-filtration chromatography, the activity was found to be distributed in many fractions, suggesting that the elicitor consists not of a single molecule but a mixture of several active substances. This result led us to examine whether or not these elicitors share a common signalling mechanism. Ca^{2+} is an important second messenger in many physiological processes in both animal and higher plant cells, and calmodulin (CAM), a Ca^{2+}-binding protein, plays a central role in many of these systems (Marme & Dieter,1983). 6-Methoxymellein production induced by oligogalacturonides was appreciably inhibited in the presence of the Ca^{2+}-channel blocker verapamil (Kurosaki et al., 1987a). The different class of inhibitors of CAM-dependent reactions, trifluoperazine and W-7 [N-(6-aminohexyl)-5-chloro-1-naphthalenesulfonamide], also caused marked inhibition. In addition, it was found that appreciable 6-methoxymellein biosynthesis was induced in carrot by treatment with Ca^{2+}-ionophore A23187. These observations strongly suggest that the increase in cytoplasmic Ca^{2+} level is an essential early event in eliciting 6-methoxymellein production. In potato and soybean, phytoalexin production is also a Ca^{2+}-dependent process, and the elicitor-induced responses were significantly inhibited by several Ca^{2+}-inhibitors (Staeb & Ebel, 1987; Zook et al., 1987).

2.3 Activation of phosphatidylinositol cycle

Further support for the hypothesis that Ca^{2+} plays a central role in regulating phytoalexin accumulation is provided by experiments in which the turnover of phosphatidylinositol was measured in the plasma membrane of elicitor-treated carrot cells (Kurosaki et al. 1987b). The carrot cells were labelled with [^{3}H]myo-inositol and, after the addition of elicitors, acid extracts of the cells were analyzed chromatographically for the production of inositol trisphosphate (IP$_3$). In elicitor-treated cells, the release of radioactive IP$_3$ increased with time and attained a maximum at 3 - 5 min after the treatment. Phospholipase activity responsible for the degradation of phosphorylated phosphatidylinositol increased correspondingly. Several reports have shown that IP$_3$ induces rapid release of Ca^{2+} from intracellular stores in animal cells (Morgan et al., 1985). Studies on plant cells have also demonstrated that exogenous IP$_3$ releases Ca^{2+} from microsomal preparations at micromolar concentrations, although only limited information is available (Drøbak & Ferguson, 1985). Schumaker and Sze (1987) observed IP$_3$-induced release of Ca^{2+} from intact vacuoles of *Avena* seedlings. Vacuoles are the most prominent organelles in plant cells, and normally contain 0.1 to 10 µM Ca^{2+}; therefore they may serve as the Ca^{2+} store. Diacyl glycerol, another of the hydrolysates of phosphorylated phosphatidylinositol, is a known activator of protein kinase C in animal cells (Michell, 1982). The present experimental results suggest that this protein kinase also participates in the expression of phytoalexin biosynthesis in carrot cells. We found that the synthetic diacylglycerol 1-oleoyl-2-acetyl-rac-glycerol, which has been shown to be intercalated into cell membranes and to activate protein kinase C, induced 6-methoxymellein production even in the absence of elicitor. A similar result was obtained for the tumor-promoting phorbol ester, phorbol 12-myristate 13-acetate, another activator of protein kinase C (Kurosaki et al. 1987b). On the other hand the addition of H-7 [1-(5-iso-quinolinesulfonyl) -2-methyl-piperazine], a specific inhibitor for protein kinase C, resulted in suppression of phytoalexin production. These observations strongly suggest that a rapid breakdown of phosphatidylinositol in the plasma membrane of carrot cells takes place upon contact with elicitor molecules, resulting in the liberation of two types of second messengers, IP_3 and diacyl glycerol.

2.4 Role of cyclic AMP as a second messenger

In contrast to Ca^{2+}, the role of cyclic AMP (cAMP) as a second messenger in plant cells is still obscure, because there is no proof of the presence of cAMP-dependent protein kinase in plant cells. The existence of cAMP itself in plant cells has been confirmed, and, more recently, various works suggest that the cyclic nucleotide is involved in physiological events in plants (Newton & Brown, 1986). We have found (Kurosaki et al., 1987a) that the addition of dibutyryl cAMP (Bt_2cAMP) to carrot cell culture causes 6-methoxymellein production even in the absence of elicitor. Addition of several reagents which are known to change the intracellular level of cAMP, namely cholera toxin, which is an activator of adenylate cyclase, and theophylline, a phosphodiesterase (PDE) inhibitor, also led to production of 6-methoxymellein, suggesting that elevation of the cAMP concentration in carrot triggers phytoalexin production in the cells. In fact, treatment of carrot cells with oligogalacturonide elicitors led to a rapid but transient increase in the concentration of intracellular cAMP. Similar observations have been reported by Bolwell et al. (1991), who tested the effect of various modulators of signal transduction processes on the induction of phenylalanine ammonia-lyase in french bean cell cultures. They found that cholera and pertussis toxins and forskolin all stimulated synthesis of the enzyme. These reagents are known to activate adenylate cyclase, either through interaction with G-protein or directly.

We examined changes in the activity of protein phosphorylation in carrot cells following treatment with either Bt_2cAMP, forskolin or Ca^{2+}-ionophore A23187 (Kurosaki & Nishi, 1993). Addition of cAMP to cell extracts prepared from these treated cells did not cause any change in phosphorylation activity, indicating that cAMP-dependent kinase activity is absent or very low in carrot cells, as well as in most of the other plants. By contrast, the activities of Ca^{2+}- and Ca^{2+}/CAM-dependent protein kinases increased markedly in both cytosolic and microsomal fractions after the treatment. Phosphorylation activity was stimulated not only by Ca^{2+}-ionophore but also by Bt_2cAMP and forskolin. Furthermore, although Bt_2cAMP and forskolin can stimulate phytoalexin production in carrot cells, the effect was severely suppressed by several Ca^{2+} channel blockers and CAM antagonists. These observations suggest that cAMP acts as second messenger by stimulation of the Ca^{2+}-cascade, rather than by activating cAMP-dependent protein kinases. This view is further supported by experimental results in which changes in the concentration of cytosolic Ca^{2+} in carrot cells were measured by a fluorescent Ca^{2+}-indicator (fluo-3) after treatment with the reagents. The Ca^{2+} level in the cytoplasm of untreated carrot cells was found to be about 0.1 μM. A marked increase in the intracellular concentration of Ca^{2+} to 0.6 - 0.8 μM was observed 3 - 6 min after the addition of Bt_2cAMP or forskolin. These results suggest that the increase in cytoplasmic cAMP level leads to the Ca^{2+}-influx into carrot cells. This conclusion was also drawn from an experiment in which the effect of cAMP on the Ca^{2+}-flux was examined using $^{45}Ca^{2+}$-loaded vesicles of plasma membrane (Kurosaki & Nishi, 1993). Plasma membranes prepared by the two-phase partitioning method are generally composed of differently oriented sealed vesicles, rightside-out and inside-out (Graef & Weiler, 1989).

Incubation of these vesicles with $^{45}Ca^{2+}$ in the presence of ATP results in selective incorporation of the radiolabeled ions into the inside-out vesicles by the plasma membrane-located Ca^{2+}-ATPase. When the $^{45}Ca^{2+}$-loaded vesicles were incubated with cAMP, a rapid release of $^{45}Ca^{2+}$ from the vesicles was observed. This discharge was specifically observed with cAMP among the nucleotides tested. These observations are consistent with the hypothesis that the cytoplasmic level of cAMP is raised by an appropriate stimulus, and the nucleotide triggers Ca^{2+}-influx without accompanying cAMP-dependent protein phosphorylation, probably through cAMP-sensitive ion channels.

2.5 Synthesis and degradation of cyclic AMP

Addition of forskolin to carrot cell culture caused an appreciable increase in adenylate cyclase activity. However, the increase was transient although the activator was present throughout the experiment (Kurosaki et al., 1993). The forskolin-stimulated activity of the enzyme in carrot cell extracts was detected only when EGTA was included in the assay mixture, and the addition of exogenous Ca^{2+} strongly inhibited the enzyme activity. The effect of various concentrations of Ca^{2+} on adenylate cyclase activity was therefore studied using buffers with the concentration of free Ca^{2+} adjusted by the EGTA-Ca^{2+} buffer system (Kurosaki et al., 1993). The activity of the cyclase was markedly affected by the free Ca^{2+} concentration, and was maintained at a high level only when the Ca^{2+} concentration was below 0.1 µM. This figure is close to the Ca^{2+} concentration in cytoplasm in the resting state of various plant species.

Constitutive activity of PDE was found in cultured carrot cells, and this activity did not depend on either Ca^{2+} or CAM. In contrast, a CAM-dependent isoform of PDE (CAM-PDE) was induced in the cells by adding forskolin or Bt$_2$cAMP to the culture (Kurosaki & Kaburaki, 1995). Induction of CAM-PDE activity in Bt$_2$cAMP-treated carrot cells was markedly inhibited in the presence of verapamil, while addition of Ca^{2+}-ionophore A23187 induced CAM-PDE. These results suggest that increased Ca^{2+}, but not cAMP, in the stimulated carrot cells triggers induction of the PDE isoenzyme. Affinity of CAM-PDE to the substrate was low compared to constitutive PDE (Km values, 0.14 and 0.07 µM, respectively); however, V for the induced PDE was approximately 2.7 times higher than for the constitutive isoenzyme.

These results suggest that synthesis and degradation of cAMP in cultured carrot cells are both controlled and switched on/off according to the concentration of Ca^{2+} in carrot cytoplasm. Adenylate cyclase activity is induced in the cells only in the resting state, and the enzyme activity is automatically inhibited when the concentration of cytoplasmic Ca^{2+} increases and reaches the level of the excitatory state. The constitutive PDE, which is insensitive to the cytoplasmic Ca^{2+} level, is important in maintenance of the resting state of carrot cells, by keeping cellular cAMP and Ca^{2+} levels very low, while CAM-PDE induced in excited cells hydrolyzes the messenger nucleotide rapidly under conditions of high cAMP and Ca^{2+}, *in vivo*, as a response-decay mechanism.

In animal cells, the cAMP-induced Ca^{2+}-influx through the nucleotide-sensitive channels is terminated by the hydrolysis of cAMP, the ligand of the channels (Ranganathan, 1994). However, in cultured carrot cells, the cytoplasmic Ca^{2+} concentration elevated by the stimulation of cAMP began decreasing even though the level of intracellular cAMP was high (Kurosaki et al., 1993). Furthermore, when a Ca^{2+}-influx was triggered by treating the cells with Bt_2cAMP, the cytoplasmic concentration of Ca^{2+} returned to its base level after a few minutes, by which time the cAMP analogue was still present at a high concentration. These results clearly indicate that, in contrast to animal cells, degradation of cAMP is not the immediate reason for the response decay of the cAMP-gated cation channel in carrot cells. We found that the discharge of Ca^{2+} from inside-out sealed vesicles of carrot plasma membrane was strongly inhibited when the suspension of the vesicles was supplemented with 1 µM free Ca^{2+}, while Ca^{2+} concentrations lower than 0.1 µM did not affect Ca^{2+}-release. In addition, the inhibited Ca^{2+}-flux across the plasma membrane was restored by the addition of CAM inhibitors and anti-CAM IgG (Kurosaki et al., 1994). These results suggest that the Ca^{2+}-influx initiated by increases in intracellular cAMP in cultured carrot cells is terminated when the cytosolic Ca^{2+} concentration reaches the threshold excitatory level in the cells. It is probable that CAM located in the plasma membrane plays an important role in the decay response of the cyclic nucleotide-gated cation channels. CAM involved in this transmembrane signaling process might be partially embedded in the lipid bilayer as reported in the pea (Collinge & Trewavas, 1989).

2.6 Regulation of Ca^{2+}-ATPase activity

As with other eukaryotic cells, maintenance of low Ca^{2+} concentration in the cytoplasm of non-stimulated higher plant cells is essential. The cytoplasmic Ca^{2+} concentration of plant cells in the resting state, as described above, is generally maintained at approximately 0.1 µM by the action of Ca^{2+}-transporting systems (Poovaiah & Reddy, 1987; Rasi-Caldogno et al., 1989) which sequester the ion into internal organelles, including endoplasmic reticulum, mitochondria, and vacuoles, or mediate its efflux to the cell exterior. It is known that Ca^{2+}-pumping ATPase at the plasma membrane plays a key role in transporting Ca^{2+} to apoplastic spaces. Characteristics of Ca^{2+}-translocating ATPase have been reported from a wide range of plants (Briskin, 1990), although some are highly variable depending on the plant species. One of the most serious controversies over properties of ATPase is the role of CAM in regulation of the enzyme; inconsistent observations on the CAM-dependence of enzyme activity have been reported from several plants (Askerlund & Evans, 1992). It is not yet clear whether this discrepancy represents genuine variation across species or is an experimental artifact. However, it seems that results depend partly on the fact that plasma membrane preparations obtained from higher plant cells sometimes contain the membranes of other organelles. A highly purified plasma membrane fraction from cultured carrot cells was prepared by the aqueous two phase-partition method (Graef & Weiler, 1989), in order to re-evaluate the role of CAM in regulating Ca^{2+}-ATPase at the plasma membrane of the cells. The Ca^{2+}-translocating activity of ATPase was considerably inhibited in the presence of different classes of CAM antagonists or anti-CAM IgG (Kurosaki & Kaburaki, 1994). This Ca^{2+}-pumping activity decreased significantly when the plasma membrane preparation was washed with EGTA-containing buffer; however, it was restored to almost the control level upon adding exogenous CAM. These results suggest that Ca^{2+}-ATPase at the plasma membrane of carrot cells is regulated by CAM, and the modulator protein associates with the enzyme in a manner dependent on the Ca^{2+} concentration. The biochemical basis of CAM-induced stimulation of Ca^{2+}-ATPase activity in carrot cells was studied further by determining the parameters of the Ca^{2+}-translocating reaction of the enzyme in the presence and absence of exogenous CAM, using EGTA-treated plasma membrane (Kurosaki & Kaburaki, 1994). The affinity of Ca^{2+}-ATPase for Ca^{2+} was considerably increased by association with CAM, and Km values decreased from 11.4 μM to 0.7 μM. These figures are close to those of CAM-dependent Ca^{2+}-ATPase at the plasma membrane in animal cells. Affinity of the enzyme for ATP was also increased in the presence of CAM, although the increase was low compared to that for Ca^{2+} (Km values of 914 and 670 μM in the absence and presence of CAM). In contrast to the affinities for the substrates, the relative V values of the ATPase were similar or slightly decreased by the addition of CAM.

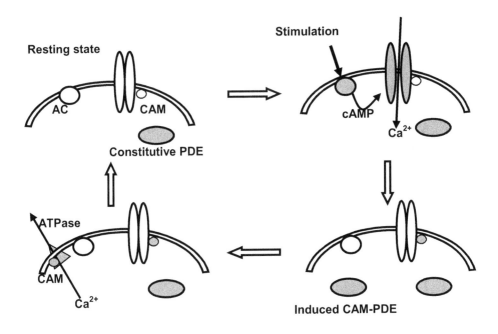

Fig. 2. Signal cross-talking between cAMP and Ca^{2+}.

It is well known that, in the excited plant cells having high Ca^{2+} concentration, CAM is activated by binding to the ion, and is able to associate with various CAM-dependent proteins. The Ca^{2+} concentration in resting plant cells, by contrast, is too low to activate CAM, resulting in the dissociation of the modulator from its target proteins, including Ca^{2+}-ATPase (Malatialy et al., 1988). The Kca of the ATPase associated with CAM is similar to that of the cytoplasmic Ca^{2+} level of excited plant cells (0.7 μM), while the Kca of the ATPase without CAM increased markedly (11.4 μM) though the cytoplasmic Ca^{2+} concentration in the resting cells is quite low. These observations suggest that Ca^{2+}-ATPase at the carrot plasma membrane plays an important role in the excited cells only as an 'acute' enzyme. However, Rasi-Caldogno et al. (1989) pointed out that Kca decreased from about 10 μM to about 0.1 μM if the level of free Ca^{2+} alone is considered. This low Km value of CAM-depleted Ca^{2+}-ATPase for Ca^{2+} is consistent with the transport protein involved in maintaining Ca^{2+} concentration at the submicromolar range as a 'house keeping' enzyme in resting cells. These results strongly suggest that, on binding of CAM, the affinity of the carrot Ca^{2+}-ATPase for Ca^{2+} is markedly increased, and this is the most important biochemical change behind the CAM-induced pumping activity of the enzyme.

The characterization of the functional proteins involved in cAMP-induced cellular events suggests that most components of these signal transduction processes are correlated, and regulate each other. A plausible scheme for signal cross-talking of the messenger nucleotide with the Ca^{2+}-cascade in the early stages of transmembrane signaling processes is as follows (Fig. 2). 1) In the resting state only constitutive PDE is active, and both adenylate cyclase and cAMP-sensitive channels are inactive; therefore cAMP and Ca^{2+} are both maintained at low levels. 2) Upon the arrival of elicitor signals on the receptor protein located at the plasma membrane, adenylate cyclase is activated, and the increased level of cAMP associates with cAMP-sensitive channels as the ligand to open the ion gates. 3) Influx of Ca^{2+} activates the Ca^{2+}-cascade leading to the expression of genes encoding the biosynthetic enzymes of the phytoalexin. In parallel, activity of adenylate cyclase is inhibited by Ca^{2+}, and the ion activates the membrane-embedded CAM to close the cAMP-dependent channels. In addition, CAM-PDE is induced to hydrolyze the messenger molecules rapidly. 4) Finally, Ca^{2+} activates the cytoplasmic CAM to enhance the activity of Ca^{2+}-translocating ATPase, causing the cells to return to the resting state.

2.7 Possible scheme for signal transduction mechanisms of elicitors

These studies all support the hypothesis that external stimuli as elicitors cause an increase in the cytoplasmic Ca^{2+} level via the phosphatidylinositol cycle and/or the adenylate cyclase system. Although an authoritative picture of this process cannot yet be given, possible signal transduction mechanisms are summarized in Fig. 3.

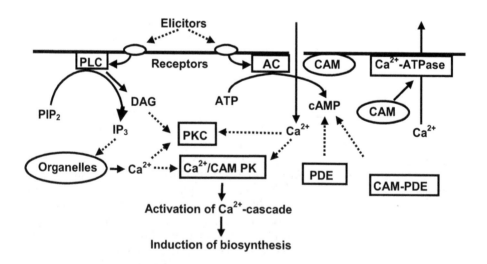

Fig. 3. Schematic presentation of signal transduction mechanisms of elicitors.

At present the data are still fragmentary, so that it is important to learn more about the biochemical nature and function of the components involved in signal transduction process in plants. Evidence has been accumulated suggesting that plant cells contain the major components of the phosphatidylinositol cycle, while the function of cAMP described here is unique. This class of signal transducing mechanism is rare (Kaplan et al., 2007), and is seldom seen in animal and microbial cells. However, a similar gating action of cAMP has been reported in olfactory transduction in animal sensory cells (Nakamura & Gold, 1987). In these cells the cAMP content increases in response to odoriferous substances, and this change induces an influx of Ca^{2+} into the cells without cAMP-dependent protein phosphorylation. Krupinski et al. (1989) have suggested that the amino acid sequence of an adenylate cyclase from the bovine brain is topographically similar to ion channels such as Ca^{2+} and K^+. Based on this assumption, Schultz et al. (1992) tested the pore-forming ability of adenylate cyclase from *Paramecium* in an artificial lipid layer, and suggested that the enzyme has a secondary function as a carrier of ions.

3. Jasmonates and plant secondary metabolism

Jasmonates, jasmonic acid and methyl jasmonate (MJ), are essential plant hormones that regulate defense responses against environmental stressors, such as drought, wounding, and microbial infection. It has been also shown (Gundlach et al., 1992; Creelman & Mullet, 1997) that the several cell physiological activities of elicitors can be sometimes replaced by jasmonic acid and MJ, and exogenous application of jasmonates to plant cells enhances accumulation of a variety of secondary metabolites.

Recent studies on the signal transduction mechanisms of jasmonates have demonstrated (Turner et al., 2002) that the active form of jasmonates is an amino acid-conjugate, jasmonoyl-isoleucine, and this adducts would associate with a protein complex that functions as the receptor of this plant hormone. It has been also shown that jasmonates-signalling cascade further links to ubiquitin-proteasome-mediated protein degradation processes, however, only very limited information is available on the detail mechanism by which jasmonates induce the biosynthesis of various secondary metabolites in plant cells.

3.1 Role of Ca^{2+} and CAM in jasmonates signaling

We have recently reported (Kasidimoko et al., 2005) that biosynthesis of a tetracyclic diterpenoid of *Scoparia dulcis*, such as scopadulcic acid A, scopadulciol and scopadulin, is stimulated by the treatment of the plant with MJ, and that this process is triggered by Ca^{2+}-influx into the cytoplasmic space of the plant cells. We also demonstrated that activation of Ca^{2+}-cascade in the signal transduction pathway is an essential requirement for MJ-induced diterpene production in *S. dulcis* (Fig. 4). As is in phytoalexin production in carrot described above, we have demonstrated that CAM plays an important role in the MJ-induced enhancement of the biosynthetic activity. The transcriptional level of the gene(s) encoding CAM had been assumed to be maintained at almost constant level. However, recent studies clearly showed that plant CAMs are composed of several isoforms, and the expression of specific CAM gene(s) is sometimes markedly induced upon the contact with appropriate stimuli or under stress conditions. For example, carrot CAM genes consist of more than fifteen isoforms, and activation of several specific genes was observed by the treatment with various elicitor-active substances (Ishigaki et al., 2004, 2005). At least eight genes encoding CAM are contained in potato, and these genes were differently expressed during the development of the plant (Takezawa et al., 1995). In tobacco cells, it was demonstrated (Yamakawa et al., 2001) that specific CAM genes are transcriptionally activated against microbial infection.

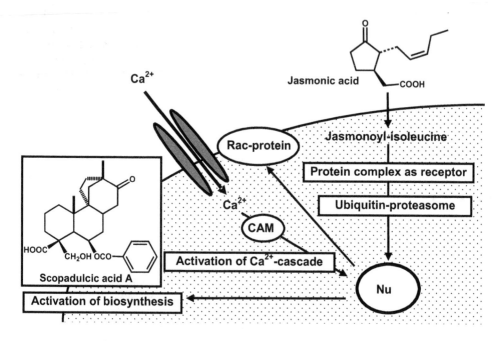

Fig. 4. Schematic presentation of signal transduction mechanisms of jasmonates.

In order to understand MJ-induced activation of diterpene biosynthesis in *S. dulcis* on the molecular basis, we attempted to isolate CAM gene homologues of the plant and examined the possible change in their expression activities (Saitoh et al., 2007). Based on the reported nucleotide sequences of CAM proteins, we isolated and selected sixteen cDNA clones encoding CAM from *S. dulcis* by means of rapid amplification of cDNA end (RACE) method. It was found that the coding regions (149 amino acids) of all of these isolated clones were completely identical, and the deduced amino acid sequence showed very high homology to those of CAMs from various biological sources. In addition, the nucleotide sequences of the 3′-untranslatable regions (UTRs) of these DNA fragments were also identical though a few gaps in the sequences were found in two of these samples. However, even in the cases, the other parts of the nucleotide sequences of either coding regions or UTRs were completely identical. These cDNA fragments were then subjected to 5′RACE, and eight clones were selected. As was in 3′RACE, the nucleotide sequences of these clones were completely identical both in coding regions and in 5′-UTRs. In genomic Southern blot hybridization analyses, only one hybridized band was observed in the DNA fragments digested by either *Eco*RV, *Hind*III or *Xho*I. It is well known that the nucleotide sequences of

CAM genes of higher plant cells showed very high identity (for example, 97-87% in *Arabidopsis thaliana* (Ling et al., 1991) and 98-86% in *Daucus carota* (Ishigaki et al., 2004, 2005). Thus, the appropriate probes are capable of hybridizing with the several restriction fragments of plant genomic DNA containing CAM genes, and usually complex patterns with multiple signals were observed. Therefore, the very simple results obtained for CAM gene(s) of *S. dulcis* should be a quite unusual case. For further characterization of CAM gene(s) in *S. dulcis*, genomic DNA of the plant was digested with *Hinf*I which is expected to hydrolyze the CAM gene at the middle point of its coding region (at 241 position of 447 nucleotides). After probing, two hybridized signals with similar intensity were visualized. These results strongly suggest that, unlike many of higher plants, CAM gene of *S. dulcis* occurs as the sole gene that encodes CAM protein in the genome of the plant.

Possible changes in the expression of CAM gene in leaf organ cultures of *S. dulcis* challenged by Ca^{2+}-ionphore A23187 or MJ were examined. The transcription of the CAM gene was transiently activated by the treatment with A23187, and a marked increase in the intensity of the band of the amplified DNA was observed after 3 h of the addition of the ionophore into the culture. After that, the expression of the gene decreased gradually and then returned to the initial level. Addition of MJ showed almost the same results, and the expression level of the CAM gene appreciably elevated after 3 to 6 h of the treatment, and it decreased thereafter. In contrast, the intensity of the band of the DNA fragments appeared to be maintained at the constant level in controls which received ethanol instead of the reagents. These results suggest that the elevation of transcriptional activity of CAM gene of *S. dulcis* is one of the early events of MJ-induced activation of Ca^{2+}-cascade in the cells, which leads to the enhancement of the biosynthetic activity of the tetracyclic diterpene compounds.

As described above, occurrence of several isoforms of CAM and multiple genes encoding the protein has been reported from various plant sources. It has been also demonstrated that a certain specific CAM gene(s) is sometimes expressed under stress conditions or by the stimulation to respond to various environmental change (Takezawa et al., 1995; Yamakawa et al., 2001). In sharp contrast to these reports, it has been shown that *S. dulcis* is a unique plant and only one gene encoding CAM protein should occur in the cells. How does the plant respond to the numerous external stimuli with only one CAM gene? We have shown that regulation of CAM activity by controlling the transcriptional level is, at least, one of the physiological mechanisms of the cells. It might be also possible that intracellular translocation of CAM to the appropriate structures or the spaces in the cells would be another mechanism in the regulation of the activity of the modulator protein (Collinge & Trewavas, 1989).

3.2 Participation of Rac/Rop GTPases in jasmonates signaling

For further elucidation of signal transduction mechanisms of MJ-enhanced diterpene biosynthesis in *S. dulcis*, we examined the possible participation of monomeric GTP-binding proteins in these processes. Monomeric GTPase proteins are involved in regulating the essential functions of eukaryotic cells, such as cell differentiation, intracellular vesicle transport, and cytoskeleton organization (Valster et al., 2000). These small GTPases are classified into several subfamilies, and, among them, Rac/Rop proteins have been shown to regulate auxin-signalling and defense responses in higher plants (Yang, 2002; Gu et al., 2004). Rac/Rop GTPase genes are usually organized as multigene family in plant cells, and it has been assumed that each member of the subfamily is functionally distinct and plays specific roles, respectively. It has been also shown that these proteins are usually activated by prenylation, and the modification with the hydrophobic groups evokes the translocation of the proteins to plasma membranes to allow the association with the target molecules called effectors. We have isolated two Rac/Rop GTPase genes, Sdrac-1 (965 bp encoding 196 amino acid residues) and Sdrac-2 (969 bp encoding 197 amino acid residues), from S. dulcis, and found that the transcriptional activities of these genes appreciably increased by the stimulation with MJ, however, in contrast, they did not respond to the treatment with Ca^{2+}-ionophore A23187 (Mitamura et al., 2009; Shite et al., 2009). These observations led us to assume that Sdrac-1 and Sdrac-2 might play roles in a certain cellular event in MJ-signalling processes which occurs between reception of the external signal and Ca^{2+}-influx across plasma membranes.

Translocation of small GTPases to membranes is usually initiated by the binding of hydrophobic groups to these proteins (Yang, 2002; Gu et al., 2004). Therefore, we tested the possibility that Rac/Rop proteins of S. dulcis are targeted to membrane structures by the stimulation with MJ. We constructed the expression vector harbouring Sdrac-1 or Sdrac-2 tagged with glutathione-S-transferase (GST), and young seedlings of Atropa belladonna germinated under sterilized conditions were transformed with Agrobacterium-mediated methods. The intracellular translocation of Sdrac-1 and Sdrac-2 proteins to cellular membranes was examined by measuring the change in GST activities in microsomal fractions prepared from the transformed belladonna. GST activity in the microsomes of the transformants was maintained at low levels even after being incubated with MJ, and was almost comparable with that of the untreated control. In contrast, enzyme activity in the membrane fraction, which was prepared from belladonna tissues transformed with GST-Sdrac-1, was considerably elevated by incubation with MJ for 5 min, and it gradually increased for at least 30 min. However, GST showed low and almost constant activities in the untreated control. A similar set of results was also obtained for belladonna tissues transformed with GST-Sdrac-2, and a marked increase in GST activity in the microsomal fraction was specifically observed in MJ-treated cells. These results strongly suggest that both Sdrac-1 and Sdrac-2, Rac/Rop GTPase proteins of S. dulcis, rapidly translocate to microsomal fractions in response to MJ stimulation.

We also attempted to elucidate the possible post-translational modifications of these monomeric GTPases with hydrophobic groups which evoke the targeting of the proteins to plant plasma membrane (Mitamura et al., 2011). In vitro modifications of Sdrac-1 and Sdrac-2 were studied using the His-tagged recombinant proteins, and the purified Sdrac proteins were incubated with [^{14}C]-isopentenyl diphosphate, geranyl diphosphate and recombinant farnesyl diphosphate synthase protein, the [^{14}C]-farnesyl diphosphate-generating system, in the presence or absence of MJ-treated cell extracts of S. dulcis. The radiolabeled prenyl chain appeared to bind to Sdrac-2 protein when the assay mixture was incubated in the presence of MJ-treated cell extracts. In contrast, it was likely that Sdrac-2 did not accept the prenyl group without the cell extracts. Addition of the heat denatured cell extracts also showed no apparent effect on the binding of isoprene units to the protein. These results strongly suggested that Sdrac-2 would bind to prenyl chain, very likely C15 chain, in the presence of prenylation enzyme(s) probably occurring in MJ-treated cell extracts of S. dulcis.

In sharp contrast, however, conjugate of Sdrac-1 and the prenyl group was not formed either in the presence or absence of the cell extracts of *S. dulcis*. It was demonstrated (Lavy et al., 2002) that, among the translate products of Rac/Rop GTPase gene homologues of *A. thaliana*, targeting of AtRAC8 to the plasma membrane is initiated by palmitoylation of this protein. Therefore, we examined the possibility whether the palmitoyl group is capable of binding to Sdrac-1 protein in response to MJ stimulation. Considerable radioactivity was exhibited by purified His-tagged Sdrac-1 when it was incubated with [^{14}C]-palmitoyl-CoA in the presence of MJ-treated cell extracts of *S. dulcis*, while much lesser amounts of the radioactivities were found to associate with recombinant Sdrac-1 in the absence of the cell extracts or in the presence of the heat denatured extracts. From these results, we concluded that Sdrac-1 cannot be prenylated, however, it was acylated in response to MJ stimulation.

This set of the experiments strongly suggests that although Sdrac-1 and Sdrac-2 are similarly translocated to the membrane fraction by binding with hydrophobic groups in response to MJ stimulation, translocation of these GTPases is initiated by distinct modification mechanisms, i.e., palmitoylation for Sdrac-1 and prenylation for Sdrac-2. A well known consensus post-translational modification site for prenylation, CXXL, occurs near the C terminal of Sdrac-2. In addition, heterogeneous prenylation sites of Rac/Rop proteins as well as the putative motif CAA in maize (Ivanchenko et al., 2000) and CTAA in *Arabidopsis* (Li et al., 2001) have been recently demonstrated. In contrast, the structural prerequisites for palmitoylation of these GTPases remain obscure. The C-terminal amino acid sequence of palmitoylated *Arabidopsis* AtRAC8 is CGKN (Lavy et al., 2002), while Sdrac-1 with the C terminal of CAIF is also acylated. Therefore, at present, it should be quite difficult to predict the mode of post-translational modification of Rac/Rop GTPase proteins, prenylation or acylation, on the bases of the amino acids sequences near C-terminal.

4. Activation of secondary metabolism by modification of signal transduction processes of plant cells

In this manuscript, we have demonstrated that the increase in cytoplasmic Ca^{2+} level and activation of Ca^{2+}-cascade in higher plant cells would be essential events in the enhancement of plant secondary metabolisms triggered by the treatment with external stimuli such as elicitors and jasmonates. We have also shown that CAM is a key modulator protein to evoke natural products biosynthesis in elicitors- or jasmonates-stimulated plant cells. As mentioned above, a series of recent studies clearly demonstrated (Takezawa et al., 1995; Yamakawa et al., 2001) that, unlike in animal cells, plant CAM proteins are encoded by several homologous genes and the specific gene(s) is sometimes expressed by various physiological stresses. We isolated fifteen clones of CAM genes from carrot, and found that, among them, the transcription level of *cam-4* was markedly increased by the treatment of the cells with oligouronide elicitor (Ishigaki et al., 2004).

We assumed that the introduction and over-expression of appropriate gene(s) encoding key protein in secondary metabolism-related signal transduction mechanism, such as CAM, would activate Ca^{2+}-cascade and maintain the cells in the excitatory state. It might be also possible that the biosynthetic activities of several defensive compounds are significantly activated in these transformed plant cells. At present, only very limited information is available about the biochemical changes in the plant cells transformed with CAM gene, however, it has been reported (Harding et al., 1997; Cho et al., 1998) that over-expression of the gene in tobacco cells results in the unusual activation of CAM-dependent functional proteins followed by the generation of active oxygen species and NO. In animal cells it was shown (Broillet, 2000) that the elevation of NO concentration appreciably enhances the synthesis of cyclic nucleotides. As described above, we showed that the increase in cytoplasmic level of cyclic nucleotides stimulates Ca^{2+}-cascade in cultured carrot cells by activating the nucleotide-sensitive cation channels. Therefore, we attempted to produce the transgenic plants in which carrot *cam-4* gene was introduced and over-expressed by the infection of transformed *Agrobacterium tumefaciens*. In the preliminary experiments, sesame *(Sesamum schinzianum* Asch.) showed the highest transformation and re-differentiation efficiencies among several plants tested, therefore, we focused on this plant as the target of the transformation.

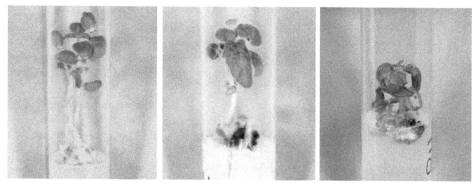

Fig. 5. Control and transformed sesame plants. Wild type (left), transformed with the empty expression vector (middle), and transformed with the vector harbouring *cam-4* gene (right).

Sesame seedlings were infected by *A. tumefaciens* transformed with pMAT vector harbouring cauliflower mosaic virus 35S promoter-*cam-4*, and the formation of crown galls was observed at the cut surfaces of the stems following incubation for 2-3 weeks. The gall tissues were harvested and then transferred onto agar medium containing an antibiotic and cytokinin for the sterilization and the formation of multiple shoots. The re-differentiated sesame plants, transformed with *cam-4* and the control for *Agrobacterium*-infection, were used for further analyses together with the wild sesame seedlings germinated under the sterilized condition (Fig. 5). The appearance of the infection-control of sesame was somewhat different from that of the wild plantlets directly germinated from seeds. However, the shape of the transformed and re-differentiated sesame was quite abnormal as compared with those of the wild and the control plants (Fig. 5). It was also confirmed that the concentration of CAM protein in the transgenic sesame was appreciably higher than those in the wild and the control plants (relative ratio was estimated to be 1: 1.1 : 2.6 as analyzed by immuno-blotting followed by densitometric scan).

In the next experiments, possible changes in the enzyme activities of defense-related secondary metabolisms and the contents of phenolic compounds in the transformed plants were examined. As the key enzymes of defense reactions, we focused on phenylalanine ammonia-lyase (PAL) and caffeic acid O-methyltransferase (COMT), the most important enzymes involved in the biosynthesis of lignin and the related compounds. PAL activity in the transgenic sesame was appreciably higher than those of the wild and the infection-control (1.9- and 2.4-fold higher levels, respectively). This marked stimulation of the catalytic activity in the transformed plant was also found in COMT, and 2.3- and 1.9-fold increases in the activities were observed. The increased ratio of these two enzyme activities in the transgenic sesame were almost comparable to the elevated ratio of the 'bulk' expression levels of CAM genes described above. It was also shown that the contents of phenolic compounds, caffeic acid and ferulic acid, in the *cam-4*-transformed sesame markedly increased (3.0– to 5.8-fold higher levels).

It was demonstrated, therefore, that the CAM gene specifically expressed for the biosynthesis of 6-methoxymellein in carrot, a polyketide compound, is capable of enhancing the production of phenylpropane derivatives in sesame. Is there any specificity in the enhancement of secondary metabolism in higher plants in which CAM gene is over-expressed? Although CAM plays roles in numerous cellular events, the structure of the protein is known to be highly conservative. Therefore, the specificity of the final cellular responses mediated by CAM is considered to be regulated by certain processes in the downstream of the signal transduction cascade. From these facts, we assume that the pathway(s) of secondary metabolism in higher plants which would be activated by the transformation with CAM genes might depend on the inherent natures of the individual plant species, such as the networks of the signalling cascade, the properties of the functional proteins mediating these processes, and the levels and/or timings of the expression of the genes participating in these cellular events.

5. Conclusion

Secondary metabolism of higher plants is appreciably activated by the treatment of the cells with appropriate external stimuli, such as elicitor-active compounds and jasmonates. It is very likely that the increase in cytoplasmic Ca^{2+} concentration followed by the activation of Ca^{2+}-cascade is an essential cellular event for the enhancement of the biosynthesis of natural products in plant cells, and CAM protein appears to play the important cell physiological roles in these processes. Series of the experiments presented in this manuscript suggest the possibility that the elucidation and engineering of signal transduction processes to maintain the plant cells at the excitatory states would be a novel method for molecular breeding of useful medicinal plants.

6. Acknowledgments

This work was supported, in part, by Grants-in-Aid from the Ministry of Education, Culture, Sports, Science and Technology of Japan, and by a Research Grant from Yamazaki Spice Promotion Foundation..

7. References

Askerlund, P. & Evans, D. E. (1992). Reconstitution and characterization of a calmodulin-stimulated Ca^{2+}-pumping ATPase purified from *Brassica oleracea* L. *Plant Physiol.*, Vol. 100, pp. 1670-1681

Bolwell, G. P., Coulson, V., Rodgers, M. W., Murphy, D. L. & Jones, D. (1991). Modulation of the elicitation response in cultured french bean cells and its implication for the mechanism of signal transduction. *Phytochemistry*, Vol. 30, pp. 397-405

Briskin, D. P. (1990). Ca-translocating ATPase of the plant plasma membrane. *Plant Physiol.*, Vol. 94, pp. 397-400

Broillet, M. C. (2000). A single intracellular cysteine residue is responsible for the activation of the olfactory cyclic nucleotide-gated channel by NO. *J. Biol. Chem.*, Vol. 275, pp. 15135-15141

Cho, M. J., Vaghy, P. L., Kondo, R., Lee, S. H., Davis, J. P., Rehl, R., Heo, W. D. & Johnson, J. D. (1998). Reciprocal regulation of mammalian nitric oxide synthase and calcineurin by plant calmodulin isoforms. *Biochemistry*, Vol. 37, pp. 15593-15597

Collinge, M. & Trewavas, A. (1989). The location of calmodulin in the pea plasma membrane. *J. Biol. Chem.*, Vol. 264, pp. 8865-8872

Condon, P. & Kuc, J. (1960). Isolation of a fungitoxic compound from carrot root tissue inocuated with *Ceratocystis fimbrata*. *J. Phytopathol.*, Vol. 50, pp. 267-270

Creelman, R. A. & Mullet, M. E. (1997). Biosynthesis and action of jasmonates in plants. *Ann. Rev. Plant Physiol. Plant Mol. Biol.*, Vol. 48, pp. 355-381

Drøbak, B. K. & Ferguson, I. B. (1985). Release of Ca^{2+} from plant hypocotyl microsomes by inositol-1,4,5-trisphosphate. *Biochem. Biophys. Res. Commun.*, Vol. 130, pp. 1241-1246

Graef, P. & Weiler, E. W. (1989). ATP-driven Ca^{2+}-transport in sealed plasma membrane vesicles prepared by aqueous two-phase partitioning from leaves of *Commelia communis*. *Physiol. Plant.*, Vol. 75, pp. 469-478

Gu, Y., Wang, Z. & Yang, Z. (2004). ROP/RAC GTPase: an old new master regulator for plant signaling. *Curr. Opin. Plant Biol.*, Vol. 7, 527-536

Gundlach, H., Muller, M. J., Kutchan, T. M. & Zenk, M. H. (1992). Jasmonic acid is a signal transducer in elicitor-induced plant cell cultures. *Proc. Nat. Acad. Sci. U.S.A.*, Vol. 89, pp. 2389–2393

Harding, S. A., Oh, S.-H. & Roberts, D. M. (1997). Transgenic tobacco expressing foreign calmodulin genes show an enhanced production of active oxygen species. *EMBO J.*, Vol. 16, pp. 1137-1144

Kaplan, B., Sherman, T. & Fromm, H. (2007). Cyclic nucleotide-gated channels in plants. *FEBS Lett.*, Vol. 581, pp. 2237-2246

Kasidimoko, N. M., Kurosaki, F., Lee, J. B. & Hayashi, T, (2005). Stimulation of calcium signal transduction involves in enhancement of production of scopadulcic acid B by methyl jasmonate in the cultured tissues of *Scoparia dulcis*. *Plant Biotechnol.*, Vol. 22, pp. 333-337

Kurosaki, F. & Kaburaki, H. (1994). Calmodulin-dependency of a Ca-pump at the plasma membrane of cultured carrot cells. *Plant Science*, Vol. 104, pp. 23-30

Kurosaki, F. & Kaburaki, H. (1995). Phosphodiesterase isoenzymes in cell extracts of cultured carrot. *Phytochemistry*, Vol. 40, pp. 685-689

Kurosaki, F., Kaburaki, H. & Nishi, A. (1993). Synthesis and degradation of cyclic AMP in cultured carrot cells treated with forskolin. *Arch. Biochem. Biophys.*, Vol. 303, pp. 177-179

Kurosaki, F., Kaburaki, H. & Nishi, A. (1994). Involvement of plasma membrane-located calmodulin in the response decay of cyclic nucleotide-gated cation channel of cultured carrot cells. *FEBS Lett.*, Vol. 340, pp. 193-196

Kurosaki, F. & Nishi, A. (1983). Isolation and antimicrobial activity of the phytoalexin 6-methoxymellein from cultured carrot cells. *Phytochemistry*, Vol. 22, pp. 669-672

Kurosaki, F. & Nishi, A. (1984). Elicitation of phytoalexin production in cultured carrot cells. *Physiol. Plant Pathol.*, Vol. 24, pp. 169-176

Kurosaki, F. & Nishi, A. (1993). Stimulation of calcium influx and calcium cascade by cyclic AMP in cultured carrot cells. *Arch. Biochem. Biophys.*,Vol. 302, pp. 144-151

Kurosaki, F., Tsurusawa, Y. & Nishi, A. (1987a). The elicitation of phytoalexins by Ca^{2+} and cyclic AMP in carrot cells. *Phytochemistry*, Vol. 26, pp. 1919-1923

Kurosaki, F., Tsurusawa, Y. & Nishi, A. (1987b). Breakdown of phosphatidylinositol during the elicitation of phytoalexin production in cultured carrot cells. *Plant Physiol.*, Vol. 85, pp. 601-604

Ishigaki, E., Asamizu, T., Arisawa, M. & Kurosaki, F. (2004). Cloning and expression of calmodulin genes regulating phytoalexin production in carrot cells. *Biol. Pharm. Bull.*, Vol. 27, pp. 1308-1311

Ishigaki, E., Sugiyama, R. & Kurosaki, F. (2005). Multiple forms of calmodulin genes in carrot treated with fungal mycelial walls. *Biol. Pharm. Bull.*, Vol. 28, pp. 1109-1112

Ivanchenko, M., Vejlupkova, Z., Quatrano, R. S. & Fowler, J. E. (2000). Maize ROP7 GTPase contains a unique, CaaX box-independent plasma membrane targeting signal. *Plant J.*, Vol. 24, pp. 79-90

Lavy, M., Bracha-Drori, K., Sternberg, H. & Yalovsky, S. (2002). A cell-specific, prenylation-independent mechanism regulates targeting of type II RACs. *Plant Cell*, Vol. 14, pp. 2431-2450

Li, H., Shen, J., Zheng, Z., Lin, Y. & Yang, Z. (2001). The Rop GTPase switch controls multiple distinct developmental processes in *Arabidopsis*. *Plant Physiol.*, Vol. 126, pp. 670-684

Ling, V., Perera, I. Y. & Zielinski, R. E. (1991). Primary structures of. *Arabidopsis* calmodulin isoforms deduced from the sequences of cDNA clones. *Plant Physiol.*, Vol. 96. pp.1196-1202

Malatialy, L., Greppin, H. & Penel, C. (1988). Calcium uptake by tonoplast and plasma membrane vesicles from spinach leaves. *FEBS Lett.*, Vol. 233, pp.196-200

Marme, D. & Dieter, P. (1983). Role of Ca and calmodulin in plants In: *Calcium and Cell Function*, W. Y. Cheug (Ed.), Vol. 4, pp. 263-311, Academic Press, New York

Michell, R. H. (1982). Stimulated inositol lipid metabolism: An introduction. *Cell Calcium*, Vol. 3, pp. 285-294

Mitamura, T., Shite, M., Yamamura, Y. & Kurosaki, F. (2009). Cloning and characterization of a gene encoding Rac/Rop-like monomeric guanosine 5'-triphosphate-binding protein from *Scoparia dulcis*. *Biol. Pharm. Bull.*, Vol. 32, pp.1122-1125

Mitamura, T., Yamamura, Y. & Kurosaki, F. (2011). Modification and translocation of Rac/Rop guanosine 5'-triphosphate-binding proteins of *Scoparia dulcis* in response to stimulation with methyl jasmonate. *Biol. Pharm. Bull.*, Vol. 36, pp. 845-849

Morgan, N. G., Rumford, G. M. & Montaque, W. (1985). Studies on the role of inositol trisphosphate in the regulation of insulin secretion from isolated rat islets of Langerhans. *Biochem. J.*, Vol. 228, pp. 713-718

Nakamura, T. & Gold, G. H. (1987). A cyclic nucleotide-gated conductance in olfactory receptor cilia. *Nature*, Vol. 325, pp. 442-444

Newton, R. P. & Brown, E. G. (1986). The biochemistry and physiology of cyclic AMP in higher plants. In: *Hormones, Receptors and Cellular Interaction in Plants*, C. M. Chadwick & D. R. Garrod (Eds.) pp. 115-154, Cambridge University Press, London

Poovaiah, B. W. & Reddy, A. S. N. (1987). Calcium messenger system in plants. *CRC Crit. Rev. Plant Sci.*, Vol. 6, pp. 47-103

Ranganathan, R. (1994). Evolutionary origins of ion channels. *Proc. Natl. Acad. Sci. U.S.A.*, Vol. 91, pp. 3484-3486

Rasi-Caldogno, F., Pugliarello, M. C., Olivari, C. & DeMichelis, M. I. (1989). Identification and characterization of the Ca^{2+}-ATPase which drives active transport of Ca^{2+} at the plasma membrane of radish seedlings. *Plant Physiol.*, Vol. 90, pp. 1429-1434

Saitoh, D., Asakura, Y., Kasidimoko, N. K., Shite, M., Sugiyama, R., Lee, J. B., Hayashi, T. & Kurosaki, F. (2007). Cloning and expression of calmodulin gene in *Scoparia dulcis*. *Biol. Pharm. Bull.*, Vol. 30, pp. 1161-1163

Schumaker, K. S. & Sze, H. (1987). Inositol 1,4,5-trisphosphate releases Ca^{2+} from vacuolar membrane vesicles of oat roots. *J. Biol. Chem.*, Vol. 262, pp. 3944-3946

Shite, M., Yamamura, Y. & Kurosaki, F. (2009). Cloning and transcriptional regulation of *Sdrac* encoding a Rac/Rop small guanosine 5′-triphosphate-binding protein gene from *Scoparia dulcis*. *Plant Biotechnol.*, Vol. 26, pp. 403-408

Staeb, M. R. & Ebel, J. (1987). Effects of Ca on phytoalexin induction by fungal elicitor in soybean. *Arch. Biochem. Biophys.*, Vol. 257, pp. 416-423

Takezawa, D., Liu, Z. H., An, G. & Poovaiah, B. W. (1995). Calmodulin gene family in potato: developmental and touch-induced expression of the mRNA encoding a novel isoform. *Plant Mol. Biol.*, Vol. 27. pp. 693-703.

Turner, J. G., Ellis, C. & Devoto, A. (2002). The jasmonate signal pathway. *Plant Cell*, Vol. 14, pp. S153-S164

Valster, A. H., Hepler, P. K. & Chernoff, J. (2000). Plant GTPases: the Rhos in bloom. *Trends Cell. Biol.*, Vol. 10, pp.141-146

Yamakawa, H., Mitsuhara, I., Ito, N., Seo, S., Kamada, H. & Ohashi, Y. (2001). Transcriptionally and post-transcriptionally regulated response of 13 calmodulin genes to tobacco mosaic virus-induced cell death and wounding in tobacco plants. *Eur. J. Biochem.* Vol. 268, pp. 3916–3929

Yang, Z. (2002). Small GTPases, versatile signaling switches in plants. *Plant Cell*, Vol. 14, pp. S375-S388

Zhao, J., Davis, L. C. & Verpoorte, R. (2005). Elicitor signal transduction leading to production of plant secondary metabolites. *Biotechnol. Adv.*, Vol. 23, pp. 283-333

Zook, M. N., Rush, J. S. & Kuc, J. A. (1987). A role for Ca^{2+} in the elicitation of rishitin and lubimin accumulation in potato tuber tissue. *Plant Physiol.*, Vol. 84, pp. 520-525

Permissions

The contributors of this book come from diverse backgrounds, making this book a truly international effort. This book will bring forth new frontiers with its revolutionizing research information and detailed analysis of the nascent developments around the world.

We would like to thank Dr. Suleiman M. Olimat, for lending his expertise to make the book truly unique. He has played a crucial role in the development of this book. Without his invaluable contribution this book wouldn't have been possible. He has made vital efforts to compile up to date information on the varied aspects of this subject to make this book a valuable addition to the collection of many professionals and students.

This book was conceptualized with the vision of imparting up-to-date information and advanced data in this field. To ensure the same, a matchless editorial board was set up. Every individual on the board went through rigorous rounds of assessment to prove their worth. After which they invested a large part of their time researching and compiling the most relevant data for our readers. Conferences and sessions were held from time to time between the editorial board and the contributing authors to present the data in the most comprehensible form. The editorial team has worked tirelessly to provide valuable and valid information to help people across the globe.

Every chapter published in this book has been scrutinized by our experts. Their significance has been extensively debated. The topics covered herein carry significant findings which will fuel the growth of the discipline. They may even be implemented as practical applications or may be referred to as a beginning point for another development. Chapters in this book were first published by InTech; hereby published with permission under the Creative Commons Attribution License or equivalent.

The editorial board has been involved in producing this book since its inception. They have spent rigorous hours researching and exploring the diverse topics which have resulted in the successful publishing of this book. They have passed on their knowledge of decades through this book. To expedite this challenging task, the publisher supported the team at every step. A small team of assistant editors was also appointed to further simplify the editing procedure and attain best results for the readers.

Our editorial team has been hand-picked from every corner of the world. Their multi-ethnicity adds dynamic inputs to the discussions which result in innovative outcomes. These outcomes are then further discussed with the researchers and contributors who give their valuable feedback and opinion regarding the same. The feedback is then collaborated with the researches and they are edited in a comprehensive manner to aid the understanding of the subject.

Apart from the editorial board, the designing team has also invested a significant amount of their time in understanding the subject and creating the most relevant covers. They scrutinized every image to scout for the most suitable representation of the subject and create an appropriate cover for the book.

The publishing team has been involved in this book since its early stages. They were actively engaged in every process, be it collecting the data, connecting with the contributors or procuring relevant information. The team has been an ardent support to the editorial, designing and production team. Their endless efforts to recruit the best for this project, has resulted in the accomplishment of this book. They are a veteran in the field of academics and their pool of knowledge is as vast as their experience in printing. Their expertise and guidance has proved useful at every step. Their uncompromising quality standards have made this book an exceptional effort. Their encouragement from time to time has been an inspiration for everyone.

The publisher and the editorial board hope that this book will prove to be a valuable piece of knowledge for researchers, students, practitioners and scholars across the globe.

List of Contributors

Manoj Goyal and B.P. Nagori
Lachoo Memorial College of Science and Technology, Pharmacy Wing, Jodhpur, Rajasthan, India

D. Sasmal
Department of Pharmaceutical Sciences, BIT Mesra, Ranchi, Jharkhand, India

A. Paul Hornby
Hedron Analytical Inc., Canada

Zhang Guo-Gang, He Ying-Cui, Liu Hong-Xia, Zhu Lin-Xia and Chen Li-Juan
College of Traditional Chinese Materia Medica, Shenyang Pharmaceutical University, Shengyang, China

Moronkola Dorcas Olufunke
Department of Chemistry, University of Ibadan, Nigeria

Anjoo Kamboj
Chandigarh College of Pharmacy, Landran, Mohali, India

María Yolanda Rios
Centro de Investigaciones Químicas, Universidad Autónoma del Estado de Morelos, Col. Chamilpa, Cuernavaca, Morelos, México

Ken Yasukawa
School of Pharmacy, Nihon University, Japan

Jennifer Billinsky, Katherine Maloney, Ed Krol and Jane Alcorn
Drug Design and Discovery Research Group, College of Pharmacy and Nutrition, University of Saskatchewan, Canada

Mei Fen Shih
Department of Pharmacy, Chia-Nan University of Pharmacy & Science, Tainan, Taiwan

Jong Yuh Cherng
Department of Chemistry & Biochemistry, National Chung Cheng University, Chia-Yi, Taiwan

Hirofumi Takigawa and Yusuke Shibuya
Biological Science Laboratories/Kao Corporation, Japan

Fumiya Kurosaki

Laboratory of Plant Resource Sciences, Graduate School of Medicine and Pharmaceutical Sciences for Research, University of Toyama, Sugitani, Toyama, Japan